guidelines for

PERINATAL CARE

Sixth Edition

American Academy
of Pediatrics

The American College
of Obstetricians
and Gynecologists

Supported in part by

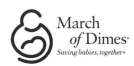

March
of Dimes
Saving babies, together

Guidelines for Perinatal Care was developed through the cooperative efforts of the American Academy of Pediatrics (AAP) Committee on Fetus and Newborn and the American College of Obstetricians and Gynecologists (ACOG) Committee on Obstetric Practice. The guidelines should not be viewed as a body of rigid rules. They are general and intended to be adapted to many different situations, taking into account the needs and resources particular to the locality, the institution, or the type of practice. Variations and innovations that improve the quality of patient care are to be encouraged rather than restricted. The purpose of these guidelines will be well served if they provide a firm basis on which local norms may be built.

Copyright © October 2007 by the American Academy of Pediatrics and the American College of Obstetricians and Gynecologists

Library of Congress Cataloging-in-Publication Data

Guidelines for perinatal care / American Academy of Pediatrics [and] the American College of Obstetricians and Gynecologists. — 6th ed.
    p. ; cm.
"Supported in part by March of Dimes."
Includes bibliographical references and index.
ISBN 978-1-58110-270-3 (AAP) – ISBN 978-1-932328-36-3 (ACOG)
    1. Perinatology—Standards—United States. I. American Academy of Pediatrics. II. American College of Obstetricians and Gynecologists. III. March of Dimes Birth Defects Foundation.
    [DNLM: 1. Perinatal Care—standards—United States—Practice Guideline. WQ 210 G955 2008]

    RG600.G85 2008
    618.3'2—dc22
                                        2007015737
    ISBN 978-1-58110-270-3 AAP
    ISBN 978-1-932328-36-3 ACOG

Orders to purchase copies of *Guidelines for Perinatal Care* or inquiries regarding content can be directed to the respective organizations.

American Academy of Pediatrics
141 Northwest Point Boulevard
PO Box 927
Elk Grove Village, IL 60009-0927

The American College of Obstetricians and Gynecologists
409 12th Street, SW
PO Box 96920
Washington, DC 20090-69020

123456/10987

Editorial Committee

Editors
Charles J. Lockwood, MD, FACOG
James A. Lemons, MD, FAAP
Associate Editors
Laura E. Riley, MD, FACOG
Lillian Blackmon, MD, FAAP

Staff
ACOG
Stanley Zinberg, MD, MS, FACOG
Beth Steele
Debra A Hawks, MPH
Sarah Smee

AAP
Jim Couto, MA

ACOG Committee on Obstetric Practice

Members, 2004–2005
Laura E. Riley, MD, FACOG (Chair)
Eleanor L. Capeless, MD (Vice Chair)
Jeanne M. Coulehan, CNM
Gary D.V. Hankins, MD, FACOG
Susan C. Hellerstein, MD, FACOG
Sarah J. Kilpatrick, MD, FACOG
Carol A. Major, MD, FACOG
Sean McFadden, MD, FACOG
Lee Self, MD, FACOG
Paul G. Tomich, MD, FACOG
Jeffrey A. Kuller, MD, FACOG (Ex Officio)
John Wachtel, MD, FACOG (Ex Officio)

Liaison Representatives
Lillian Blackmon, MD
Joshua A, Copel, MD
David J. Birnbach, MD
Hani Atrash, MD
William Callaghan, MD
Catherine Y. Spong, MD
Katharine D. Wenstrom, MD
Phill H. Price, MD

Members, 2005–2006
Gary D.V. Hankins, MD, FACOG (Chair)
Sarah J. Kilpatrick, MD, FACOG (Vice Chair)
Angela L. Bell, MD, FACOG
Jeanne M. Coulehan, CNM
Susan C. Hellerstein, MD, FACOG
Jack Ludmir, MD, FACOG
Carol A. Major, MD, FACOG
Sean McFadden, MD, FACOG
Susan M. Ramin, MD, FACOG
Russell R. Snyder, Col, MC USAF
William N.P. Herbert, MD, FACOG (Ex Officio)
John Wachtel, MD, FACOG (Ex Officio)

Liaison Representatives
Ann R. Stark, MD
Joshua A. Copel, MD
David J. Birnbach, MD
Hani Atrash, MD
William M. Callaghan, MD
Catherine Y. Spong, MD
Gary A. Dildy III, MD
Phill H. Price, MD

Members, 2006–2007
Gary D.V. Hankins, MD, FACOG (Chair)
Sarah J. Kilpatrick, MD, FACOG (Vice Chair)
Katia M. Apollon, MD, FACOG
Angela L. Bell, MD, FACOG
Jeanne M. Coulehan, CNM

Liaison Representatives
Ann R. Stark, MD
Joshua A. Copel, MD
Samuel Hughes, MD
Hani Atrash, MD
William M. Callaghan, MD

contents

preface

The sixth edition of *Guidelines for Perinatal Care* is a user-friendly guide that provides updated and expanded information from the fifth edition. This edition maintains the focus of the last edition on reproductive awareness and regionally based prenatal care services but with an added focus of patient safety and quality improvement.

Guidelines for Perinatal Care represents a cross section of different disciplines within the perinatal community. It is designed for use by all personnel who are involved in the care of pregnant women, their fetuses, and their neonates in community programs, hospitals, and medical centers. An intermingling of information in varying degrees of detail is provided to address their collective needs. The result is a unique resource that complements the educational documents listed in Appendix I, which provide more specific information. Readers are encouraged to refer to the appendix for related documents to supplement those listed at the end of each chapter.

The sixth edition of *Guidelines for Perinatal Care* includes new information on levels of perinatal care, maternal transport, dental care during pregnancy, human immunodeficiency virus (HIV), childbearing after 50 years of age, obesity, multiple gestation, patient safety, hyperbilirubinemia, breastfeeding, and newborn screening. There also is a new and revised ACOG Antepartum Record and Postpartum Form in Appendix A.

Both the American Academy of Pediatrics (AAP) and the American College of Obstetricians and Gynecologists (ACOG) will continue to update information presented here through policy statements and recommendations that both organizations issue periodically, particularly with regard to rapidly evolving technologies and areas of practice, such as genetics, treatment of HIV infection, and immunization recommendations.

Guidelines for Perinatal Care is published as a companion document to ACOG's *Guidelines for Women's Health Care*, which is in its third edition.

Although each book is developed with the aid of a separate committee, their contents are coordinated to provide a comprehensive reference to all aspects of women's health care with minimal duplication.

The most current scientific information, professional opinions, and clinical practices have been used to create this document, which is intended to offer guidelines, not strict operating rules. Local circumstances must dictate the way in which these guidelines are best interpreted to meet the needs of a particular hospital, community, or system. For instance, the term *readily available*, used to designate acceptable levels of care, should be defined by each institution within the context of its resources and geographic location. Emphasis has been placed on identifying those areas to be covered by specific, locally defined protocols rather than on promoting rigid recommendations.

The content of this newest edition of *Guidelines for Perinatal Care* has undergone careful review to ensure accuracy and consistency with the policies of both groups. The guidelines are not meant to be exhaustive, nor do they always agree with those of other organizations; however, they reflect the latest recommendations of AAP and ACOG. The recommendations of AAP and ACOG are based on the best understanding of the data and consensus among authorities in the discipline. The text was written, revised, and reviewed by members of the AAP Committee on Fetus and Newborn and the ACOG Committee on Obstetric Practice; consultants in a variety of specialized areas also contributed to the content. The pioneering efforts of those who developed the previous editions also must be acknowledged. To each and every one of them, our sincere appreciation is extended.

introduction

Throughout its prior five editions, *Guidelines for Perinatal Care* has focused on improving the outcomes of pregnancies and reducing maternal and perinatal mortality and morbidity by suggesting sound paradigms for providing perinatal care. Its strong advocacy of regionalized perinatal systems, including effective risk identification, care in a risk-appropriate setting, and maternal or neonatal transport to tertiary care facilities when necessary, has had a demonstrable effect on perinatal outcomes. The current edition incorporates evidence-based data to further refine optimal regionalized care. This edition also makes evidence-based recommendations on the use of safe and effective diagnostic and therapeutic interventions in both maternal–fetal medicine and neonatology.

The full gamut of high-quality perinatal care is covered by this sixth edition of *Guidelines for Perinatal Care*, from the principles of preconception counseling and the provision of antepartum and intrapartum care in routine and complex settings to guidelines for routine and complex neonatal and postpartum care. Examples include evaluation of the efficacy of prenatal diagnostic techniques, use of antenatal steroids to accelerate fetal maturation, intrapartum antibiotic chemoprophylaxis to prevent neonatal group B streptococcal sepsis, antibiotics for preterm premature rupture of membranes, and surfactant therapy for newborn respiratory distress syndrome.

This edition also contains updated recommendations for the conduct of perinatal care in a hospital setting, covering the breadth of care from nurse staffing guidelines to housekeeping techniques. The importance of establishing effective quality improvement initiatives within every department and hospital is highlighted in this edition. Quality improvement focuses on improving the systems of health care, which translates into better outcomes for individual patients. Providing optimal patient care and caring entails a patient-centered approach, wherein patients and families are recognized and respected as true partners in their health care. Excellent communication provided in an empathic manner is the foundation of such care.

Communication between caregivers is equally important. In its 2001 report, *Crossing the Quality Chasm*, the Institute of Medicine identified six performance characteristics that could affect better health for people; these included patient safety and patient-centered care, with effective and seamless communication between and among caregivers as essential (1). This edition of *Guidelines for Perinatal Care* provides extensive commentary on the need for procedures and policies to ensure such communication to improve patient care and enhance patient safety.

Buffeted by the professional liability insurance crisis, a growing regulatory burden, and accelerating consumer demands, obstetricians and their neonatal colleagues have much to gain by striving to prevent medical errors, which is perhaps the most important initiative to enhance patient safety. Whereas many, if not most, legal claims against obstetricians are unfounded, there can be no doubt that medical errors do occur during the provision of perinatal care. Ironically, the defensive medical practices that have arisen in response to the professional liability insurance crisis, such as ordering more diagnostic tests, prescribing more medications, and referring patients to specialists in unnecessary circumstances, may enhance the likelihood of harm because they increase the opportunity to miss abnormal laboratory test results, make medication errors, or fail to accurately communicate recommendations (2).

Indeed, communication failures among obstetric care providers are noted in up to one third of adverse outcomes (3). This may be an underestimate because the Joint Commission (formerly the Joint Commission on Accreditation of Healthcare Organizations [JCAHO]) has reported that communication lapses are present in 65% of "sentinel events." Two thirds of these communication errors result from disruption in the flow of critical information between or among caregivers. Again, excessive ordering of tests, medications, and consultations can compound the problem by obscuring abnormal values, medication errors, or consultant recommendations.

There are many constraints to effective communication among perinatal care providers. This edition of *Guidelines for Perinatal Care* addresses many of these issues. However, all facilities providing perinatal care must attend to local impediments to communication, including rudimentary or absent electronic order entry, laboratory reporting, and patient record systems; variations in individual practice styles and configurations; and even the physical layout of obstetric and neonatal care areas. Another impediment to smooth communication and patient safety is the growing national nursing shortage, coupled with deteriorating hospital finances. This is leaving fewer nurses to care for sicker patients in an ever more complex environment.

A number of novel solutions have been proposed to further enhance the safety and efficacy of perinatal care. Many centers have implemented Crew Resource Management strategies. This innovative system is used by the U.S. military and the Federal Aviation Administration "to detect, avoid, trap, or mitigate the effects of human error and, therefore, prevent fatal accidents" (4). Applied to the perinatal setting, Crew Resource Management breaks down nursing, physician, laboratory, and pharmacy care silos through team training and implementation of interacting perinatal care teams that make frequent rounds, anticipate potential problems, facilitate access to critical laboratory data, and confirm the timely administration of medications at their correct dosages. The teams also improve care "hand-offs" and ensure compliance with jointly developed policies and procedures. Team members are trained to speak a common language when describing electronic fetal heart rate patterns and obstetric and neonatal complications.

Some practices and institutions have implemented 24-hour labor and delivery coverage by "laborists." These physicians work in shifts and are dedicated solely to the management of laboring patients. Some laborists focus only on the care of their practice's patients, whereas others provide care to patients belonging to a group of collaborating practices. In large centers, laborists may be dedicated to providing back-up or contingency care for other on-site providers, coordinating multiple care teams, and triaging access to anesthesia or operating rooms.

In concert with team training, many hospitals also are redesigning labor floors and neonatal intensive care units to facilitate patient flow and provider communication. Hospitals' information systems are being updated, and electronic medical records embedded with patient safety features increasingly are being deployed by practices and hospitals. Assuming these patient-safety initiatives prove beneficial following rigorous investigation, we predict that the seventh and subsequent editions of this book will contain significant new recommendations regarding team training, communication, electronic records, and the use of laborists.

References

1. Institute of Medicine (US). Crossing the quality chasm: a new health system for the 21st century. Washington, DC: National Academy Press; 2001.

2. Studdert DM, Mello MM, Sage WM, DesRoches CM, Peugh J, Zapert K, et al. Defensive medicine among high-risk specialist physicians in a volatile malpractice environment. JAMA 2005;293:2609–17.

3. White AA, Pichert JW, Bledsoe SH, Irwin C, Entman SS. Cause and effect analysis of closed claims in obstetrics and gynecology. Obstet Gynecol 2005;105:1031–8.

4. Sachs BP. A 38-year-old woman with fetal loss and hysterectomy. JAMA 2005;294:833–40.

chapter 1

Organization of Perinatal Health Care

Health Care Delivery System

One of the great success stories in the field of health care delivery has been the organization of perinatal health care on a regional basis beginning in the 1970s and 1980s. Regional organization of perinatal care was endorsed in a 1976 report by the March of Dimes Foundation, *Toward Improving the Outcome of Pregnancy*, which was prepared by the Committee on Perinatal Health, an ad-hoc committee of representatives appointed by participating professional organizations with support from the March of Dimes Foundation. The importance of regional organization was further emphasized in a second March of Dimes Foundation report by the Committee on Perinatal Health in 1993, *Toward Improving the Outcome of Pregnancy: The 90s and Beyond*. A regional system of perinatal health care should address not only the management of labor and delivery and neonatal care but also the care received by the mother before and during the early stages of pregnancy. A health care system that is responsive to the needs of families, and especially women, requires strategies to:

- Improve access to services
- Identify risks early
- Provide linkage to the appropriate level of care
- Ensure compliance, continuity, and comprehensiveness

Structural, financial, and cultural barriers to care need to be identified and eliminated. The regional organization must evolve within the framework of the general health care delivery system while avoiding unnecessary duplication of services. Four aspects can be identified that are essential to the successful regional perinatal health care system: 1) access to comprehensive perinatal health care services, 2) education of the public about reproductive health, 3) family-centered health care, and 4) accountability for all components of the health care delivery system.

Comprehensive Perinatal Health Care Services

The integration of clinical activities, level I (basic) through level III (subspecialty), within one geographical region potentially provides timely access to care at the appropriate level for the entire population. The primary goal of providing the appropriate level of care is facilitated by early and ongoing risk assessment to prevent, recognize, and treat conditions associated with maternal and infant morbidity and mortality. A secondary goal is to improve referral and consultation among institutions that provide different levels of care. When populations needing reproductive health care are widely dispersed, both geographically and economically, a carefully structured, well-organized system of supportive services becomes necessary to ensure access to appropriate care for all pregnant women and newborn infants. Networks and other forms of vertically integrated systems should be structured to provide all the necessary services, including health care, transportation, public and professional education, research, and outcome evaluations with data organized in standard format. All components are necessary to minimize perinatal mortality and morbidity while using resources efficiently.

Education of the Public About Reproductive Health

Insight into the broad social and medical implications of pregnancy and awareness of reproductive risks, health-enhancing behaviors, and family-planning options are essential to improving the outcomes of pregnancy. Education about reproductive health must be integrated more effectively into the health care system and society at large. An Institute of Medicine report, *The Best Intentions, Unintended Pregnancy and the Well-Being of Children and Families,* emphasizes that in the United States:

- Approximately 60% of pregnancies are unintended, either mistimed or unwanted altogether.

- Unintended pregnancies occur in all segments of society.

- A woman with an unintended pregnancy is less likely to seek early prenatal care and is more likely to expose the fetus to noxious substances.

- An unwanted pregnancy is at higher risk of producing a low birth weight neonate with other complications throughout childhood.

- Approximately one half of unintended pregnancies end in abortion.

That less than one half of pregnancies in the United States are planned suggests the need for a new approach to reproductive education. Because unintended pregnancies and reproductive health hazards—including the use of alcohol, tobacco, and other drugs—occur across all socioeconomic groups, the target group for reproductive education must be all women of childbearing age. Reproductive health screening should be implemented by all health care providers serving women in their reproductive years. A sample form that may be useful in facilitating appropriate selective reproductive health screening is shown in Table 1–1.

Every encounter with the health care system, including those involving adolescents and men, should be viewed as an opportunity to reinforce awareness of reproductive health issues. New messages regarding responsible reproductive health practices and innovations in marketing techniques may be required to change attitudes and behaviors among women and men.

In communicating with both the patient and the public, it is important to realize that a large portion of the population has low levels of functional literacy, which may compromise the quality of care received, contribute to poor health outcomes, and increase the risk of medical liability litigation. This problem must be addressed on a public health basis, but its effects also can be minimized by careful use of simplified language on written documents, such as consent forms and patient instructions, and in conversation with the patient. Whenever possible, interpreter services must be provided to assist with important discussions if patients are not fluent in English or if they are hearing impaired. Reasonable steps are required to ensure meaningful access to interpreter services. Various options may be available, including hiring interpreters as office staff, using appropriate community resources, or using translation telephone services.

Table 1–1. Health Screening for Women of Reproductive Age

Selective Reproductive Health Screening (Menarche to Menopause)	Done	Referred
Reproductive awareness		
Pregnancy prevention counseling	❏	❏
Prepregnancy and nutrition counseling	❏	❏
Medical diseases (counsel regarding effects on future pregnancies)		
Diabetes mellitus	❏	❏
Hypertension	❏	❏
Epilepsy	❏	❏
Other chronic illness	❏	❏
Infectious diseases (counsel, test, or refer)		
Sexually transmitted diseases, including human immunodeficiency virus (HIV)	❏	❏
Hepatitis A	❏	❏
Hepatitis B (immunize if at high risk)	❏	❏
Rubella (test; if nonimmune, immunize)	❏	❏
Varicella	❏	❏
Teratogens and genetics (counsel regarding effects on future pregnancies)		
Hemoglobinopathy	❏	❏
Medication and vitamin use (eg, isotretinoin and vitamin A [retinoic acid])	❏	❏
Self or prior child with congenital defect	❏	❏
Family history of genetic disease	❏	❏
Environmental exposure at home or in workplace	❏	❏
Behavior (counsel regarding effects on future pregnancies)		
Alcohol use	❏	❏
Tobacco use	❏	❏
Use of illicit substances (eg, cocaine or crack)	❏	❏
Social support		
Safety (eg, domestic violence)	❏	❏
Personal resources (eg, transportation or housing)	❏	❏

Modified from March of Dimes Birth Defects Foundation, Committee on Perinatal Health. Toward improving the outcome of pregnancy: the 90s and beyond. White Plains (NY): March of Dimes Birth Defects Foundation; 1993.

Family-Centered Health Care

The health care system should be oriented toward providing family-centered health care because the family often is the primary source of support for individuals receiving health services. Health care providers should engage the parents as coproviders and decision-making partners and should seek to ensure that every encounter builds on the patient's strengths, preserves their dignity, and enhances their confidence and competence. Such an approach incorporates family perspectives, offers real choices, and respects the decisions made by the parents for themselves and their children. All counseling should be sensitive to cultural diversity, and a skilled translator should be used when the primary language of the patient is not that of the health care provider.

Hospital and program leaders should communicate the concepts of family-centered care consistently and clearly to staff, students, families, and communities through statements of vision, mission, and philosophy and through institutional policies and actions. Providing an environment that is supportive of the family's key role in promoting the health of its members is important in successful health promotion. This includes respecting the choices, values, and cultural backgrounds of expectant and new mothers and other family members; communicating honestly and openly; promoting opportunities for mutual support and information sharing; and collaborating in the development and evaluation of services.

Family-centered practices can help expectant and new parents become nurturing caregivers. Efforts should be made throughout the neonatal course to minimize the separation of newborns and families. Economic interests and decisions should never take priority over the best interests of the newborn, the mother, the family, and the community in keeping the family together. When separation of the family unit is necessitated by the requirement for a higher level of care for the mother or newborn, the responsibility for maintaining communication and involvement of the family in care decisions should be shared by the entire care team. Whenever medically feasible, a mother whose newborn infant has been transferred to another hospital should be discharged or transferred to the same facility. Staff interactions and unit policies at every level should consistently reinforce the importance of parents and other family members to the health and well-being of their newborns. Families' strengths and capabilities should be the foundation on which to build competency and confidence in caregiving abilities. Preserving an individual sense of personal responsibility and identity is important for the optimum outcome of pregnancy and family life.

Accountability

Accountability for actions is a fundamental principle of health care provision applicable to all components of a health care delivery system and is a valuable attribute of professional practice that benefits all patients. This accountability includes, but is not limited to, the care of individual patients by individual health care providers. Patients and their families have a shared partnership for their health care. Within the perinatal health care delivery system, accountability and responsibility must be required equally of all participants, including patients, families, perinatal health care programs and systems, government agencies, insurers, and health maintenance organizations, all of whose actions and policies influence the delivery of patient care and thereby influence outcomes. Accountability includes developing meaningful quality-improvement programs, monitoring medical errors, and working to ensure patient safety. Access to high-quality care for all patients is a responsibility that requires a coordinated system with involvement, commitment, and accountability of all parties.

Clinical Components of Regionalized Perinatal Services

A regionally coordinated system, focusing on levels of hospital-based perinatal care, has been shown to be effective and to result in improved outcomes for women and their newborns. Such a system can be extended to encompass preconception evaluation and early-pregnancy risk assessment in both ambulatory and hospital-based settings.

Preconception Care

Regional perinatal health care programs and systems should enhance the positive effect of antepartum care on outcomes by placing additional emphasis on preconception care through educational programs. Clinical details of preconception care for perinatal health care providers are presented in "Preconception Care" in Chapter 4. All women of childbearing age should be provided access, structure, and support for preconception care and family-planning consultation.

All health care providers have an obligation to provide information and counseling about sexuality, the medical and psychosocial risks of pregnancy, and reproductive health care options in accordance with state and federal statutes and regulations to all adolescents in their practices. In addition, every opportunity during preventive-care visits should be taken to provide education to parents, especially mothers, emphasizing the adverse medical and social consequences of adolescent pregnancy.

Ambulatory Prenatal Care

The goals for regional coordination of ambulatory prenatal care are to ensure appropriate care for all women, to ensure good use of available resources, and to improve the outcome of pregnancies. Prenatal care can be delivered more effectively and efficiently by defining the capabilities and expertise (basic, specialty, and subspecialty) of providers and ensuring that pregnant women receive risk-appropriate care (Table 1–2). Developments in maternal–fetal risk assessment and diagnosis, as well as interventions to change behavior, make early and ongoing prenatal care an effective strategy to improve pregnancy outcomes.

Early and ongoing risk assessment should be an integral component of perinatal care. Early identification of high-risk pregnancies allows prevention and treatment of conditions associated with morbidity and mortality. Risk assessment facilitates development of a plan of care, including referral and consultation as appropriate, among providers of basic, specialty, and subspecialty prenatal care on the basis of the patient's circumstances and the capability of the individual providers.

The content and timing of prenatal care should be varied according to the needs and risk status of the woman and her fetus. Use of community-based risk assessment tools, such as a standardized prenatal record (see "ACOG Antepartum Record" in Appendix A), by all providers within a perinatal care region helps to ensure appropriate implementation of risk assessment and intervention activities. All prenatal health care providers should be able to identify a full range of medical and psychosocial risks and either provide appropriate care or make appropriate referrals (see Appendixes B and C).

Prenatal care may involve the services of many types of health care providers, including the early involvement of pediatricians and neonatologists as well as other specialists. Consultation with a neonatologist to discuss the pediatric implications with the mother and her partner is particularly important when fetal risks or problems have been identified.

Table 1-2. Ambulatory Prenatal Care Provider Capabilities and Expertise

Level of Prenatal Care	Capabilities	Provider Types
Basic (level I)	Risk-oriented prenatal care record, physical examination and interpretation of findings, routine laboratory assessment, assessment of gestational age and normal progress of pregnancy, ongoing risk identification, mechanisms for consultation and referral, psychosocial support, childbirth education, and care coordination (including referral for ancillary services, such as transportation, food, and housing assistance)	Obstetricians, family physicians, certified nurse midwives, and other advanced-practice nurses with experience, training, and demonstrated competence
Specialty (level II)	Basic care plus fetal diagnostic testing (eg, biophysical tests, amniotic fluid analysis, basic ultrasonography), expertise in management of medical and obstetric complications	Obstetricians
Subspecialty (level III)	Basic and specialty care plus advanced fetal diagnoses (eg, targeted ultrasonography, fetal echocardiography); advanced therapy (eg, intrauterine fetal transfusion and treatment of cardiac arrhythmias); medical, surgical, neonatal, and genetic consultation; and management of severe maternal complications	Maternal-fetal medicine specialists and reproductive geneticists with experience, training, and demonstrated competence

Modified from March of Dimes Birth Defects Foundation, Committee on Perinatal Health. Toward improving the outcome of pregnancy: the 90s and beyond. White Plains (NY): March of Dimes Birth Defects Foundation; 1993.

In-Hospital Perinatal Care

In *Toward Improving the Outcome of Pregnancy*, the Committee on Perinatal Health of the March of Dimes Foundation designated three levels of perinatal care: levels I, II, and III. Although this designation remains in use among many institutions and public agencies, such as state maternal–child health programs, the second March of Dimes Foundation Committee on Perinatal Health report in 1993 recommended replacing numerical designations with the functional, descriptive designations of basic, specialty, and subspecialty care. Since then, financial and marketing pressures, as well as community demands, have led some hospitals to raise their perinatal care service-level designation without attention to regional coordination concerns. This tendency conflicts with the traditional concept of regional organization, in which single level III or sub-specialty care centers had the sole capability to provide complex patient care and usually, but not always, assumed regional responsibilities for transport, outreach education, research, and quality improvement for a specific population or geographic area. However, these regional services still are provided by many level III centers. Among other educational services provided to the level I and II centers in the region, the level III center should assist these centers with establishing and maintaining fetal and infant mortality review programs. Attempts to share responsibilities among hospitals have not been uniformly successful. Sometimes differing levels of perinatal care services have developed within a single hospital—usually a basic or specialty obstetrics service in conjunction with a subspecialty neonatology service. This imbalance or lack of coordination in the provision of services may be a product of a growing competitive health care market and efforts by insurers and health plans to control the costs of health care. Such competitive forces frequently have led to the unnecessary duplication of services within a single community or geographic region, with the potential to result in poorer patient outcomes and, ironically, increased cost.

Careful documentation of birth-weight specific neonatal mortality rates by hospital of birth has shown that the survival of premature, very low birth weight infants is highest when births occur in hospitals with larger neonatal intensive care units. This finding has been reported in the United States and other countries. In addition, multiple reports regarding the outcomes of neonatal surgery support the concentration of resources and patients in a few highly specialized centers for neonatal surgery. Given the weight of the evidence, it must be emphasized that inpatient perinatal health care services should be organized within individual regions or service areas in such a manner that there is a concentration of care for the highest-risk pregnant women and their fetuses and neonates in the highest level perinatal health care centers.

Distinction must be made between the perinatal care services level that characterizes an institution or hospital and the level of care provided within individual patient-care units of a hospital. The former applies to the total organization of perinatal health care services and the additional responsibilities associated with participation in a coordinated, regional system of care. The latter is based on the individual needs of the perinatal patient, postpartum woman, and neonate (see "Physical Facilities" in Chapter 2 for a detailed description). The determination of the appropriate level of care to be provided by a given hospital should be guided by prevailing local health care regulations, national professional organization guidelines, and identified regional perinatal health care service needs. In the case of neonatal services, level of care should be assigned according to the expanded classification system developed by the American Academy of Pediatrics and published in 2004.

The expected capabilities of basic, specialty, and subspecialty levels of inpatient perinatal health care services are shown in Table 1–3, listed by both functional and numerical designations for the various levels of care services (see Chapter 2, "Inpatient Perinatal Care Services").

Level I units (well-newborn nurseries) provide a basic level of newborn care to infants at low risk. They have the capability to perform neonatal resuscitation at every delivery and to evaluate and provide routine postnatal care for healthy newborn infants. In addition, they can stabilize and care for late preterm infants (35–37 weeks of gestation) who remain physiologically stable and can stabilize newborn infants who are less than 35 weeks of gestation or who are ill until they can be transferred to a facility at which specialty neonatal care is provided.

Care in a specialty-level facility should be reserved for stable or moderately ill newborns with problems that are expected to resolve rapidly and who would not be anticipated to need subspecialty-level services on an urgent basis. These situations usually occur as a result of relatively uncomplicated preterm labor or preterm rupture of membranes at 32 weeks of gestation or later.

Currently, some hospitals with specialty-level obstetric services also provide some elements of neonatal intensive care; such disproportionate service capability is not encouraged. In particular, the availability of pediatric subspecialties, such as pediatric cardiology, pediatric surgery, pediatric anesthesiology, and pediatric radiology, may be limited. However, in some states, geographic distances or demographics necessitate perinatal care programs that allow for hos-

Table 1–3. Capabilities of Providers in Hospitals Delivering Basic, Specialty, and Subspecialty Care

Level of Care	Capabilities	Provider Types
Level I (basic)	Surveillance and care of all patients admitted to the obstetric service, with an established triage system for identifying patients at high risk who should be transferred to a facility that provides specialty or subspecialty care	Family physicians, obstetricians, pediatricians
	Proper detection and initial care of unanticipated maternal–fetal problems that occur during labor and delivery	
	Capability to begin an emergency cesarean delivery within 30 minutes of the decision to do so	
	Availability of appropriate anesthesia, radiology, ultrasonography, and laboratory and blood bank services on a 24-hour basis	
	Care of postpartum conditions	
	Resuscitation and stabilization of all neonates born in the hospital	
	Evaluation and continuing care of healthy neonates in a nursery or with their mothers until discharge	
	Adequate nursery facilities and support for stabilization of small or ill neonates before transfer to a specialty or subspecialty facility	
	Consultation and transfer arrangements	
	Accommodations and policies that allow families, including their other children, to be together in the hospital following the birth of an infant	
	Data collection, storage, and retrieval	
	Quality improvement programs, including efforts to maximize patient safety	
Level II (specialty)	Provision of basic care services as described previously and, in addition, provision of the following enhanced services:	Obstetricians, pediatricians, sometimes neonatologists
	• Care of appropriate women at high risk and fetuses, both admitted and transferred from other facilities	
	• Stabilization of severely ill newborns before transfer	
	• Treatment of moderately ill, larger preterm and term newborns	

(continued)

Table 1–3. Capabilities of Providers in Hospitals Delivering Basic, Specialty, and Subspecialty Care *(continued)*

Level of Care	Capabilities	Provider Types
Level III (subspecialty)	Provision of comprehensive perinatal health care services for both directly admitted and transferred women and neonates of all risk categories, including basic and specialty care services as described previously Evaluation of new technologies and therapies	Maternal–fetal medicine specialists, neonatologists
Regional subspecialty perinatal health care center	Provision of comprehensive perinatal health care services at and above those of subspecialty care facilities Responsibility for regional perinatal health care service organization and coordination, including the following areas: • Maternal and neonatal transport • Regional outreach support and education programs • Development and initial evaluation of new technologies and therapies • Training of health care providers with specialty and subspecialty qualifications and capabilities • Analysis and evaluation of regional data, including those on perinatal complications and outcomes	Maternal–fetal medicine specialists, neonatologists, other subspecialists, including obstetric, pediatric, and surgical subspecialists

pitals to be approved for advanced care capability in the neonatal unit above that for the perinatal service as a whole. Additional institutional requirements are stipulated for approval at the advanced level. Under such oversight, higher-level neonatal care capability is acceptable. In general, each hospital should have a clear understanding of the categories of perinatal patients that can be managed appropriately in the local facility and those that should be transferred to a higher-level facility. Preterm labor and impending delivery at less than 32 weeks of gestation usually warrant maternal transfer to a subspecialty (level III) center. Infants whose mothers could not be transferred before delivery usually should be transferred after stabilization following delivery.

The services provided by a subspecialty care facility vary markedly from those at a specialty facility. Subspecialty care services include expertise in both maternal–fetal medicine and neonatology. Both usually are required for management of pregnancies with threatened maternal complications at less than 32 weeks of gestation. Fetuses that may require immediate, complex care should be delivered at a subspecialty care center. In circumstances in which subspecialty-level maternal care is needed, the level of care subsequently needed by the neonate may prove to be at the basic or specialty level. It is difficult to predict accurately all neonatal risks and outcomes before birth. Appropriate assessment and consultation should be used, considering the potential risks for the woman as well as her infant.

Not all subspecialty perinatal health care hospitals must act as regional centers; however, regional organization of perinatal health care services requires that there be coordination in the development of specialized services, professional continuing education to maintain competency, and the collection of data on long-term outcomes to evaluate both the effectiveness of delivery of perinatal health care services and the safety and efficacy of new therapies. Experience has shown that these functions usually are best achieved when responsibility is concentrated in a single regional center with both perinatal and neonatal subspecialty services. In some cases, regional coordination may be provided adequately by the collaboration of a children's hospital with a subspecialty perinatal facility that is in close geographic proximity.

Expanded Classification System for Levels of Neonatal Care

In 2004, the American Academy of Pediatrics published an expanded system for classification of levels of neonatal care. This system builds on the previous categories of basic, specialty, subspecialty, and regional subspecialty care. Whereas the previous system applies to both obstetric and neonatal care, the expanded system applies to only neonatal care. No similar expanded classification system exists for obstetric care. The categories of this new system are listed as follows:

- Level I neonatal care (basic)
- Level II neonatal care (specialty)
  - Level IIA: similar to previous level II
  - Level IIB: additional capability to provide mechanical ventilation for up to 24 hours or continuous positive airway pressure
- Level III (subspecialty) neonatal intensive care unit
  - Level IIIA has the following additional capabilities:
    Provide comprehensive care for infants born at more than 28 weeks of gestation and weighing more than 1,000 g

Provide sustained mechanical ventilation but not more advanced life support

Perform minor surgical procedures, such as placement of a central vein catheter or repair of an inguinal hernia

— Level IIIB has the following additional capabilities:

Comprehensive care for infants born at 28 weeks of gestation or less and weighing 1,000 g or less.

Advanced respiratory support, such as high-frequency ventilation and inhaled nitric oxide

Advanced imaging, with interpretation on an urgent basis, including computed tomography, magnetic resonance imaging, and echocardiography

Prompt on-site access to a full range of pediatric medical subspecialists

Pediatric surgical subspecialists and pediatric anesthesiologists on site or at a closely related institution to perform major surgery

— Level IIIC has all the capabilities of a level IIIB neonatal intensive care unit but also can provide:

Extracorporeal life support

Open-heart surgery for repair of complex, congenital cardiac malformations

Maternal and Newborn Postdischarge Care

Perinatal health care at all levels should include ambulatory care of the woman and the neonate after hospital discharge. Increasing economic pressure for early discharge and decreased length of hospital stay after delivery has increased the importance of organization and coordination of continuing care as well as the need for evaluation and monitoring of outcomes. Postdischarge care for an infant who has survived a complicated perinatal course should include care by a pediatrician with expertise and experience in caring for such infants. Neonatal intensive care unit graduates also should be enrolled in an organized follow-up program that tracks and records medical and neurodevelopmental outcomes to allow later analysis. Such a follow-up program is an essential component of subspecialty neonatal services. Service components for follow-up care for women are discussed in Chapter 5 and for neonates in Chapter 7 and Chapter 8.

Workforce: The Distribution and Supply of Perinatal Care Providers

The distribution and supply of physicians providing perinatal health care services has been changing. Although the number of physicians has increased substantially over the past 20 years, the percentage of all physicians who provide obstetric care has declined. Published data indicate that there currently are sufficient physician specialists in neonatal care. However, obstetricians who provide care for high-risk patients, maternal–fetal medicine specialists, and neonatologists are unevenly distributed among geographic areas and types of facilities. Good data on the number of obstetricians who provide care for high-risk patients and neonatologists needed to serve a given population are lacking. A team approach to perinatal health care delivery is essential to improving the outcome of pregnancy. Certified nurse midwives, physician assistants, advanced practice nurses, respiratory therapists, perinatal social workers, lactation consultants, and other professionals also are important providers of perinatal services.

Strategies aimed at increasing recruitment of perinatal health care providers are needed, particularly in rural and urban medically underserved areas. More than 2,000 federal Health Professional Shortage Areas have been designated; most of the people in need of services in these areas are women of childbearing age and young children. Lack of sufficient funding to support perinatal health care services contributes to the number of underserved women.

Examples of regional programs that have been successfully used to increase access to care include liability cost relief, locum tenens programs, satellite practice models, financial incentives to establish or maintain a practice, innovative approaches to continuing education, and programs to provide technical support. The National Health Service Corps and state scholarship and loan repayment programs for the education of health care professionals, which include a special requirement for service in underserved areas, provide another important incentive. Such programs should be strengthened, adequately funded, and encouraged to give priority to perinatal health care providers.

Data Collection and Documentation

Outcomes have been a concern of perinatal health care providers for decades. Care has been monitored and improved by focusing on specific outcomes, such as maternal, newborn, and neonatal mortality. The public, including the media, parents, government agencies, and interested parties such as foundations, also has played an important and appropriate role in focusing concerns. The fact that the low birth weight rate is increasing, despite public funding of both research and patient-care programs for several decades, points to the need for continual reassessment of care components and delivery systems.

A regional perinatal health care program must be able to track the results of patient care using standard measures and indicators; this provides an important way to evaluate the success of health service delivery. Significant progress has been made in methods for collecting data and gathering vital statistics (eg, prenatal records and linked birth and death certificates). The National Center for Health Statistics standard certificates and reports for birth, death, and fetal death should be followed (Appendix D). The concept of key indicators has been used to signal inadequate access to early and continuous perinatal care and to predict or measure poor pregnancy outcome. For example, rates of unintended pregnancy; use of prenatal care services; and fetal, neonatal, and maternal mortality are possible measures of access and outcome at different points along the continuum of perinatal health care delivery. New and improved tools in evaluative clinical sciences should be used to monitor performance and provide the basis for improvement in clinical care and outcomes. Perinatal health care providers and facilities must play an active role by participating in regional data collection, developing standardized data collection tools, supporting analysis, and using the resulting information for individual, institutional, and professional quality improvement. Thorough and systematic collection of data on long-term outcomes is essential to evaluate changes in perinatal care delivery systems as well as new technologies and therapies.

In addition to an individual hospital's or perinatal region's efforts to track outcomes and mortality sentinel events, two useful programs provide an opportunity for continuous quality improvement efforts to review fetal, infant, and maternal deaths.

The Fetal and Infant Mortality Review (FIMR) process is a broad type of analysis that is valuable at the community level. The FIMR process brings together key members of the community, including prenatal and pediatric providers, public health professionals, social service agency representatives, grief professionals, consumer advocates, consumers, and others. They review deidentified information from individual cases of fetal and infant death to identify factors associated with those deaths, determine if they represent service system problems that require change, develop recommendations for change, and assist in the implementation of change.

A recent national evaluation of FIMR has documented that the process is an effective perinatal-systems initiative. Currently, FIMR is being implemented in 200 communities in 40 states. The entire FIMR evaluation report can be viewed on the Johns Hopkins University web site (www.med.jhu.edu/wchpc [Appendix E]). For more information about the FIMR process or to learn if there is a FIMR program in your community, go to www.NFIMR.org. The National Fetal and Infant Mortality Review Program (NFIMR) is a collaborative effort between the American College of Obstetricians and Gynecologists and the federal Maternal and Child Health Bureau, Health Resources and Services Administration.

Although maternal deaths attributable to pregnancy remain relatively rare, it is important that each death be identified and carefully reviewed at the state level. The lessons learned from reviews of these deaths need to be shared with those who have the opportunity to influence policies and practices related to the systems of care in place for preconception, interconception, and pregnant and postpartum women.

Resources

American College of Obstetricians and Gynecologists. Patient Communication. In: Special issues in women's health. Washington, DC: ACOG; 2005. p. 3–9.

Blackmon L. The role of the hospital of birth on survival of extremely low-birthweight, extremely preterm infants. Neoreviews 2003;4:e147–52.

American College of Obstetricians and Gynecologists. Cultural competency, sensitivity, and awareness in the delivery of health care. In: Special issues in women's health. Washington, DC: ACOG; 2005. p. 11–20.

Chien LY, Whyte R, Aziz K, Thiessen P, Matthew D, Lee SK. Improved outcome of preterm infants when delivered in tertiary care centers. Obstet Gynecol 2001;98: 247–52.

Cifuentes J, Bronstein JM, Phibbs CS, Phibbs RH, Schmitt SK, Carlo WA. Mortality in low birth weight infants according to level of neonatal care at hospital of birth. Pediatrics 2002;109:745–51.

Committee on Perinatal Health. Toward improving the outcome of pregnancy: recommendations for the regional development of maternal and perinatal health services. White Plains (NY): National Foundation—March of Dimes; 1976.

Congressional Budget Office. Factors contributing to the infant mortality ranking of the United States. CBO Staff Memorandum. Washington, DC: CBO; 1992. Available at: http://www.cbo.gov/ftpdocs/62xx/doc6219/doc05b.pdf. Retrieved December 15, 2006.

Evidenced-based quality improvement in neonatal and perinatal medicine. Pediatrics 1999;103(suppl).

Halamek LP. The advantages of prenatal consultation by a neonatologist. J Perinatol 2001;21:116–20.

Horbar JD. The Vermont Oxford Network: evidence-based quality improvement for neonatology. Pediatrics 1999;103(suppl):350–9.

Howell EM, Richardson D, Ginsburg P, Foot B. Deregionalization of neonatal intensive care in urban areas. Am J Public Health 2002;92:119–24.

The importance of preconception care in the continuum of women's health care. American College of Obstetricians and Gynecologists. ACOG Committee Opinion No. 313. Obstet Gynecol 2005;106:665–6.

Institute of Medicine. Including children and pregnant women in health care reform. Summary of two workshops. Washington, DC: National Academy Press; 1992.

Institute of Medicine (US). The best intentions: unintended pregnancy and the well-being of children and families. Washington, DC: National Academy Press; 1995.

Institute of Medicine (US). Health literacy: a prescription to end confusion. Washington, DC: National Academies Press; 2004.

Makuc DM, Haglund B, Ingram DD, Kleinman JC, Feldman JJ. Health service areas for the United States. Vital Health Stat 2 1991;(112):1–102.

March of Dimes Birth Defects Foundation. Toward improving the outcome of pregnancy: the 90s and beyond. White Plains (NY): MDBDF; 1993.

Paul DA, Epps S, Leef KH, Stefano JL. Prenatal consultation with a neonatologist prior to preterm delivery. J Perinatol 2001;21:431–7.

Phibbs CS, Bronstein JM, Boxton E, Phibbs RH. The effects of patient volume and level of care at the hospital of birth on neonatal mortality. JAMA 1996;276:1054–9.

Pollack LD. An effective model for reorganization of perinatal services in a metropolitan area: a descriptive analysis and historical perspective. J Perinatol 1996;16:3–8.

Public Health Service (US). Caring for our future: the content of prenatal care. A report of the Public Health Service Expert Panel on the Content of Prenatal Care. Washington, DC: Department of Health and Human Services; 1989.

Richardson DK, Gray JE, Gortmaker SL, Goldmann DA, Pursley DM, McCormick MC. Declining severity adjusted mortality: evidence of improving neonatal intensive care. Pediatrics 1998;102:893–9.

Stark AR. Levels of neonatal care. American Academy of Pediatrics Committee on Fetus and Newborn. Pediatrics 2004;114:1341–7.

Stevenson DK, Quaintance CC. The California Perinatal Quality Care Collaborative: a model for national perinatal care. J Perinatol 1999;19:249–50.

Wall SN, Handler AS, Park CG. Hospital factors and nontransfer of small babies: a marker of deregionalized perinatal care? J Perinatol 2004;24:351–9.

chapter 2

Inpatient Perinatal Care Services

This chapter outlines recommendations regarding medical expertise, nursing ratios, staffing guidelines, support services, perinatal outreach education, and physical facilities required for providing hospital-based perinatal care. These components have been defined for facilities providing level I (basic), level II (specialty), and level III (subspecialty) care. Regionalized systems are recommended to ensure that each newborn infant is delivered and cared for in a facility appropriate for his or her health care needs and to facilitate the achievement of optimal outcomes. Within regionalized systems, electronic communications, including the use of electronic medical records, are important to ensuring quality care.

Personnel

Factors critical to planning and evaluating the quality and level of personnel required to meet patients' needs in perinatal settings include the mission, philosophy, geographic location, and design of the facility; the patient population; the scope of practice; the qualifications of staff; and obligations for education or research. Perinatal care programs at level I, level II, and level III hospitals should be coordinated jointly by medical and nursing directors for obstetric and pediatric services.

Medical Providers

Credentialing and granting privileges to members of its medical staff are among the most important responsibilities of any health care facility. Credentialing is a multifaceted process that involves verification of licensure, education, training, medical liability coverage, experience, and specialty board certification. Other criteria for effective credentialing include review of official source data, such as the National Practitioner Data Bank, data from other facilities where the individual has privileges, and references from peers. Hospitals must query the National Practitioner Data Bank at the time of application for clinical privileges and every 2 years, as well as when the hospital wants to expand existing privileges.

The more difficult, yet critical, aspect of the credentialing process is the actual determination of which requested privileges should be granted. The granting of privileges is based on training, experience, and demonstrated clinical competence. For obstetric providers, care may be stratified into different levels of complexity. Core privileges represent areas grouped together that require similar education, training, or skill to be performed. The concept also may be referred to as "bundling" of privileges.

Other key elements of the credentialing process that may be considered by a facility include the following:

- New appointees may be granted privileges for a provisional period of no less than 12 months, during which time the appointee must have admitted a minimum number of patients or performed a predetermined number of surgical procedures to demonstrate competence.

- Appointees in good standing should have a quality improvement file maintained at all times that should be reviewed every 2 years, or at the time of reappointment, for trends; sentinel events; and issues with specific diagnoses, procedures, or behaviors, including complaints or compliments.

New equipment or technology may improve health care outcomes, provided that practitioners and other hospital staff use the tools as specified for the conditions for which they are designed. Problems can arise when physicians or staff perform procedures or use equipment for which they are not trained. The board should consider granting privileges for new skills only when the appropriate training has been completed and documented and the competency level has been achieved with adequate supervision.

For pediatric providers, the credentials required and the privileges extended will depend on the level of care that is provided. Verification of training, experience, and current clinical competence is similar to that for obstetric providers.

Specific definitions of levels of care are recommended based on the functional capability of facilities to provide increasing complexity of quality care to newborns according to their degree of risk and severity of illness. These are identified as level I (basic), level II (specialty), and level III (subspecialty) (see "In-Hospital Perinatal Care" in Chapter 1). The obstetric service within a facility should be matched with the level of neonatal care that can be provided.

Level I (Basic) Care Facility

The perinatal care program at a hospital providing basic care should be coordinated jointly by the chiefs of the obstetric, pediatric, nursing, and midwifery services. This administrative approach requires close coordination and unified policy statements. The coordinators of perinatal care at a basic care hospital are responsible for developing policy, maintaining appropriate guidelines, and collaborating and consulting with the professional staff of hospitals providing specialty and subspecialty care in the region. In hospitals that do not separate these services, one person may be given the responsibility for coordinating perinatal care.

A qualified physician or certified nurse midwife should attend all deliveries. Collaborative practice involving a multidisciplinary team is encouraged. This team may consist of obstetrician–gynecologists and certified nurse midwives as well as other health care professionals who function within the context of their educational preparation and scope of practice. For example, certified nurse midwives are educated in the disciplines of nursing and midwifery and possess evidence of certification meeting the requirements of the American College of Nurse-Midwives. Certified nurse midwives may provide care for low-risk women in the antepartum, intrapartum, and postpartum periods; manage normal newborns; and provide primary gynecologic services in accordance with state laws or regulations. Obstetrician–gynecologists' training, credentials, and responsibilities place them in the role of team leaders, but various other providers are needed for unique contributions that are valuable and important to the quality of patient outcomes. Clinical practice relationships between obstetrician–gynecologists and certified nurse midwives should provide for mutually agreed-on, written medical guidelines and protocols for clinical practice that define the individual and shared responsibilities of certified nurse midwives and obstetrician–gynecologists, or other physicians with obstetric hospital privileges, in the delivery of health care services and for ongoing communication that defines appropriate consultation between obstetrician–gynecologists and certified nurse midwives. These guidelines also should provide for informed consent about the involvement of obstetrician–gynecologists, other physicians with obstetric hospital privileges, certified nurse midwives, and other health care providers in the services offered. The obstetrician should be informed of the patient's condition and progress as appropriate for the situation.

Hospitals should ensure the availability of skilled personnel for perinatal emergencies. Anesthesia personnel with credentials to administer obstetric anesthesia should be available on a 24-hour basis. The nursery at a level I facility should have the personnel and equipment to perform neonatal resuscitation. At least one person whose primary responsibility is for the newborn and who is capable of initiating neonatal resuscitation should be present at every delivery. Either that person or someone else who is immediately available should have the skills required to perform a complete resuscitation, including endotracheal intubation and administration of medications. This resuscitation should be performed according to the American Heart Association and American Academy of Pediatrics Neonatal Resuscitation Program. When required, one or two additional persons should be available to assist with neonatal resuscitation (see "Neonatal Resuscitation" in Chapter 7).

Personnel and equipment should be available to evaluate and provide postnatal care of healthy newborn infants, to stabilize and provide care for infants born at 35–37 weeks of gestation who remain physiologically stable, and to stabilize newborns born at less than 35 weeks of gestation or ill newborns until they are transferred to a facility that can provide the appropriate level of neonatal care.

Level II (Specialty) Care Facility

A level II (specialty) nursery is organized with the personnel and equipment to provide care to infants born at more than 32 weeks of gestation and weighing more than 1,500 g who have physiologic immaturity, such as apnea of prematurity, inability to maintain body temperature, or inability to take oral feedings; who are moderately ill with problems that are expected to resolve rapidly and are not anticipated to need subspecialty services on an urgent basis; or who are convalescing from intensive care.

Level II care is subdivided into two categories that are differentiated by the ability to provide assisted ventilation. Level IIA nurseries do not have the capability to provide assisted ventilation, except on a limited basis until the infant can be transferred to a higher-level facility. Level IIB nurseries can provide mechanical ventilation for brief durations (less than 24 hours) or continuous positive airway pressure. They must have the personnel (eg, physicians, specialized nurses, respiratory therapists, radiology technicians, laboratory technicians) and equipment (eg, portable chest radiograph, blood gas laboratory) continuously available to provide ongoing care as well as to address emergencies. When the nursery has an infant on a ventilator, specialized personnel should be available on site to manage respiratory emergencies. At a hospital with a level II nursery, a board-certified obstetrician–gynecologist with special interest, experience, and, in some situations, a subspecialty in maternal–fetal medicine, should be chief of the obstetric service. In a level IIB hospital, a board-certified pediatrician with subspecialty certification in neonatal–perinatal medicine should be chief of the neonatal care service. These physicians should coordinate the hospital's perinatal care services and, in conjunction with other medical, anesthesia, nursing, respiratory therapy, and hospital administration staff, develop policies concerning staffing, procedures, equipment, and supplies.

Care of neonates at high risk should be provided by appropriately qualified physicians. A general pediatrician should have the expertise to assume responsibility for acute, although less critical, care of newborns; understand the need for proper continuity of care and be capable of providing it; and share responsibility with a consulting neonatologist for the development and delivery of effective services for newborns at risk in the hospital and community. In collaboration with a physician, care may be provided by qualified advanced-practice nurses who have formal education in acute care and training in the care of critically ill newborns in level II or III neonatal intensive care units (NICU), as well as at least 600 supervised clinical hours and experience in the care of these newborns at high risk.

The director of obstetric anesthesia services should be board certified in anesthesia and should have training and experience in obstetric anesthesia. Anesthesia personnel with privileges to administer obstetric anesthesia should be available according to hospital policy. Policies regarding the provision of obstetric anesthesia, including the necessary qualifications of personnel who are to administer anesthesia and their availability for both routine and emergency deliveries, should be developed.

The hospital staff also should include a radiologist and a clinical pathologist who are available 24 hours per day. Specialized medical and surgical consultation also should be available.

Level III (Subspecialty) Care Facility

A level III (subspecialty) NICU has continuously available personnel and equipment to provide life support for as long as needed and to provide comprehensive care for newborn infants at extremely high risk and those with complex and critical illnesses.

Level IIIA NICUs can provide care for newborns with a birth weight of more than 1,000 g and a gestational age of more than 28 weeks. Continuous life support can be provided but is limited to conventional mechanical ventilation. Minor surgical procedures can be performed. Level IIIB NICUs care for infants with extreme prematurity (28 weeks of gestation or less) or extremely low birth weight (1,000 g or less) or who have severe or complex illnesses. Advanced respiratory support, including high-frequency ventilation and inhaled nitric oxide, and physiologic monitoring equipment must be available. Level IIIC NICUs, which may be located at children's hospitals, have the capabilities of level IIIB NICUs and also are located within an institution with the capability of providing extracorporeal membrane oxygenation and performing surgical repair of complex congenital cardiac malformations that require cardiopulmonary bypass. Because of the degree of risk involved, advanced fetal interventions, such as intrauterine fetal transfusions and fetal–placental surgery, should be performed at level IIIB or IIIC facilities.

The director of the maternal–fetal medicine service of a hospital providing subspecialty care should be a full-time, board-certified obstetrician with subspecialty certification in maternal–fetal medicine. The director of the newborn intensive care unit should be a full-time, board-certified pediatrician with subspecialty certification in neonatal–perinatal medicine. As codirectors of the perinatal service, these physicians are responsible for maintaining practice guidelines and, in cooperation with nursing and hospital administration, are responsible for developing the operating budget; evaluating and purchasing equipment; planning, developing, and coordinating in-hospital and outreach educational programs; and participating in the evaluation of perinatal care. If they are in a regional center, they should devote their time to providing and supervising patient care services, research, and teaching, and they should coordinate the services provided at their hospital with those provided at level I (basic) and level II (specialty) hospitals in the region.

Other maternal–fetal medicine specialists and neonatologists who practice in the subspecialty care facility should have qualifications similar to those of the chief of their service. A maternal–fetal medicine specialist and a neonatologist should be continuously available for consultation 24 hours per day. Personnel qualified to manage obstetric or neonatal emergencies should be in-house.

Advanced obstetric and neonatal diagnostic imaging facilities with interpretation on an urgent basis should be available 24 hours per day. Level IIIB and IIIC NICUs require urgent access for consultation to a broad range of pediatric, rather than adult, medical subspecialists, including cardiology, neurology, hematology, genetics, nephrology, metabolism, endocrinology, gastroenterology–nutrition, infectious diseases, pulmonology, immunology, pathology, and pharmacology. Pediatric surgical subspecialists (eg, general pediatric surgeons; cardiovascular surgeons; neurosurgeons; and orthopedic, ophthalmologic, urologic, plastic, and otolaryngologic surgeons) should be available on site or at a closely related institution for consultation and care. Evidence indicates that management of neonates and young children by adult subspecialists, rather than pediatric subspecialists, results in greater costs, longer hospital stays, and potentially greater morbidity.

A board-certified anesthesiologist with special training or experience in maternal–fetal anesthesia should be in charge of obstetric anesthesia services at a level III (subspecialty) care hospital. Personnel with privileges in the administration of obstetric anesthesia should be available in the hospital 24 hours per day. Pediatric anesthesiologists should be available for all neonatal surgical procedures.

Nurse and Physician Assistant Providers

Delivery of safe and effective perinatal nursing care requires appropriately qualified registered nurses in adequate numbers to meet the needs of each patient. The number of staff and level of skill required are influenced by the scope of nursing practice and the degree of nursing responsibilities within an institution. Nursing responsibilities in individual hospitals vary according to the level of care provided by the facility, practice procedures, number of professional registered nurses and ancillary staff, and professional nursing activities in continuing education and research. Intrapartum care requires the same labor intensiveness and expertise as any other intensive care and, accordingly, perinatal units should have the same adequately trained personnel and fiscal support.

Trends in medical management and technologic advances influence and may increase the nursing workload. Each hospital should determine the scope of nursing practice for each nursing unit and specialty department. The scope of practice should be based on national nursing guidelines for the specialty area of practice and should be in accordance with state laws and regulations. A multidisciplinary committee, including representatives from hospital, medical, and nursing administrations, should follow published professional guidelines, consult state nurse practice acts and any accompanying regulations, identify the types and numbers of procedures performed in each unit, delineate the direct and indirect nursing care activities performed, and identify the activities that are to be performed by nonnursing personnel.

Trends in neonatal care have resulted in an increased use of advanced-practice nurses and physician assistants (PAs). An advanced-practice neonatal nurse is prepared, according to nationally recognized standards, by the completion of an educational program of study and supervised practice beyond the level of basic nursing. As of January 1, 2000, this preparation must include the attainment of a master's degree in the nursing specialty. Graduates from previous years who currently are credentialed advanced-practice neonatal nurse or certificate-prepared (nongraduate) neonatal nurse practitioners should be allowed to maintain their practice and are encouraged to complete a formal graduate education. Included in this category are the following nursing professionals:

- Neonatal clinical nurse specialist—A neonatal clinical nurse specialist is a registered nurse with a master's degree who, through study and supervised practice at the graduate level, has become expert in the theory and practice of neonatal nursing. Responsibilities of the neonatal clinical nurse specialist include serving as a resource for neonatal nurses, neonatal nurse practitioners, and other care providers; establishing and evaluating standards of patient care within a unit; assessing and identifying educational needs of the family, nursery, and community; designing and implementing appropriate educational programs on the basis of identified needs; providing consultation to others in the nursery, hospital, or community; and initiating research projects, participating in data collection, and implementing changes on the basis of research findings.

- Neonatal nurse practitioner—A neonatal nurse practitioner is a registered nurse with clinical expertise in neonatal nursing who has obtained a master's degree or completed an educational program of study and supervised practice beyond the level of basic nursing in the specialty with supervised clinical experience in the management of newborns and their families. These nurses manage a caseload of neonatal patients with consultation, collaboration, and medical supervision. Using their acquired knowledge of pathophysiology, pharmacology, and physiology, neonatal nurse practitioners exercise independent judgment in the assessment and diagnosis of newborns and in the performance of certain delegated procedures. Similar to advanced-practice neonatal nurses, neonatal nurse practitioners are involved in education, consultation, and research. Any advanced-practice nurses caring for neonates must demonstrate completion of a formal neonatal educational program with at least 600 precepted clinical hours in an accredited postmaster's degree neonatal nurse practitioner program.

- Physician assistants—Physician assistants are health care professionals licensed to practice medicine with physician supervision. Within the physician–PA relationship, PAs exercise autonomy in medical decision making and provide a broad range of diagnostic and therapeutic services. A PA's responsibilities also may include education, research, and administrative services. Physician assistants are educated and trained in programs accredited by the Accreditation Review Commission on Education for the Physician Assistant. Graduation from an accredited PA program and passage of the national certifying examination are required for state licensure. A number of postgraduate PA programs also have been established to provide practicing PAs with advanced education in medical specialties. The responsibilities of a PA depend on the practice setting, education and experience of the PA, and on state laws and regulations. Regardless of background training, the following guidelines are recommended:

  — Physician supervision should be provided by a neonatologist in NICUs. In basic and specialty units, a board-certified pediatrician with special interest and experience in neonatal medicine may provide supervision.

  — The PA is responsible for maintaining clinical expertise and knowledge of current therapy by participating in continuing medical education and scholarly activities.

  — To maintain their national certification, PAs must log 100 hours of continuing medical education every 2 years and sit for a recertification examination with the National Commission on Certification of Physician Assistants every 6 years.

- The term neonatal nurse clinician is imprecise and should no longer be used.

The spectrum of duties performed by an advanced-practice neonatal nurse will vary according to the institution and may be determined by state regulations. Each of these roles currently requires advanced education and a master's degree. Nationally recognized certification examinations exist for each category of advanced-practice neonatal nurse. Credentialing to practice currently is governed by individual states. Inpatient care privileges are granted by individual institutions. Each institution should develop a procedure for the initial granting and subsequent maintenance of privileges, ensuring that the proper professional credentials are in place. Each institution must ensure that the advanced-practice nurse has the formal education to function within the neonatal scope of practice. That procedure is best developed by the collaborative efforts of the nursing administration and the medical staff governing body. The following guidelines are recommended:

- Medical care provided by an advanced-practice neonatal nurse in a NICU should be supervised by a neonatologist. In level I and level II units, a board-certified pediatrician with special interest and experience in neonatal medicine may provide supervision.

- The advanced-practice neonatal nurse should collaborate and consult with other health care professionals.

- The advanced-practice neonatal nurse should demonstrate graduation from an accredited neonatal program that provides didactic and precepted clinical experiences in neonatal critical care according to the National Association of Neonatal Nurses education standards.

- The advanced-practice neonatal nurse should be certified by a nationally recognized organization in the neonatal specialty and should maintain that certification.

- The advanced-practice neonatal nurse should maintain clinical expertise and knowledge of current therapy by participating in continuing education and other scholarly activities.

- The advanced-practice neonatal nurse should comply with hospital policy regarding credentialing and recredentialing.

Recommended nurse/patient ratios for perinatal services are shown in Table 2–1. Additional personnel are necessary for indirect patient-care activities. Close evaluation of all factors involved in a specific case is essential for establishing an acceptable nurse/patient ratio. Variables such as birth weight, gestational age, and diagnosis of patients; patient turnover; acuity of patients' conditions; patient or parent education needs; bereavement care; mixture of skills of the staff; environment; types of delivery; and use of anesthesia must be taken into account in determining appropriate nurse/patient ratios. The efficiency of nursing care can be enhanced by a team approach.

Level I (Basic) Care Facility

Perinatal nursing care at a basic care facility should be under the direction of a registered nurse. The registered nurse's responsibilities include directing peri-

Table 2-1. Recommended Registered Nurse/Patient Ratios for Perinatal Care Services

Registered Nurse/Patient Ratio	Care Provided
Intrapartum	
1:2	Patients in labor
1:1	Patients in second stage of labor
1:1	Patients with medical or obstetric complications
1:2	Oxytocin induction or augmentation of labor
1:1	Coverage for initiating epidural anesthesia
1:1	Circulation for cesarean delivery
Antepartum–Postpartum	
1:6	Antepartum and postpartum patients without complications
1:2	Patients in postoperative recovery
1:3	Antepartum and postpartum patients with complications but in stable condition
1:4	Newborns and those requiring close observation
Newborns	
1:6-8*	Newborns requiring only routine care
1:3-4	Normal mother-newborn couple care or breastfeeding care
1:3-4	Newborns requiring continuing care
1:2-3	Newborns requiring intermediate care
1:1-2	Newborns requiring intensive care
1:1	Newborns requiring multisystem support
1:1 or greater	Unstable newborns requiring complex critical care

*This ratio reflects traditional well-newborn nursery care. If it is necessary to separate the well mother and newborn couple and return the newborn to a central nursery, the mother-newborn registered nurse still is responsible for the mother-newborn couple. Another registered nurse should provide care for the newborn in the central nursery. At least one registered nurse should be available at all times in each occupied basic care nursery when newborns physically are present in the nursery. In special care and subspecialty care nurseries, a minimum of two registered nurses, with training and expertise in neonatal nursing, should be in immediate attendance (National Association of Neonatal Nurses. Minimum staffing in NICUs. NANN Position Statement 3009. Glenview [IL]: NANN; 1999. Available at http://www.nann.org/files/public/articles/309.doc. Retrieved June 10, 2002). Direct care of newborns in the nursery may be provided by ancillary personnel under the registered nurse's direct supervision. Adequate staff is needed to respond to acute and emergency situations at all times.

natal nursing services, guiding the development and implementation of perinatal policies and procedures, collaborating with medical staff, and consulting with hospitals that provide level II (specialty) and level III (subspecialty) care in the region.

For antepartum care, it is recommended that a registered nurse whose responsibilities include the organization and supervision of antepartum, intrapartum, and neonatal nursing services be on duty. The presence of one or more registered nurses or licensed practical nurses with demonstrated knowledge and clinical competence in the nursing care of women, fetuses, and newborns during labor, delivery, and the postpartum and neonatal periods is suggested. Ancillary personnel, supervised by a registered nurse, may provide support to the patient and attend to her personal comfort.

Intrapartum care should be under the direct supervision of a registered nurse. Responsibilities of the registered nurse include initial evaluation and admission of patients in labor; continuing assessment and evaluation of patients in labor, including checking the status of the fetus, recording vital signs, monitoring the fetal heart rate, performing obstetric examinations, observing uterine contractions, and supporting the patient; determining the presence or absence of complications; supervising the performance of nurses with less training and experience and of ancillary personnel; and staffing of the delivery room at the time of delivery. A licensed practical nurse or nurse assistant, supervised by a registered nurse, may provide support to the patient and attend to her personal comfort.

Postpartum care of the woman and her newborn should be provided by a registered nurse whose responsibilities include initial and ongoing assessment, newborn care education, support for the attachment process and breastfeeding, preparation for healthy parenting, preparation for discharge, and follow-up of the woman and her newborn within the context of the family. This registered nurse should have training and experience in the recognition of normal and abnormal physical and emotional characteristics of the mother and her newborn. Again, a licensed practical nurse or nurse assistant, supervised by a registered nurse, may provide support to the mother and attend to her personal comfort in the postpartum period.

In the level I nursery, the registered nurse directly observes the neonate during the stabilization period after birth. The nurse monitors the infant's adaptation to extrauterine life and then, ideally, assists in the transition of the newborn to rooming in with the mother. The neonatal nurse also can practice in a newborn nursery, taking care of healthy newborns.

Level II (Specialty Care Facility)

Specialty care hospitals should have a director of perinatal and neonatal nursing services who has overall responsibility for inpatient activities in the respective obstetric and neonatal areas. This registered nurse should have demonstrated expertise in obstetric or neonatal care.

In addition to fulfilling nursing responsibilities of level I hospitals, nursing staff in the labor, delivery, and recovery areas should be able to identify and respond to the obstetric and medical complications of pregnancy, labor, and delivery. A registered nurse with advanced training and experience in routine and high-risk obstetric care should be assigned to the labor and delivery area at all times. In the postpartum period, a registered nurse should be responsible for providing support for women and families with newborns who require intensive care and for facilitating visitation and communication with the NICU.

Licensed practical nurses and unlicensed personnel who have appropriate training in perinatal care and are supervised by a registered nurse may provide assistance with the delivery of care, provide support to the patient, assist with lactation support, and attend to the woman's personal comfort.

All nurses caring for ill newborns must possess demonstrated knowledge in the observation and treatment of newborns, including cardiorespiratory monitoring. Furthermore, the registered nursing staff of a level II nursery in a specialty care hospital takes on a greater responsibility for monitoring the premature newborn or the newborn who is having difficulty in adapting to extrauterine life. The neonatal nurse at this level cares for premature or term newborns who are ill or injured from complications at birth. The neonatal nurse provides the newborn with frequent observation and monitoring and should be able to monitor and maintain the stability of cardiopulmonary, neurologic, metabolic, and thermal functions; assist with special procedures, such as lumbar puncture, endotracheal intubation, and umbilical vessel catheterization; and perform emergency resuscitation. The nurse should be specially trained and able to initiate, modify, or stop treatment when appropriate, according to established protocols, even when a physician or advanced practice nurse is not present. In units where neonates receive mechanical ventilation, medical, nursing, or respiratory therapy, staff (ie, medical staff or nursing staff) with demonstrated ability to intubate the trachea, manage assisted ventilation, and decompress a pneumothorax should be available continually (see Table 2–1). The nursing staff should be formally trained and validated in neonatal resuscitation. The unit's medical director, in conjunction with other personnel, should define and supervise the delegated medical functions, processes, and procedures performed by various categories of personnel.

Level III (Subspecialty) Care Facility

The director of perinatal and neonatal nursing services at a level III (subspecialty) hospital should have overall responsibility for inpatient activities in the maternity–newborn care units. This registered nurse should have experience and training in obstetric or neonatal nursing or both, as well as in the care of patients at high risk. Preferably, this individual should have an advanced degree.

For antepartum care, a registered nurse should be responsible for the direction and supervision of nursing care. All nurses working with antepartum patients at high risk should have evidence of continuing education in maternal–fetal nursing. An advanced-practice nurse who has been educated and prepared at the master's level should be on staff to coordinate education.

For intrapartum care, a registered nurse should be in attendance within the labor and delivery unit at all times. This registered nurse should be skilled in the recognition and nursing management of complications of labor and delivery.

For postpartum care, a registered nurse should be in attendance at all times. This registered nurse should be skilled in the recognition and nursing management of complications in women and newborns.

Registered nurses in the NICU should have specialty certification or advanced training and experience in the nursing management of neonates at high risk and their families. They also should be experienced in caring for unstable neonates with multi-organ system problems and in specialized care technology. The neonatal nurse in a level III NICU provides direct care for the premature or term infant who requires complex care, including an infant requiring intensive life-support techniques, such as mechanical ventilation. In level IIIB and IIIC units, the nurse also should be able to provide care for infants requiring inhaled nitric oxide therapy and high-frequency ventilation. The nurse in a level IIIC unit also should be able to provide care for infants requiring extracorporeal membrane oxygenation. The nurse in level IIIB and IIIC units also should be able to care for the chronically technology-dependent infant.

An advanced-practice nurse should be available to the staff for consultation and support on nursing care issues. Additional nurses with special training are required to fulfill regional center responsibilities, such as outreach and transport (see "Transport Procedure" and "Outreach Education" in Chapter 3).

The obstetric and neonatal areas may be staffed by a mix of professional and technical personnel. Assessment and monitoring activities should remain the responsibility of a registered nurse or an advanced-practice nurse in obstetric–neonatal nursing, even when personnel with a mixture of skills are used.

Support Providers

All Facilities

Personnel who are capable of determining blood type, crossmatching blood, and performing antibody testing should be available on a 24-hour basis. The hospital's infection control personnel should be responsible for surveillance of infections in women and neonates, as well as for the development of an appropriate environmental control program (see "Infection Control" and "Environmental Control" in Chapter 10). A radiologic technician should be readily available 24 hours per day to perform portable X-rays. Availability of a postpartum care provider with expertise in lactation is essential. The need for other support personnel depends on the intensity and level of sophistication of the other support services provided. An organized plan of action that includes personnel and equipment should be established for identification and immediate resuscitation of neonates in need of intervention (see "Neonatal Resuscitation" in Chapter 7).

Level II (Specialty) and Level III (Subspecialty) Care Facilities

The following support personnel should be available to the perinatal care service of level II (specialty) and level III (subspecialty) hospitals:

- At least one full-time, master's degree-level, medical social worker for every 30 beds who has experience with the socioeconomic and psychosocial problems of both women and fetuses at high risk, ill neonates, and their families. Additional medical social workers are required when there is a high volume of medical or psychosocial activity.

- At least one occupational or physical therapist with neonatal expertise

- At least one individual skilled in evaluation and management of neonatal feeding and swallowing disorders (eg, speech-language pathologist)

- At least one registered dietitian or nutritionist who has special training in perinatal nutrition and can plan diets that meet the special needs of both women and neonates at high risk

- Qualified personnel for support services, such as diagnostic laboratory studies, radiologic studies, and ultrasound examinations (these personnel should be available 24 hours per day)

- Respiratory therapists who can supervise the assisted ventilation of neonates with cardiopulmonary disease
- Pharmacy personnel with pediatric expertise who can work to continually review their systems and processes of medication administration to ensure that patient care policies are maintained
- Personnel skilled in pastoral care, available as needed

The hospital's engineering department should include air-conditioning, electrical, and mechanical engineers and biomedical technicians who are responsible for the safety and reliability of the equipment in all perinatal care areas.

Education

In-Service and Continuing Education

The medical and nursing staff of any hospital providing perinatal care at any level should maintain knowledge about and competency in current maternal and neonatal care through joint in-service sessions. These sessions should cover the diagnosis and management of perinatal emergencies, as well as the management of routine problems and family-centered care. The staff of each unit should have regular multidisciplinary conferences at which patient care problems are presented and discussed.

The staff of regional centers should be capable of assisting with the in-service programs of other hospitals in their region on a regular basis. Such assistance may include periodic visits to those hospitals as well as periodic review of the quality of patient care provided by those hospitals. Regional center staff should be accessible for consultation at all times. The medical and nursing staff of hospitals providing level II (specialty) and level III (subspecialty) care should participate in formal courses or conferences. Regularly scheduled conferences may include the following subjects:

- Review of the major perinatal conditions, their medical treatment, and nursing care
- Review of electronic fetal monitoring, including maternal–fetal outcomes, toward a goal of standardizing nomenclature and patient care
- Review of perinatal statistics, the pathology related to all deaths, and significant surgical specimens
- Review of current imaging studies
- Family-centered care

- Review of perinatal complications and outcomes
- Review of patient satisfaction data, complaints, and compliments

Perinatal Outreach Education

Design and coordination of a program for perinatal outreach education should be provided jointly by neonatal and obstetric physicians and advanced-practice neonatal nurses. Responsibilities should include assessing educational needs; planning curricula; teaching, implementing, and evaluating the program; collecting and using perinatal data; providing patient follow-up information to referring community personnel; writing reports; and maintaining informative working relationships with community personnel and outreach team members.

Ideally, a maternal–fetal medicine specialist, a certified nurse–midwife, an obstetric nurse, a neonatologist, and a neonatal nurse should be members of the perinatal outreach education team. Other professionals (eg, a social worker, respiratory therapist, occupational and physical therapist, or nutritionist) also may be assigned to the team. Each member should be responsible for teaching, consulting with community professionals as needed, and maintaining communication with the program coordinator and other team members.

Each subspecialty care center in a regional system may organize an education program that is tailored to meet the needs of the perinatal health professionals and institutions within the network. The various educational strategies that have been found to be effective include seminars, audiovisual and media programs, self-instruction booklets, and clinical practice rotations. Perinatal outreach education meetings should be held at a routine time and place to promote standardization and continuity of communication among community professionals and regional center personnel. As mandated by the subspecialty boards and the Accreditation Council for Graduate Medical Education, a level III (subspecialty) center that has a fellowship training program should have an active research program.

Quality Improvement and Patient Safety

Continuous Quality Improvement

The Joint Commission (formerly the Joint Commission on Accreditation of Healthcare Organizations [JCAHO]) has promoted assessment of quality and patient safety in hospitals and other health care organizations for many years. There are three terms that apply to this process:

- Quality assessment: the retrospective analysis of data (outcomes)
- Quality improvement (QI): the improvement of identified problems
- Continuous quality improvement (CQI): an ongoing, systematic process to continually improve care.

Continuous quality improvement starts from the premise that although most medical care is good, it always can be better. The goal is to reduce variations in care and improve performance. Continuous quality improvement accepts that good care depends upon more than just the judgment of the individual. The assessment of quality care focuses on the following dimensions:

- Structure
- Process
- Outcomes

In order to provide the structure, there must be adequate space, equipment, staffing, policies, procedures, and guidelines. Process refers to the steps that are taken to ensure good outcomes. Finally, even with adequate structures and an efficient process, quality care requires that the desired outcomes be achieved. All of these components—structures, processes, and outcomes, with an emphasis on patient safety—are the focus of a well-designed CQI program.

A CQI program requires effective, responsive leadership from both medical staff and administration. The chair of the department ultimately is responsible for QI activities. When physicians accept these leadership positions, their primary purpose is to establish an environment in which QI can thrive.

Peer review is a quality assessment process in which a retrospective analysis of cases is undertaken using outcomes data to assess adherence to guidelines or other standards of care. Although initial screening may be done by nonphysicians, true peer review is performed by peer physicians with similar background and training. Peer review may result in recommendations of individual practice changes or more global changes resulting from the QI process.

A departmental peer review committee may include the following members, with consideration given to the vice chair of the department serving as the committee chair:

- Representative physicians with varying levels of clinical experience (junior and senior staff) within the department

- Representative subspecialists, when available
- House staff member, when appropriate
- The department chair (ex officio)

Small hospitals may face difficulty conducting peer review because of competitive interests or interpersonal problems that have a real or perceived effect on the efficacy of the review. Therefore, it may be helpful to develop a relationship with another hospital to conduct peer review. An alternative would be to use the services of an outside, independent reviewer. In either case, it is important to remember that responsibility for peer review and QI rests with the hospital medical staff and, ultimately, the governing board.

A CQI program also requires tools to assess and determine overall performance. The department may choose to apply or develop clinical guidelines for high-volume, resource-intensive, or costly diagnoses or procedures. Guidelines may take the form of a multidisciplinary plan of care or a simple decision tree. Clinical pathways are intended to improve outcomes and efficiency by reducing unwanted variation and complexity. A pathway is not a standard but a guideline for care. Deviations may occur but should be well documented. All disciplines involved in a pathway, including nursing, physicians, nutrition, social work, and case management, must be involved in the design and implementation of the pathway.

Continuous quality improvement programs must focus on measurable dimensions of care when selecting indicators to track for identifying processes in need of improvement (Box 2–1).

In its report *Crossing the Quality Chasm*, the Institute of Medicine set forth a list of performance characteristics that, if addressed and improved, would lead to better health and function for the people of the United States (see Resources). There are six specific qualities of good care that can be helpful in designing a QI program. The Institute of Medicine said that health care should be:

- Safe—avoiding injuries to patients from the care that is intended to help
- Effective—providing services based on scientific knowledge to all who could benefit and refraining from providing services to those not likely to benefit (avoiding underuse and overuse)
- Patient centered—providing care that is respectful of and responsive to individual patient preferences, needs, and values, and ensuring that patient values guide all clinical decisions

Box 2–1. Indicators to Track for Identifying Processes in Need of Improvement

Characteristics to consider when developing indicators

- Is the indicator clearly and accurately defined?
- Can the indicator be broken down into smaller parts that may be assessed individually?
- Can the indicator be measured or quantified?
- What is the method used to track the indicator?
- How frequently does the indicator occur?
- How frequently should the indicator be measured?
- What is the severity of outcome to the patient or system?
- What is the economic effect?
- What is the liability effect?
- Is there an opportunity for improvement?
- How does the indicator compare to other institutions (benchmarks)?

Examples of obstetric quality indicators

- Unplanned maternal readmission within 14 days (outcome)
- In-hospital initiation of antibiotics 24 hours or more following term vaginal delivery (process)
- Unplanned removal, injury, or repair of organ during operative procedure (process)
- Excessive maternal blood loss (process)
- Maternal length of stay in excess of 1 day more than the local standard after vaginal or cesarean delivery (outcome)
- Delivery unattended by the "responsible" physician (to be defined by each institution) (outcome)
- Cesarean delivery for uncertain fetal status (outcome)
- Cesarean delivery for failure to progress (outcome)
- Deaths of infants weighing 500 g or more, subcategorized by intrahospital neonatal deaths, total stillborns, and intrapartum stillborns (outcome)
- Delivery of an infant at less than 32 weeks of gestation in an institution without a neonatal intensive care unit (outcome)
- Transfer of a neonate to a neonatal care unit in another institution (outcome)
- Elective induction of a patient less than 39 weeks of gestation without fetal lung maturity assessment (process)

American College of Obstetricians and Gynecologists. Quality Improvement in Women's Health Care. Washington, DC: ACOG; 2000.

- Timely—reducing waits and sometimes harmful delays for those who receive and those who provide care
- Efficient—avoiding waste, in particular, waste of equipment, supplies, ideas, and energy
- Equitable—providing care that does not vary in quality because of personal characteristics such as gender, ethnicity, geographic location, and socioeconomic status

Patient Safety

Patient safety shares many characteristics with a well-designed CQI model. However, patient safety emphasizes a systems analysis of medical errors and minimizes individual blame and retribution.

The Joint Commission recognizes the importance of patient safety. Beginning in 2003, the Joint Commission created the first set of National Patient Safety Goals. These goals, derived from Sentinel Event Alerts and other sources, are designed to be explicit, evidence based, and measurable. Each year, existing goals are modified based on public comment and the experience of reviewers and new goals are added. In this way, over time, the Joint Commission will develop a compendium of recommended practices that will improve patient safety (www.jcaho.org/accredited+organizations/patient+safety/npsg.htm).

The American College of Obstetricians and Gynecologists and the American Academy of Pediatrics also have a long-standing commitment to patient safety and quality. To improve patient care and reduce medical errors, they encourage all health care providers to promote the following four principles in all practice settings.

1. Commit to a culture of patient safety

   A culture of patient safety continuously evolves and should be the framework for every effort to reduce medical errors. Patient safety focuses on systems of care, not individuals. Confidential reporting and analysis of errors and near misses will reveal areas that require remediation to provide improved patient safety. State and federal laws may have an effect on the level of confidentiality and the manner of reporting.

   A culture of patient safety starts at the top with strong leadership that provides the necessary human and financial resources to achieve patient safety. Additionally, a culture of safety recognizes the importance of team function in optimizing individual performance.

2. Implement safe medication practices

Medication errors are one of the most common types of preventable adverse events. Automated systems for prescribing and dispensing medication can greatly reduce these errors, but there are many "low-tech" solutions that can be implemented rapidly with minimal cost:

- Improve legibility of written orders

- Avoid nonstandard abbreviation as recommended by the Joint Commission (www.jointcommission.org/patientsafety/DoNot UseList/)

- Always use a leading 0 for doses less than 1 unit (eg, 0.1 not .1) and never use a trailing 0 after a decimal point (eg, 1 mg not 1.0 mg): "always lead, never follow"

- All verbal orders should be written by the individual receiving the order then read back to the prescriber, and an effort should be made to eliminate verbal orders

3. Reduce likelihood of surgical errors

The American College of Obstetricians and Gynecologists and the American Academy of Pediatrics, along with other specialty societies and other organizations, have endorsed the Joint Commission's Universal Protocol to Prevent Wrong Site, Wrong Procedure, and Wrong Patient Surgery. The Joint Commission now requires this protocol as part of a preoperative "time out" involving all members of the operating room team, including the patient (www.jointcommission. org/PatientSafety/UniversalProtocol).

4. Improve communication

Physicians should be aware that complete and accurate communication of medical information is important in reducing preventable medical errors. Improving communication skills merits the same attention as improving clinical skills.

According to information gathered from the Joint Commission, in collecting sentinel event information, the most common cause of preventable adverse outcomes is communication error. Optimal communication to improve patient safety has many dimensions including:

- Communication with patient and family

- Communication among all those caring for the patient

- Availability of information necessary for coordination of care

The key to a good patient–clinician relationship is the ability to listen, explain, and empathize. This is particularly important if the patient is under stress, which negatively affects her ability to grasp important messages. The U.S. Preventive Services Task Force defines shared decision making as a process in which both the patient and clinician share information, participate in the decision-making process, and agree on a course of action (www.ahrq.gov/clinic/3rduspstf/shared/sharedba.htm).

Another factor potentially limiting communication is health literacy, which is unrelated to level of education or social status. In order to have a meaningful discussion with an individual about her health care, it is imperative that one recognize and address the patient's level of understanding and knowledge. Consider the following options to improve communication, elevate the level of understanding, and improve health literacy:

- Actively listen to the patient and understand her concerns and issues.

- Learn to recognize when the patient does not comprehend.

- Have the patient bring a family member or friend when difficult and crucial discussions are held.

- Have the patient recount her understanding of the information that was presented to her.

- Use several formats and repeat material and information in different ways to increase understanding and comprehension.

- Do not rush encounters.

A culture of patient safety fosters open communication and welcomes input from team members at every level. Care must be taken to ensure that hierarchical systems do not hamper free communication among clinicians. Competing clinical demands, interruptions, and distractions are inherent in clinical practice. It requires specific effort to ensure that issues are understood and that meaningful information is transferred. Certain clinical communications should be verified, such as reading back medication orders. Inaccurate information and missing clinical data can result in serious medical errors and patient injury. Relevant communications should be documented appropriately.

A very important part of communication is when and how to disclose medical errors. The National Patient Safety Foundation has stated: "When a health care injury occurs, the patient and the family or representative are entitled to a prompt explanation of how the injury occurred and its short- and long-term effects. When an error contributed to the injury, the patient and the family or representative should receive a truthful and compassionate explanation about the error and the remedies available to the patient. They should be informed that the factors involved in the injury will be investigated so that steps can be taken to reduce the likelihood of similar injury to other patients" (www.npsf. org/html/statement.html).

Patient safety is an explicit principle that must be embraced as a core value in patient care. This is an ongoing process that requires health care professionals to continually strive to learn from problems, identify system deficiencies, redesign processes, and implement change in their daily practice. Patient-centered care, open communication, and teamwork provide the foundation for optimal patient care and safety.

Physical Facilities

The physical facilities in which perinatal care is provided should be conducive to care that meets the unique physiologic and psychosocial needs of parents, neonates, and families (see "Family-Centered Care" in Chapter 1). Special facilities should be available when deviations from the norm require uninterrupted physiologic, biochemical, and clinical observation of patients throughout the perinatal period. Labor, delivery, and newborn care facilities should be located in close proximity to each other. When these facilities are distant from each other, provisions should be made for appropriate transitional areas.

The following recommendations are intended as general guidelines and should be interpreted with consideration given to local needs. Individual limitations of physical facilities for perinatal care may impede strict adherence to these recommendations. Furthermore, every facility will not have each of the functional units described. Provisions for individual units should be consistent with a regional perinatal care system and state and local public health regulations.

Obstetric Functional Units

The patient's personal needs, as well as those of her newborn and family, should be considered when obstetric service units are planned. The service should be consolidated in a designated area that is physically arranged to prohibit unrelated traffic through the service units. The obstetric facility should incorporate the following components of maternity and newborn care:

- Antepartum care for patient stabilization or hospitalization before labor

- Fetal diagnostic testing (eg, nonstress and contraction stress testing, biophysical profile, amniocentesis, and ultrasound examinations)
- Labor observation and evaluation for patients who are not yet in active labor or who must be observed to determine whether labor has actually begun; hospital obstetric services should develop a casual, comfortable area ("false-labor lounge") for patients in prodromal labor
- Labor
- Delivery
- Postpartum maternal and newborn care

Where rooms are suitably sized, located, and equipped, some or all of the components of maternity care listed previously can be combined in one or more rooms. For example, to maximize economy and flexibility of staff and space, many hospitals have successfully combined functions into labor–delivery–recovery (LDR) rooms or labor–delivery–recovery–postpartum (LDRP) rooms. Single-room maternity care services use LDRP rooms for intrapartum care and for postpartum care of both the woman and her neonate, a model that supports breastfeeding.

The following facilities should be available to both antepartum and postpartum units and, in appropriate circumstances, may be shared:

- Unit director and head nurse's office
- Nurses' station
- Medical records area
- Conference room
- Patient education area
- Staff lounge, locker rooms, and on-call sleep rooms
- Examination and treatment room(s)
- Secure area for storage of medications
- Instrument cleanup area
- Area and equipment for bedpan cleansing
- Sitz bath facilities
- Kitchen and pantry
- Workroom and storage area
- Sibling visiting area

Nonobstetric Patients

The labor and delivery area should be used for nonobstetric patients only during periods of low occupancy. The obstetric department, in conjunction with the hospital administration, should establish written policies according to state and local regulations indicating which nonobstetric patients may be admitted to the labor and delivery suite. Under all circumstances, however, labor and delivery patients must take precedence over nonobstetric patients in this area. Clean gynecologic operations may be performed in the delivery rooms if patients are adequately screened to eliminate infectious cases and if enough personnel are present to prevent any compromise in the quality of obstetric care.

Labor

The room provided for a woman in labor should be private. Each woman should have direct access to a private toilet and handwashing area in her room. Ideally, each room should have a shower or bathtub and a window.

Areas used for women in labor should have the following equipment:

- Sterilization equipment (if there is no central sterilization equipment)
- X-ray view box
- Stretchers with side rails
- Equipment for pelvic examinations
- Emergency drugs
- Suction apparatus, either operated from a wall outlet or portable equipment
- Cardiopulmonary resuscitation cart (maternal and neonatal)
- Protective gear for personnel exposed to body fluids
- Warming cabinets for solutions and blankets
- A labor or birthing bed and a footstool
- A storage area for the patient's clothing and personal belongings
- Sufficient work space for information management systems
- One or more comfortable chairs
- Adjustable lighting that is pleasant for the patient and adequate for examinations
- An emergency signal and intercommunication system
- Adequate ventilation and temperature control

- Equipment to measure and monitor blood pressure
- Mechanical infusion equipment
- Fetal monitoring equipment
- Oxygen outlets
- Access to at least one shower for use by patients in labor
- A writing surface for medical records, computer hookup for medical record purposes, or both
- Storage facilities for supplies and equipment

The room should have adequate space for support persons, personnel, and equipment, and room for the patient to ambulate in labor. Labor rooms should have a single bed and require a minimum of 100 net sq ft. Labor rooms used for intensive care of patients at high risk in hospitals with no designated high-risk units should be planned with a minimum of 160 net sq ft and should have at least two oxygen and two suction outlets. Design or renovation should include planning for information management systems at bedside and at work-stations and for computer management of medical information.

Patients with significant medical or obstetric complications should be cared for in a room that is specially equipped with cardiopulmonary resuscitation equipment and other monitoring equipment necessary for observation and special care. This room is best located in the labor and delivery area and should meet the physical standards of any other intensive care room in the hospital. When patients with significant medical or obstetric complications receive care in the labor and delivery area, the capabilities of the unit should be identical to those of an intensive care unit.

Delivery

Delivery can be performed in a properly sized and equipped delivery, LDR, or LDRP room. Where delivery rooms are used, they should be close to the labor rooms to afford easy access and to provide privacy to women in labor. A comfortable waiting area for families should be adjacent to the delivery suite, and restrooms should be nearby.

Traditional delivery rooms and cesarean delivery rooms are similar in design to operating rooms. Vaginal deliveries can be performed in either room; cesarean delivery rooms are designed especially for that purpose and, therefore, are larger. The traditional delivery room should be 350 net sq ft with a 9-ft ceiling. A cesarean delivery room should be 400 net sq ft. Each room should be well lit and environmentally controlled to prevent chilling of the woman and the neonate. The World Health Organization recommends that delivery rooms be kept at 25°C or higher to prevent hypothermia, especially in low birth weight, premature infants. Cesarean deliveries should be performed in the obstetric unit or designated operating unit, and postpartum sterilization capabilities should be available in that area when appropriate. We encourage at least one family member to be present at the time of cesarean delivery.

Each delivery room should be maintained as a separate unit that has the following equipment and supplies necessary for normal delivery and for the management of complications:

- Birthing bed that allows variations in position for delivery
- Instrument table and solution basin stand
- Instruments and equipment for vaginal delivery and repair of lacerations
- Solutions and equipment for the intravenous administration of fluids
- Equipment for administration of all types of anesthesia, including equipment for emergency resuscitation of the patient
- Individual oxygen, air, and suction outlets for the mother and neonate
- An emergency call system
- Good lighting
- Mirrors for patients to observe the birth (optional)
- Wall clock with a second hand
- Equipment for fetal heart rate monitoring
- Neonatal resuscitation and stabilization unit (as defined in "Neonatal Functional Units" in this chapter)
- Scrub sinks strategically placed to allow observation of the patient

Trays containing drugs and equipment necessary for emergency treatment of both the patient and the neonate should be kept in the delivery room area. Equipment necessary for cardiopulmonary resuscitation also should be easily accessible.

A workroom should be available for washing instruments. Instruments should be prepared and sterilized in a separate room; alternatively, these services may be performed in a separate area or by a central supply facility. There also should be a room for the storage and preparation of anesthetic equipment.

Postpartum and Newborn Care

The postpartum unit should be flexible enough to permit the comfortable accommodation of patients when the patient census is at its peak and allow the use of beds for alternate functions when the patient census is low. Postpartum rooms ideally should be occupied by a single family. Ideally, the room is equipped for newborn care, and the patient and her neonate are admitted to the room together. Each room in the postpartum unit should have a hand-washing sink and, if possible, a toilet and shower. When this is not possible and it is necessary for patients to use common facilities, patients should be able to reach them without entering a general corridor. When the patient is breast-feeding, the room should have a handwashing sink, a mobile bassinet unit, and supplies necessary for the care of the newborn. Siblings may visit in the patient's room or in a designated space in the antepartum or postpartum area.

Larger services may have a specific recovery room for postpartum patients and a separate area for patients at high risk. The equipment needed is similar to that needed in any surgical recovery room and includes equipment for monitoring vital signs, suctioning, administering oxygen, and infusing fluids intravenously. Cardiopulmonary resuscitation equipment must be immediately available. Equipment for pelvic examinations also should be available.

Combined Units

Comprehensive obstetric and neonatal care can be provided for women at both low risk and high risk and their healthy newborns in a conventional obstetric unit that uses different rooms for labor, delivery, recovery, and newborn care; in an LDR unit that uses different rooms for intrapartum, postpartum, and newborn care; or in single-room maternity care services where an LDRP room is used for all stages of maternity and newborn care. Registered nurses who are cross-trained in antepartum care, labor and delivery, postpartum care, and neonatal care should staff this unit, increasing the continuity and quality of care.

Each LDR and LDRP room is a single-care room containing a toilet and shower with optional bathtub. A lavatory should be located in each room for scrubbing, handwashing, and neonate bathing. A window with an outside view is desirable in the LDR or LDRP room. Each room should contain a birthing bed that is comfortable during labor and can be readily converted to a delivery bed and transported to the cesarean delivery room when necessary. A bassinet for the infant should be readily available. Separate oxygen, air, and suction facilities should be provided in two separate locations for the woman and the neonate. Gas outlets and wall-mounted equipment should be easily accessible but may be covered with a panel. Either a ceiling mount or a portable delivery light may be used, depending on the preference of the medical staff. An area within the room, but distinct from the patient's area, should be provided for neonate stabilization and resuscitation.

Proper care of the patient requires sufficient space for a sphygmomanometer, stethoscope, fetal monitor, infusion pump, and regional anesthesia administration, as well as resuscitation equipment at the head of the bed. Proper care requires access to the newborn from three sides and quick transport to the nursery should the need arise. The family area should be farthest from the entry to the room, and there should be a comfortable area for the support person.

Equipment needed for labor, delivery, newborn resuscitation, and newborn care should be stored either in the room or in a nearby central storage or supply area and should be immediately available to the LDR or LDRP room. For ease of movement, space below the foot of the bed should be adequate to accommodate staff and equipment brought into the room. Standard major equipment held in this area for delivery should include a fetal monitor, delivery case cart, linen hamper, and portable examination lights. A unit equipped for neonatal stabilization and resuscitation (described in "Neonatal Functional Units" in this chapter) should be available during delivery.

The workable size of an LDR or LDRP room is 256 net sq ft with room dimensions of 16 ft by 16 ft, excluding the toilet and shower. This room should be able to accommodate 6–8 people comfortably during the childbirth process. A minimum 5-ft clear space at the foot of the bed should be available for the providers to occupy during delivery.

Bed Need Analysis

Historically, the calculation of the number of patient rooms needed for all phases of the birth process was based on a simple ratio involving the number of births, the average length of stay, and the accepted occupancy level. To best estimate patient room needs, each delivery service should thoroughly analyze functions, philosophies, and projections that will determine the types and quantities of rooms needed. An analysis of the present patterns of care should be reviewed, and consideration should be given to the following types of information:

- Projected birth rates
- Projected cesarean delivery rates
- Occupancy projections that address "peaks and valleys" in the census

- Present (and projected) number of women in the unit during peak periods, as well as the length and frequency of the peak periods
- Numbers and types of high-risk births
- Anticipated lengths of stay for women during labor, delivery, and recovery
- Anticipated changes in technology

One planning method is to carefully analyze the activities that will occur in each type of room. For example, LDR or LDRP rooms should not be used routinely to accommodate care such as outpatient testing when another room would provide a more appropriate setting. Rooms that allow adequate privacy are recommended for the entire birth process, from labor through discharge.

Planning the number of LDR or LDRP rooms requires that consideration be given to these additional questions:

- Will patients scheduled for cesarean delivery use LDR or LDRP rooms or other types of patient rooms for their preoperative, recovery, and postpartum stays?
- Are the LDR or LDRP rooms to be used for other purposes, such as triage or short-term observation for false labor or antepartum admission? If so, the length of stay and volume of all these activities must be considered in the calculation of bed need.

Once the data have been accumulated, the following normative formula can be used to calculate the number of rooms needed by type of room (note that patient episodes—cases or activities—is used rather than the number of births):

$$\frac{\text{Number of patient episodes}}{\text{(considering all activities, such as admission, observation, and transitional care, in this room)}}{365 \text{ days} \times \text{occupancy for the room type}} \times \text{Mean overall length of stay}$$

This formula will provide, at best, only a crude estimate of bed needs. For more precise estimates, computerized simulation models are available commercially. However, many of these software packages are expensive and require a significant investment of time for adequate training and use. Often this software will be purchased by a hospital planning department and models developed for each service as needed. Alternatively, some expert consulting firms that specialize in maternal–child services can provide an on-site assessment of obstetric capacity and perform a bed-need analysis using their own proprietary simulation software.

Neonatal Functional Units

All neonatal services in a birthing hospital should have facilities available to perform the following functions:

- Resuscitation and stabilization
- Admission and observation
- Normal newborn nursery care
- Isolation
- Visitation
- Supporting service areas

Level II and III NICUs require facilities for intermediate and intensive care. These may be separate or continuous. Consistency of nursing care provided and efficient staffing may be enhanced by having a mix of neonatal patients in a single area. Local circumstances should be considered in the design and management of these care areas.

Resuscitation and Stabilization

The resuscitation area should be illuminated to at least 100 foot-candles at the neonate's body surface and should contain the following items:

- Overhead source of radiant heat that can be regulated by the newborn's skin temperature
- Noncompressible resuscitation and examination mattress that allows access on three sides
- Wall clock
- Flat working surface for medical records
- Table or flat surface for trays and equipment
- Oxygen, pulse oximeters, blenders, compressed air, suction catheters
- Dry, preferably warmed, towels
- Resuscitation equipment, including bulb syringe, suction catheters, laryngoscope, endotracheal tubes and tape, meconium aspirator, ventilation bags and masks for term and preterm neonates, stethoscope, and vascular access catheters

- Syringes, medications, and solution(s) for volume expansion
- Equipment for examination, immediate care, and identification of the neonate
- Protective gear to prevent exposure to body fluids

The resuscitation area usually is within the delivery, LDR, or LDRP rooms, although it may be in a designated contiguous, separate room. If resuscitation takes place in the delivery, LDR, or LDRP room, the area should be large enough to allow for proper resuscitation of the newborn without interference with the care of the mother. Items contaminated with maternal blood, urine, and stool should be kept physically distant from the neonatal resuscitation area. The thermal environment for infant resuscitation should be optimized by use of an infant warmer or by increasing the room temperature to what is customary for patient rooms or operating suites. When delivery of a preterm baby is anticipated, the temperature of the room should be increased. After the neonate has been stabilized, if the mother wishes to hold her newborn, a radiant heater or prewarmed blankets should be available to keep the neonate warm. Although some newborns requiring resuscitation may remain with their mothers after stabilization, they will require increased vigilance in monitoring for abnormal temperature, cardiorespiratory instability, hypoglycemia, apnea, and cyanosis. Nursing protocols addressing these issues are required. Qualified nursing staff should be available to monitor the newborn during this period.

A resuscitation area should be allotted a minimum of 40 net sq ft of floor space if it is within a delivery, LDR, or LDRP room. A separate resuscitation room should have approximately 150 net sq ft of floor space. The area should have adequate suction, oxygen, and compressed-air outlets to accommodate simultaneous resuscitation of twins and should contain at least six electrical outlets. A separate resuscitation room also should have an electrical outlet to accommodate a portable X-ray machine, if needed. Electrical outlets should conform to regulations for areas in which anesthetic agents are administered.

Admission and Observation (Transitional and Stabilization Care)

The admission and observation area (for evaluating the neonate's condition in the first 4–8 hours after birth) should be near or adjacent to the delivery and cesarean delivery room and preferably part of a recovery room, LDR room, LDRP room, or other area for maternal recovery. Physical separation of the mother and her newborn during this period should be avoided. This evaluation may take place within one or more areas, including the room in which the mother is recovering, the LDR or LDRP room, or the newborn nursery. In some hospitals, the newborn nursery is the primary area for transitional care, both for neonates born within the hospital and for those born outside the hospital. No special or separate isolation facilities are required for neonates born at home or in transit to the hospital.

An estimated 40 net sq ft of floor space is needed for each neonate in the admission and observation area. The capacity required depends on the size of the delivery service and the duration of close observation. The number of observation stations required depends on the birth rate and the length of stay in the observation area. There should be a minimum of two observation stations. The admission and observation area should be well lit and should contain a wall clock and emergency resuscitation equipment similar to that in the designated resuscitation area. Outlets also should be similar to those in the resuscitation area.

The physician's and nurse's assessment of the neonate's condition determines the subsequent level of care. When the admission and observation is in an LDR or LDRP room, the neonate remains in the room with the mother for breastfeeding. Healthy neonates are never separated from their healthy mothers, and they are kept with their mothers in the LDR or LDRP rooms at all times. In services where the mother must be transferred from the room in which she delivers to a postpartum room, the newborn also is admitted to the postpartum room. Some neonates require transfer to an intermediate or intensive care area.

Newborn Nursery

Within each perinatal care facility there may be several types of units for newborn care. These units are defined by the content and complexity of care required by a specific group of infants.

Routine care of apparently normal term and some late preterm neonates who have demonstrated successful adaptation to extrauterine life may be provided either in the newborn nursery or in the area where the woman is receiving postpartum care. The nursery should be close to the postpartum area. In a multifloor maternity unit, there should be a newborn nursery on each floor.

The number of bassinets in the newborn nursery should exceed the number of obstetric beds to accommodate multiple births, extended neonatal hospitalization, maternal illness, cesarean delivery, and fluctuations in demand. The bed requirement for the newborn nursery should be estimated by using data on the mean length of stay and annual number of liveborn, normal, term neonates. The use of combination LDR and LDRP rooms and rooming-in of newborns with mothers may substantially alter nursery bed requirements.

Because relatively few staff members are needed to provide care in the newborn nursery and because no bulky equipment is needed, 30 net sq ft of floor space for each neonate should be adequate. Bassinets should be at least 3 ft apart in all directions, measured from the edge of one bassinet to the edge of the neighboring bassinet. The newborn care area may be one room (in a small hospital) or one or more rooms (in larger hospitals). One registered nurse is recommended for every 6–8 neonates, and the nurse should be available in each newborn-occupied area at all times (Table 2–1). Therefore, individual rooms should have accommodations for 6–8, 12–16, or 18–24 neonates. During decreased patient occupancy, central nurseries use nursing staff inefficiently. Direct care of those newborns remaining in the nursery may be provided by licensed practical nurses and unlicensed nursing personnel under the registered nurse's direct supervision.

The newborn nursery should be well lit, have a large wall clock and a sink for handwashing, and be equipped for emergency resuscitation. One pair of wall-mounted electrical outlets is recommended for every two neonatal stations. One oxygen outlet, one compressed-air outlet, and one suction outlet are recommended for every four neonatal stations. Cabinets and counters should be available within the newborn care area for storage of routinely used supplies, such as diapers, formula, and linens. If circumcisions are performed in the nursery, an appropriate table with adequate lighting is required. Electrical outlets to power portable X-ray machines are highly recommended.

Levels of Care

Several levels of care may be provided in the same nursery units or in different areas of the same hospital. It is important to distinguish between specific units and the levels of care provided in each unit. As in the resuscitation and stabilization area and the admission and observation area, equipment for emergency resuscitation is required in all neonatal care areas. Recommendations regarding the intensity of care are made in the following paragraphs.

Newborn Nursery. In addition to providing care for healthy infants, a newborn nursery can provide care for infants born at 35–37 weeks of gestation who are physiologically stable. These neonates are not ill but may require frequent feeding and more hours of nursing than do normal term neonates. In hospitals with level II or III NICUs, these infants should be cared for in an area close to these care areas so that neonates who have received intermediate or intensive care but no longer require these levels of care may be transferred to this step-down unit for convalescence. Because the care of neonates in this area requires appropriate equipment as well as more personnel than are needed in the newborn nursery, more space is needed per patient unit. There should be 50 net sq ft of floor space for each patient station, with approximately 4 ft between bassinets or incubators. Each neonatal station should have six electrical outlets, one oxygen outlet, one compressed-air outlet, and one suction outlet. In addition, the equipment and supplies required in the newborn nursery should be available in this area. Provisions should be made for the comfort of parents or personnel who feed neonates in both incubators and bassinets. Nursing care provider to patient ratios may be 1:3 or 1:4.

Intermediate Care. Sick neonates who do not require intensive care but who require 6–12 hours of nursing care each day should be taken to an intermediate care area. This area also may be used for convalescing neonates who have returned to specialty facilities from an outside intensive care unit.

The neonatal intermediate care area should be close to the delivery and cesarean delivery room and the intensive care area and away from general hospital traffic. It should have radiant heaters or incubators for maintaining body temperature, as well as infusion pumps, cardiopulmonary monitors, and equipment for ventilatory assistance. Newborns requiring complex care, such as assisted ventilation, should be moved to an intensive care area.

At least 120 net sq ft of floor space is needed for each patient station in intensive care, although less may be adequate for intermediate care. There should be at least 4 ft between incubators, bassinets, or radiant heaters. Space needed for other purposes (eg, desks, counters, cabinets, corridors, and treatment rooms) should be added to the space needed for patients. Neonates receiving intermediate care may be housed in a single large room or in two or more smaller rooms. In the latter case, each room should accommodate some multiple of three to four newborn stations because one registered nurse is required for every three to four neonates who require intermediate care. Large rooms allow greater flexibility in the use of equipment and assignment of personnel but offer less privacy for parental involvement in newborn care.

Aisles should be wide enough to accommodate passage of personnel and equipment. Aisles should be 5 ft wide in multiple-bed rooms and 8 ft wide in single-patient rooms or fixed-cubicle partitions.

Eight electrical outlets, two oxygen outlets, two compressed-air outlets, and two suction outlets should be provided for each patient station. In addition, the area should have a special outlet to power the neonatal unit's portable X-ray machine. All electrical outlets for each patient station should be connected to both regular and auxiliary power. An oxygen tank for emergency use should be stored but readily available for each newborn receiving wall-supplied oxygen.

All equipment and supplies for resuscitation should be immediately available within the intermediate care unit. These items may be conveniently placed on an emergency cart.

Intensive Care. Constant nursing and continuous cardiopulmonary and other support for severely ill newborns should be provided in the intensive care area. Because emergency care is provided in this area, laboratory and radiologic services should be readily available 24 hours per day. The results of blood gas analyses should be available shortly after sample collection. In many centers, a laboratory adjacent to the intensive care unit provides this service.

The neonatal intensive care area should be near the delivery area and cesarean delivery room(s) and should be easily accessible from the hospital's ambulance entrance. It should be located away from routine hospital traffic. Intensive care may be provided in a single area or in two or more separate rooms.

The number of nursing, medical, and surgical personnel required in the neonatal intensive care area is greater than that required in less acute perinatal care areas. The nurse to patient ratio should be 1:2 or 1:1, depending on acuity. In some cases, such as during extracorporeal life support, additional nursing personnel are required. In addition, the amount and complexity of equipment required also are considerably greater. Therefore, incubators or overhead warmers should be separated by at least 8 ft and aisles should be 8 ft wide. The area should have 150 net sq ft of floor space for each neonate, plus space for desks, cabinets, and corridors. In addition, the educational responsibilities of a subspecialty facility require that the design of its neonatal intensive care area include space for instructional activities and office space for files on the region's perinatal experience.

Each patient station needs at least 20 simultaneously accessible electrical outlets, 3–4 oxygen outlets, 3–4 compressed-air outlets, and 3–4 vacuum outlets. Like those in the intermediate care area, all electrical outlets for each patient station should be connected to both regular and auxiliary power. In addition, each room should have a special outlet to power the portable X-ray machine housed in the NICU. An oxygen tank for emergency use should be stored but readily available for each newborn receiving wall-supplied oxygen. It is recommended that provisions should be made at each bedside to allow data transmission to a remote location.

Equipment and supplies in the intensive-care area should include all those needed in the resuscitation and intermediate-care areas. Immediate availability of emergency oxygen is essential. In addition, equipment for long-term ventilatory support should be provided. Respirators should be equipped with nebulizers or humidifiers with heaters. Continuous, on-line monitoring of oxygen concentrations, body temperature, heart rate, respiration, oxygen saturation, and blood pressure levels should be available; transcutaneous oxygen tension and transcutaneous carbon dioxide tension monitoring may be desirable. Supplies should be kept close to the patient station so that nurses are not away from the neonate unnecessarily and may use their time and skills efficiently. A central modular supply system can enhance efficiency.

In some cases, certain surgical procedures (eg, ligation of a patent ductus arteriosus) are performed in an area in or adjacent to the NICU. Specific procedures addressing preparatory cleaning, physical preparation of the unit, presence of other newborns, venting of volatile anesthetics, and quality assessment should be documented in writing. Equipment, facilities, and supplies for this area, as well as procedures, must conform to or be comparable to those required for similar procedures in the surgical department of the hospital. The latter includes adequate air exchange (at least six air changes per hour).

Visitation

Parents should have access to their newborns 24 hours per day at all levels of care within all functional units, and they should be encouraged to participate in the care of their newborns (see "Visiting Policies" in Chapter 7). Generally, parents can be with their healthy newborns in the mother's room.

Special provisions may be necessary when neonates are in intermediate- or intensive-care units. In these situations, women often are discharged from the hospital before their newborns and sometimes must travel long distances to be with them. Several systems have been developed to meet the needs of parents and their newborns under these circumstances (eg, rooms for parents in the hospital, adjacent facilities outside the hospital provided by the hospital, or other lodgings nearby). A period of mother–newborn rooming-in before discharge is highly desirable when special care is needed. In addition, intensive- and intermediate-care units require special areas that are appropriately furnished for the counseling of parents, the breastfeeding of newborns, and the support of grieving women and families.

Supporting Service Areas

Utility Rooms. Both clean and soiled utility rooms are needed in neonatal care areas. A separate clean utility room is used for storing breast milk and storing and preparing formulas, medications, and supplies frequently needed for the care of neonates in all functional units. The use of ready-mixed formulas, unit-dose medications, and disposable supplies and equipment has decreased the need for clean utility rooms; storage areas and clean working surfaces within each functional unit may replace them. Separate storage areas should be available for foodstuffs, medications, and clean supplies. Utility rooms should not have direct lighting because some of the formulas, medications, and supplies may be light sensitive.

A utility room for storing used and contaminated material before it is removed from the care area is highly desirable. It should have negative air pressure, with 100% of its air exhausted to the outside. There should be a two-door zone, one providing direct access from within the unit and another from outside the unit. This room should contain a countertop and a sink with hot and cold running water that is turned on and off by hands-free controls, soap and paper towel dispensers, and a covered waste receptacle with foot control. A separate deep sink with hot and cold running water should be available for cleaning equipment before it is returned to the central service department for resterilization.

Storage Areas. A three-level storage system is desirable. The first storage area should be the central supply department of the hospital. The second storage area should be adjacent to or within the patient care areas. In this area, routinely used supplies, such as diapers, formula, linen, cover gowns, medical records, and information booklets, may be stored. Generally, space is required in this area only for the amount of each item used between deliveries from the hospital's central supply department (eg, daily or three times weekly). The third area is needed for the storage of items frequently used at the neonate's bedside.

The bedside cabinet storage area should be approximately 8 net cu ft for each bed–patient unit in the newborn nursery, 16 net cu ft for each bed–patient unit in the intermediate-care area, and 24 net cu ft for each bed–patient unit in the intensive-care area. The newborn nursery requires approximately 3 net cu ft per patient for secondary storage of items such as linen and formula. In the resuscitation and stabilization area, the admission and observation area, and the continuing-, intermediate-, and intensive-care areas, there should be approximately 8 net cu ft per patient for secondary storage of syringes, needles, intravenous infusion sets, and sterile trays needed in procedures such as umbilical vessel catheterization, lumbar puncture, and thoracotomy.

Large equipment items (eg, bassinets, warmers, radiant heaters, phototherapy units, and infusion pumps) should be stored in a clean, enclosed storage area in close proximity to, but not within, the immediate patient care area. Approximately 6 net sq ft of floor space for equipment is required for each patient in the newborn nursery, 18 net sq ft for each patient in the intermediate-care area, and 30 net sq ft for each patient in the intensive-care area. Easily accessible electrical outlets are desirable in this area for recharging equipment.

Treatment Rooms. Many facilities have developed areas for resuscitation and stabilization, admission and observation, intermediate care, and intensive care in which each patient station constitutes a treatment area. This largely has eliminated the need for a separate treatment room for procedures such as lumbar punctures, intravenous infusions, venipuncture, and minor surgical procedures. A separate treatment area may be necessary, however, if neonates in the newborn nursery or the postpartum family unit are to undergo certain procedures (eg, circumcision). The facilities, outlets, equipment, and supplies in the treatment area should be similar to those of the resuscitation area. The amount of space required depends on the procedures performed.

Scrub Areas

At the entrance to each nursery, there should be a scrub area that can accommodate all personnel and families entering the area. It should have a sink that is large enough to prevent splashing, with faucets operated by hands-free controls. A backsplash should be provided to prevent standing or retained water. Waterless antiseptics also often are available at these sinks. Sinks for handwashing should not be built into counters used for other purposes. Soap and towel dispensers and appropriate trash receptacles should be available. The scrub areas also should contain racks, hooks, or lockers for storing clothing and personal items, as well as cabinets for clean gowns, a receptacle for used gowns, and a large wall clock with a sweep second hand for timing handwashing.

Scrub sinks should have foot-operated, knee-operated, or photoelectric-operated faucets and should be large enough to control splashing and to prevent retained water. These sinks should be provided at a minimum ratio of one for at least every 6–8 patient stations in the newborn nursery and one for every 3–4 patient stations in the intermediate- or intensive-care area. In addition, one scrub sink is needed in the resuscitation and stabilization area, and one is needed for every 3–4 patient stations in the admission and observation area.

Nursing Areas

Space should be provided at the bedside not only for patient care but also for instructional and medical record activities. A flat writing surface (eg, a clipboard) is needed.

A nurses' medical record area or desk for tasks such as compiling more detailed records, completing requisitions, and handling specimens is useful. Physicians also may perform medical record and clerical activities in this area. Maintaining medical records should be considered an unclean procedure, and personnel who have been working in medical records should wash their hands before they have further contact with a neonate.

The unit director or nurse manager should have an office close to the newborn-care areas. Nurses' dressing rooms preferably should be adjacent to a lounge and should contain lockers, storage for clean and soiled scrub attire, toilets, and showers.

Education Areas

A conference room suitable for educational purposes is highly desirable, particularly for level II and III facilities. It should be in or adjacent to the maternal–newborn areas.

Clerical Areas

The control point for patient-care activities is the clerical area. It should be located near the entrance to the neonatal care areas so that personnel can supervise traffic and limit unnecessary entry into these areas. It should have telephones and communication devices that connect to the various neonatal care areas and the delivery suite. In addition, patients' medical records, computer terminals, and hospital forms may be located in the clerical area.

General Considerations

Newborn Security

Security devices should be part of an overall security program to protect the physical safety of newborns, families, and staff. Both the NICU and normal nurseries should be designed to minimize the risk of newborn abduction.

Policies and procedures for visitation, transfer, and discharge of neonates should include identification and verification of the neonate and designated attendants and visitors.

Disaster Preparedness and Evacuation Plan

An overall disaster preparedness plan is essential for all areas of the hospital and all personnel. A plan addressing natural and terrorist disasters should be in place for each perinatal care area (ie, antepartum care, labor and delivery, postpartum care, the normal newborn nursery, intermediate care, and intensive care). This should include an evacuation plan; a relocation plan; triage principles; immediate measures for utilities and water supply; emergency supply of medical gases, essential medications, and equipment; and the role of each staff in the plan. A floor plan that indicates designated evacuation routes should be posted in a conspicuous place in each unit. The policy and floor plan should be reviewed with the staff at least annually.

Safety and Environmental Control

Because of the complexities of environmental control and monitoring, a hospital environmental engineer must ensure that all electrical, lighting, air composition, and temperature systems function properly and safely. A regular maintenance program should be specified to ensure that systems continue to function as designed after initial occupancy.

The environmental temperature in newborn-care areas should be independently adjustable, and control should be sufficient to prevent hot and cold spots, particularly when heat-generating equipment (eg, a radiant warmer) is in use. The air temperature should be kept at 22–26° C (72–78° F). Humidity should be kept between 30–60% and should be controlled through the heating and air-conditioning system of the hospital. Condensation on wall and window surfaces should be avoided.

A minimum of six air changes per hour is recommended, and a minimum of two changes should be outside air. The ventilation pattern should inhibit particulate matter from moving freely in the space, and intake and exhaust vents should be placed so as to minimize drafts on or near the patient beds. Ventilation air delivered to the NICU should be filtered at 90% efficiency.

Fresh-air intake should be located at least 25 ft from exhaust outlets of ventilating systems, combustion equipment stacks, medical or surgical vacuum systems, plumbing vents, or areas that may collect vehicular exhausts or other noxious fumes.

Radiation exposure to newborns, families, and staff is another safety concern. Radiation exposure to personnel is negligible at a distance of more than 1 ft lateral to the primary vertical roentgen beam. Care should be taken to ensure that only the patient being examined is in the primary beam. It is unnecessary for families or personnel to leave the area during the roentgen exposure.

Illumination

Ambient lighting levels in newborn intensive-care rooms should be adjustable through a range of at least 10–600 lux (approximately 1–60 ft-c) as measured at each bedside. Both natural and artificial light sources should have controls that allow immediate darkening of any bed position sufficient for transillumination or ultrasonography when necessary. Artificial light sources should have a visible spectral distribution similar to that of daylight but should avoid unnecessary ultraviolet or infrared radiation by the use of appropriate lamps, lenses, or filters. Appropriate general lighting levels for NICUs have not been established.

Newly constructed or renovated NICUs should be able to provide ambient lighting at levels recommended by the Illuminating Engineering Society (10–20 ft-c). In most cases, these levels are adequate.

Continuous reduced lighting to low levels appears to have no demonstrable clinical benefit. The benefits of exposing NICU patients to diurnal variation in ambient lighting, including reduction of nighttime levels to as low as 0.5 ft-c, are uncertain. However, avoidance of chaotic lighting and the approximation of a diurnal cycle seem a reasonable approach. Lighting should be sufficient to evaluate skin color and perfusion.

Nurseries should have the capability for adjustable illumination. Multiple switching can be helpful in this regard, but unless a master switch also is provided, this method can pose serious difficulties when rapid darkening of a room is required to permit transillumination.

Because perception of skin tones is critical in the NICU, light sources must be as balanced and as free of glare or ceiling reflections as possible.

Until better data are available, the output of ultraviolet radiation by fluorescent fixtures (including phototherapy lights) in patient care areas should be minimized by plastic or glass shields that filter out most ultraviolet radiation. Separate procedure lighting that provides no more than 1,000–1,500 lux (100–150 ft-c) of illumination to the patient bed should be available at each patient-care station.

Lighting should minimize shadows and glare, and it should be controlled with a rheostat so that it can be provided at less-than-maximal levels whenever possible. Light should be highly framed so that newborns at adjacent bed stations will not experience any increase in illumination. Temporary increases in illumination necessary to evaluate a newborn or to perform a procedure should be possible without increasing lighting levels for other newborns in the same room.

High levels of light necessary to perform a procedure may represent a danger to the developing retina. Given the lack of safety standards, it may be prudent to design directable lighting so that the procedure light can be framed away from the eyes of patients during use.

Illumination of support areas within the NICU, including medical records areas, medication preparation areas, reception desks, and handwashing areas, should conform to the specifications of the Illuminating Engineering Society. Illumination should be adequate in the areas of the NICU where staff perform important or critical tasks. In locations where these functions overlap with patient care areas (eg, close proximity of the nurse medical records area to patient beds), the design should permit separate light sources with independent controls so that the very different needs of sleeping newborns and working nurses can be accommodated to the greatest possible extent.

Windows

Windows provide an important psychologic benefit to staff and families in the NICU. Properly designed natural light is the most desirable illumination for nearly all nursing tasks, including updating medical records and evaluating newborn skin tone. However, placing newborns too close to external windows can cause serious problems with temperature control and glare, so providing windows in the NICU requires careful planning and design.

At least one source of natural light should be visible from each patient-care area. External windows in patient-care rooms should be glazed, with insulating glass to minimize heat gain and loss. They should be situated at least 2 ft away from any part of a patient bed to minimize radiant heat loss from the newborn. All external windows should be equipped with shading devices that are easily controlled to allow flexibility at various times of day. These shading devices should be either contained within the window or easily cleanable.

Interior Finish

Off-white or pale-beige walls minimize distortion of staff's color perception in patient-care areas. This advantage can be nullified by the use of inappropriate fluorescent lighting. Brighter colors may be used elsewhere. Windows in neonatal-care areas should have opaque shades that make it possible to darken the area for procedures such as transillumination.

Oxygen and Compressed-Air Outlets

Newborn-care areas should have oxygen and compressed air piped from a central source at a pressure of 50–60 psi. An alarm system that warns of any critical reduction in line pressure should be installed. Reduction valves and mixers should produce adjustable concentrations of 21–100% oxygen at atmospheric pressure for head hoods and 50–60 psi for mechanical ventilators.

Acoustic Characteristics

Newborn bed areas and the spaces opening onto them should be designed to produce minimal background noise and to contain and absorb much of the transient noise that arises within the nursery. The ventilation system, monitors, incubators, suction pumps, mechanical ventilators, and staff produce considerable noise, and the noise level should be monitored intermittently. The construction and redesign of neonatal care areas should include acoustic absorption units or other means to ensure that the combination of continuous background sound and transient sound in any bed space or patient care area does not exceed an hourly L_{eq} of 50 dB and an hourly L_{10} of 55 dB, both A-weighted slow response. The L_{max} (transient sounds) should not exceed 70 dB, A-weighted slow response. Staff members should take particular care to avoid noise pollution in enclosed patient spaces (eg, incubators). Care should be taken to avoid spaces shaped so as to focus or amplify sound levels, thus creating "hot spots" that exceed the maximum recommended noise levels.

Electrical Outlets and Electrical Equipment

All electrical outlets should be attached to a common ground. All electrical equipment should be checked for current leakage and grounding adequacy when first introduced into the neonatal care area, after any repair, and periodically while in service. Current leakage allowances, preventive maintenance standards, and equipment quality should meet the standards developed by the Joint Commission. Personnel should be thoroughly and repeatedly instructed on the potential electrical hazards within the neonatal care areas.

Resources

Advanced practice in neonatal nursing. American Academy of Pediatrics Committee on Fetus and Newborn. Pediatrics 2003;111:1453–4.

American Institute of Architects. Guidelines for design and construction of hospital and health care facilities. Washington, DC: AIA; 2001.

American Medical Association
Advancing Quality Improvement in Patient Care
515 N. State Street
Chicago, IL 60610
(800) 621-8335
www.ama-assn.org/go/quality

American Nurses Association, National Association of Neonatal Nurses. Neonatal nursing: scope and standards of practice. Silver Spring (MD): ANA; Glenview (IL): NANN; 2004.

Berwick DM. Continuous improvement as an ideal in health care. N Engl J Med 1989;320:53–6.

"Do not use" abbreviations. ACOG Committee Opinion No. 327. American College of Obstetricians and Gynecologists. Obstet Gynecol 2006;107:213–4.

Graven SN. Sound and the developing infant in the NICU: conclusions and recommendations for care. J Perinatol 2000;20:S88–93.

Institute for Healthcare Improvement
Establish a Rapid Response Team
20 University Road, 7th Floor
Cambridge, MD 02138
(866) 787-0831
www.ihi.org/IHI/Topics/CriticalCare/IntensiveCare/Changes/
EstablishaRapidResponseTeam.htm

Institute of Medicine (US). Crossing the quality chasm: a new health system for the 21st century. Washington, DC: National Academy Press; 2001.

Joint Commission on Accreditation of Healthcare Organizations. Universal protocol for preventing wrong site, wrong procedure, wrong person surgery. Oakbrook Terrace (IL): JCAHO; 2003. Available at: http://www.jointcommission.org/PatientSafety/Universal Protocol. Retrieved January 3, 2007.

Laffel G, Blumenthal D. The case for using industrial quality management science in health care organizations. JAMA 1989;262:2869–73.

Managing Obstetrical Risk Efficiently
The Society of Obstetricians and Gynecologists of Canada
780 Echo Drive
Ottawa, ON K1 5R7
(613) 730-2416
www.moreob.com

March of Dimes Birth Defects Foundation. Toward improving the outcome of pregnancy: the 90s and beyond. White Plains (NY): MDBDF; 1993.

Mirmiran M, Ariagno RL. Influence of light in the NICU on the development of circadian rhythms in preterm infants. Semin Perinatol 2000;24:247–57.

National Association of Neonatal Nurses. Minimum staffing in NICUs. NANN Position Statement No. 3009. Glenview (IL): NANN; 1999.

National Association of Neonatal Nurses. Use of assistive personnel in providing care to the high-risk infant. NANN Position Statement No. 3013. Glenview (IL): NANN; 1999.

National Patient Safety Foundation. Talking to patients about health care injury: statement of principle. North Adams (MA): NPSF; 2000. Available at: www.npsf.org /html/statement.html. Retrieved January 3, 2007.

Partnering with patients to improve safety. ACOG Committee Opinion No. 320. American College of Obstetricians and Gynecologists. Obstet Gynecol 2005;106: 1123–5.

Patient safety in obstetrics and gynecology. ACOG Committee Opinion No. 286. American College of Obstetricians and Gynecologists. Obstet Gynecol 2003;102: 883–5.

Sheridan SL, Harris RP, Woolf SH. Shared decision making about screening and chemoprevention: a suggested approach from the U.S. Preventive Services Task Force. Shared Decision-Making Workgroup of the U.S. Preventive Services Task Force. Am J Prev Med 2004; 26;56–66. Available at: www.ahrq.gov/clinic/3rduspstf/shard/sharedba.htm. Retrieved January 3, 2007.

Stark AR. Levels of neonatal care. American Academy of Pediatrics Committee on Fetus and Newborn [published erratum appears in Pediatrics 2005;115:1118]. Pediatrics 2004;114:1341–7.

White RD. Recommended standards for newborn ICU design. Committee to establish recommended standards for newborn ICU design. J Perinatol 2003;19:S1–12.

chapter 3

Interhospital Care of the Perinatal Patient

One of the goals of regionalized perinatal care is for women and neonates at high risk to receive care in facilities that provide the required level of specialized care. Because all hospitals cannot provide all levels of perinatal care, interhospital transport of pregnant women and neonates is an essential component of a regionalized perinatal system. It is accepted medical practice to transfer a neonate to a hospital able to provide the services needed or anticipated to be needed if the birth hospital cannot provide that level of service. Similarly, women who are at risk for complications that pose significant risk for adverse outcomes or whose neonates are likely to require intensive support should be considered candidates for referral during the antepartum period. Neonates born to women transported during the antepartum period have better survival rates and decreased risks of long-term sequelae than those transferred after birth.

Because of the recent focus and interpretations of the Emergency Medical Treatment and Labor Act (EMTALA) and the accepted need for interhospital transport of pregnant women, both facilities and professionals providing health care to pregnant women need to understand their obligations under the law.

Federal law requires all Medicare-participating hospitals to provide an appropriate medical screening examination for any individual seeking medical treatment at an emergency department to determine whether the patient has an emergency medical condition (Appendix F). Some states have similar statutory requirements. These laws also place strict requirements on the transfer of these patients. However, there have been misinterpretations of these laws that have been barriers to optimal health care. For example, a woman having contractions is not considered to be having an emergency medical condition if there is adequate time for her safe transfer before delivery or if the transfer will not pose a threat to the health or safety of the woman or the fetus. There also has been confusion concerning the new Health Insurance Portability and Accountability Act (HIPAA). Although this law does establish strict criteria regarding personal health information, it does not restrict the sharing of information between hospitals and health care providers caring for perinatal patients.

Guidelines for Air and Ground Transport of Neonatal and Pediatric Patients provide more extensive information regarding the transfer of the neonatal patient and address the EMTALA interpretations of 2003 and the HIPAA regulations.

Program Components

There are three types of perinatal patient transport. These types of transport are used for patients who have to be transferred between facilities.

1. Maternal transport—A pregnant woman is transferred during the antepartum or intrapartum period for special care of the woman or the neonate or both.

2. Neonatal transport—One of the following situations:
    - A team is sent from one hospital, often a regional center, to the referring hospital to evaluate and stabilize the neonate at the referring hospital and then transfer the neonate to the team's hospital.
    - A team is sent from the referring hospital with a neonate who is being transferred to another hospital for specialized or intensive care.
    - A team is sent from one hospital to the referring hospital to evaluate and stabilize the neonate and then transfer the neonate to a third hospital. Such a transfer may be necessary because of bed constraints or the need for specialized care available only at the third hospital.

3. Return transport—A woman or her neonate, after receiving intensive or specialized care at a referral center, is returned to the original referring hospital or to a local hospital for continuing care after the problems that required the transfer have been resolved. This should be done in consultation with the referring physician.

    To ensure optimal care of patients at high risk, the following components should be part of a regional referral program:
    - Formal transfer agreements between participating hospitals that clearly outline the responsibilities of each facility

- A method of risk identification and assessment of problems that are expected to benefit from consultation and transport
- Assessment of the perinatal capabilities and determination of conditions necessitating consultation, referral, or transfer by the medical staff of each participating hospital
- Resource management to maximize efficiency, effectiveness, and safety
- Adequate financial and personnel support
- A reliable, accurate, and comprehensive communication system between participating hospitals and transport teams
- Determination of responsibility for each of these functions

An interhospital transport program should provide 24-hour service. It should include a receiving or program center responsible for ensuring that patients at high risk receive the appropriate level of care, a dispatching unit to coordinate the transport of patients between facilities, an appropriately equipped transport vehicle, and a specialized transport team. The program also should have a system for providing a continuum of care by various providers, including the personnel and equipment required for the level of care needed, as well as outreach education and program evaluation.

Responsibilities

Each of the functional components of an interhospital transport program has specific responsibilities. If the transport is done by the referring hospital, the referring physician and hospital retain responsibility until the transport team arrives with the patient at the receiving hospital. If the transport team is sent by the receiving hospital, the receiving physician or designee assumes responsibility for patient care from the time the patient leaves the referring hospital. It should be emphasized that during the preparation for transport by the transport team, the referring physician and hospital retain responsibility for the patient unless there have been other prior agreements. Transport services should work with their referring hospital to delineate clearly the primary medical responsibility for the patient when the patient is still within the referring hospital but is being cared for by the transport team. Regardless of the site of origin of the transport team, qualified staff should accompany the patient to the receiving hospital.

Medical–Legal Aspects

Many legal details of perinatal transport are not well defined and are subject to interpretation. In addition, many transport teams provide service in more than one state and therefore must comply with the laws of the state in which they are practicing and cannot be guided solely by their home state or area. Legal consult should be sought when developing a service to ensure compatibility with existing laws, and periodic review is encouraged to maintain compliance with laws and regulations. It is clear that all involved parties (eg, the referring hospital and personnel, the receiving hospital and personnel, and the transportation carriers or corporations) assume a number of responsibilities for which they are accountable:

- Each transport system must comply with the standards and regulations set forth by local, state, and federal agencies.

- Informed consent for transfer, transport, and admission to and care at the receiving hospital should be obtained before the transport team moves the patient. All federal and state laws regulating patient transfer must be followed. The completed consent form should be signed by the patient or parent or guardian and witnessed; a copy should be placed in the patient's medical record. If the neonatal patient requires an emergency procedure before the parents' arrival at the receiving facility, the informed consent for this procedure should be obtained before departure from the referring facility if this action will not adversely delay the transport.

- Consent for any surgical procedures should be obtained by surgical staff by telephone if parents are not at the receiving facility.

- Formal agreements between hospitals should be developed to outline procedures for transport and responsibilities for patient care.

- Hospital medical staff policies should delineate the level of capability of their perinatal units, which conditions should prompt consultation, and which patients should be considered for transfer.

- Relevant personal identification must be provided for the patient to wear during transport.

- Patient care guidelines, standing orders, and verbal communication with the designated transport physician are to be used to initiate and maintain patient-care interventions during transport.

The professional qualifications and actions of the transport team are the responsibility of the institution that employs the team. Insurance must be adequate to protect both patients and transport team members.

Director

The director of the transport program should be either a subspecialist in maternal–fetal medicine or neonatology or, in selected cases, an obstetrician–gynecologist or pediatrician with special expertise in these subspecialty areas. The program director's responsibilities include:

- Training and supervising staff
- Ensuring appropriate review of all transport records
- Developing and implementing patient-care protocols
- Developing and maintaining standardized patient records and a database to track the program
- Establishing a program for performance improvement
- Identifying trends and effecting improvements in the transport system by regularly reviewing the following elements:
  — Reviewing operational aspects of the program, such as response times, effectiveness of communications, and equipment issues
  — Reviewing evaluation forms completed by the referring and receiving hospitals soon after each transport
- Developing protocols for programs that use multiple modes of transportation (ground, helicopter, airplane)
- Determining which mode of transport should be used and any conditions, such as weather, that would preclude the use of a particular form of transport
- Developing alternative plans for care of the patient if a transport cannot be accomplished
- Ensuring that proper safety standards are followed during transport
- Requiring the transportation services to follow established guidelines regarding maintenance and safety

The director may delegate specific responsibilities to other persons or groups but retains the responsibility of ensuring that these functions are addressed appropriately.

Referring Hospital

Referring physicians should be familiar with the transport system, including how to gain access to and appropriately use its services. The referring physician is responsible for evaluating the patient's condition and initiating stabilization procedures before the transport team arrives. Within the referring hospital, the transport team continues resuscitation and care in collaboration with the referring physician and staff. Transfer generally is performed when the infant is clinically stable, although there are circumstances when ongoing stabilization is necessary during the transfer to the accepting hospital.

Each patient should be accompanied by a maternal or neonatal transport form when being transferred. This form should contain general information about the patient, including the reason for referral, the transport mode, and any additional information that may enhance understanding of the patient's needs. Also provided should be relevant neonatal medical information that maximizes the opportunity for appropriate and timely care and minimizes duplication of tests and diagnostic procedures at the receiving hospital. The newborn must have appropriate identification bands in place.

The following items should be sent with a neonate:

- Properly labeled, red-topped tubes of clotted maternal and umbilical cord blood with label identification consistent with the newborn identification bands

- Copies of all relevant maternal antepartum, intrapartum, and postpartum records

- All recent or new diagnostic or clinical information for the neonate, including imaging studies

Responsibility for care of the newborn should be delineated between the referring team and the transport team. Parental consent should be obtained for transfer to and treatment of the neonate at the receiving hospital. The referring physician should personally transfer care to the transport team or should designate another physician to transfer care. A report on the neonate's care should be provided by the referring hospital's nursing staff to the appropriate transport team member.

Receiving Center

The receiving center is responsible for the overall coordination of the regional program. It should ensure that interhospital transport is organized in a way that ensures that patients will receive the appropriate level of care.

Contingency plans should be in place to avoid a shortage of beds for patients needing tertiary care. These plans should include provisions for accepting or transferring patients among the cooperating centers or to an alternate receiving center, rather than only the receiving center affiliated with the referral center, when special circumstances warrant (eg, patient census or need for specialized services, such as extracorporeal membrane oxygenation).

The receiving center is responsible for providing referring physicians with:

- Access by telephone on a 24-hour basis to communicate with receiving obstetric and neonatal units
- Follow-up on the neonate by telephone, letter, or fax, provided all federal, state, and local requirements are met
- A complete summary, including diagnosis, an outline of the hospital course, and recommendations for ongoing care for each patient at discharge
- Ongoing communication and follow-up

Dispatching Units

Dispatching units are responsible for the following activities:

- Providing rapid coordination of vehicles and staff
- Serving as a communication link between the transport team and the referring and receiving hospitals
- Communicating the transport team's estimated time of arrival at the referring hospital to pick up the patient so that any planned therapeutic or diagnostic interventions can be completed in time
- Communicating the patient's estimated time of arrival at the receiving center so that all resources can be mobilized and ready
- Coordinating any connections that need to be made between air transport and ground ambulances

Personnel

The transport team collectively should have the expertise necessary to provide supportive care for a wide variety of emergency conditions that can arise with women and neonates at high risk. Team members may include physicians, neonatal nurse practitioners, registered nurses, respiratory therapists, and emergency medical technicians. The composition of the transport team should be consistent with the expected level of medical need of the patient being transported. Transport personnel also should be thoroughly familiar with the transport equipment to ensure that any malfunction en route can be handled without the assistance of hospital maintenance staff.

Equipment

Safe and successful patient transfer depends on the equipment available to the transport team. The kinds and amounts of equipment, medications, and supplies needed by the transport team depend on the type of transport (maternal or neonatal), the distance of the transfer, the type of transport vehicle used, and the resources available at the referring medical facility. The transport equipment and supplies should be based on the needs of the most seriously ill patients to be transported and should include essential medications and special supplies needed during stabilization and transfer.

The transport team generally needs the following items to perform its functions:

- Equipment for monitoring physiologic functions (heart rate, blood pressure levels [invasive or noninvasive], temperature [skin or axillary], respiratory rate, noninvasive pulse oximetry, and transcutaneous oxygen or carbon dioxide)

- Resuscitation and support equipment (intravenous pumps, suction apparatus, mechanical ventilators, and newborn incubators)

- Portable medical gas tanks attached to a flowmeter, with or without a blender that can be easily integrated with vehicle or building sources of pressurized gas during transport if patients dependent on ventilators are transported

- Electrical equipment that is capable of alternating current or extended direct-current operation or both and is compatible with the sources in the transport vehicle or medical facility

Additional specialized equipment and supplies may be needed for individual clinical situations.

The performance characteristics of transport equipment should be tested for the most severe environmental conditions of air or ground transport that may be encountered. Equipment performance may be altered by a harsh electromagnetic environment, altitude changes, vibration, forces of acceleration, or extremes of temperature and humidity. Hospital-based equipment may cause electromagnetic interference with aircraft navigation or communication systems. Altered performance of medical or aircraft systems could affect the safety of the transport team and the patient.

All equipment should be tested to ensure accuracy and safety in flight. The Federal Aviation Administration and the U.S. Food and Drug Administration have no comprehensive testing guidelines. The comprehensive testing programs of the U.S. Department of Defense have discovered flaws in hospital-based medical equipment that could affect safety when used in air transport. The U.S. Army Aeromedical Research Laboratory at Fort Rucker in Alabama has tested medical equipment for helicopter use, and the Armstrong Laboratory at Brooks Air Force Base in Texas has tested equipment for airplanes. These laboratories report on completed equipment tests and conduct new evaluations. The following organizations also can offer assistance in choosing medical equipment suitable for use in aircraft:

Association of Air Medical Services
526 King Street, Suite 415
Alexandria, Virginia 22314-3143
Tel: (703) 836-8732, Fax: (703) 836-8920
www.aams.org

Emergency Care Research Institute
5200 Butler Pike
Plymouth Meeting, PA 19462-1298
Tel: (610) 825-6000, Fax: (610) 825-1275
www.ecri.org

Federal Aviation Administration
800 Independence Avenue, SW
Washington, DC 20591
Tel: (866) 835-5322
www.faa.gov

National Aeronautics and Space Administration
Washington, DC 20546-0001
Tel: (202) 358-0001, Fax: (202) 358-3469
www.nasa.gov

Professional Aeromedical Transport Association
4627 Beverly Boulevard
Los Angeles, CA 90004
Tel: (323) 468-1611, Fax: (323) 463-0433

Several factors should be considered in selecting vehicles for an interhospital transport system. Ground transportation is most appropriate for short-range transport. The use of airplanes allows for coverage of a large referral area but is more expensive, requires skilled operators and specially trained crews, and may actually prolong the time required for response and transport over relatively short distances because of the time needed to prepare for flight and the time required for transport to and from the airport. Helicopters can shorten response and transport times over intermediate distances or in highly congested areas but are very expensive to maintain and operate.

The decision to use aircraft in a patient-transport system requires special commitments from the director and members of the transport team. The pilot's decisions need to be based solely on flight safety. Therefore, the pilot should be included in appropriate decision making and should have the authority to change, modify, or cancel the mission for safety reasons.

Transport Procedure

Interhospital transport should be considered if the necessary resources or personnel for optimal patient outcomes are not available at the facility currently providing care. The resources available at both the referring and the receiving hospitals should be considered. The risks and benefits of transport, as well as the risks and benefits associated with not transporting the patient, should be assessed. Transport may be undertaken if the physician determines that the well-being of either the woman, the fetus, or the newborn will not be adversely affected or that the benefits of transfer outweigh the foreseeable risks. The staff of the referring hospital should consult with the receiving hospital as soon as the need for transport of a woman or her neonate is considered.

Transportation of patients to an alternate receiving center solely because of third-party payer issues (eg, conflicts between managed care plans and referring and receiving hospital affiliations) should be strongly discouraged and may be illegal in certain situations. All transfers should be based on medical need. When faced with preterm labor, transport of the mother in labor is recommended if time allows. Preterm labor is a valid reason for transport within the context of the EMTALA.

If the patient to be transported is pregnant, pretreatment evaluation should include the following:

- Maternal vital signs
- Fetal assessment via electronic fetal monitoring
- Fetal position
- Maternal cervical examination, if contracting

It may be necessary to stabilize the mother before transport. Initiation of blood pressure medication, intravenous fluids, or tocolytics may be started at the referring hospital. The level of care to be provided in the referring hospital is dependent on the time required for transport, method of transport, and maternal medical condition. This level of care should be determined locally between the referring and receiving hospitals' medical personnel.

If the patient to be transferred is a neonate, the family should be given an opportunity to see and touch the neonate before the transfer. A transport team member should meet with the family to explain what the team will be doing en route to the receiving hospital. The patient, personnel, and all equipment should be safely secured inside the transport vehicle.

Patient Care and Interactions

The following important components of patient care during transport should be implemented:

- Patients should be observed continuously.
- Vital signs should be monitored and recorded.
- Ventilator pressures and inspired oxygen percentages should be monitored.
- Uterine activity of maternal patients and fetal heart rates should be monitored.
- Neonatal patients should be kept in a neutral thermal environment and should receive appropriate respiratory support and additional monitoring, such as assessment of oxygen saturation and blood glucose, as clinically indicated.
- Intravenous fluids and medications should be given, monitored, and recorded as required.
- The team should be prepared to perform lifesaving invasive procedures, such as placment of a chest tube and intubation, on neonatal patients.

On arrival at the receiving hospital, the following activities are recommended:

- The receiving staff should be prepared to address any unresolved problems or emergencies involving the transported patient.
- The transport team should report the patient's history and clinical status to the receiving staff.

- The receiving staff should inform the patient's family, as well as the referring physician and staff at the referring hospital, of the condition of the patient on arrival to the receiving hospital and periodically thereafter.

- On completion of the patient transfer, the transport team or other designated personnel should immediately restock and reequip the transport vehicle in anticipation of another call.

Return Transport

Patients whose conditions have stabilized and who no longer require specialized services should be considered for return transport. Transporting the patient back to the referring hospital is important for the following reasons:

- It allows the family to return to their home, often permitting more frequent interactions between the family and the patient.

- It involves the providers who ultimately will be responsible for the continuing care of the patient earlier in the care process.

- It preserves specialized services for patients who require them and allows for a better distribution of resources.

- It enhances the integrity of the regionalized care system and emphasizes the partnership between the hospitals in the system.

Economic barriers, including those imposed by managed care organizations, that restrict or raise barriers to this movement of patients are detriments to optimal patient care. Every effort should be made to eliminate these artificial constraints.

Transfer is best accomplished after detailed communication between physicians and nursing services at both hospitals outlining the patient's care requirements and the anticipated course of the patient to ensure that the hospital receiving the return transport can provide the needed services. These services must not only be available but they must be provided in a consistent fashion and be of the same quality as those that the patient is receiving in the regional center. Further, if special equipment or treatment is required at the hospital receiving the patient, arrangements for these should be made before the patient is transferred. Lastly, there also must be an understanding that if problems arise that cannot be managed in an appropriate manner at the receiving hospital, the patient will be returned to the regional center, or the regional center will participate in developing an alternative care plan.

It is important that parents consent to the return transfer of the newborn and understand the benefits to them and their neonate. Their comfort with this process will be enhanced if they realize that the regional center and the referring hospital are working together in a regionalized system of care, that there is frequent communication between the staffs of the two hospitals, that there will be continuing support after the return transport, and that the patient will be returned to the regional center if necessary. It also may be helpful if parents visit the facility to which the neonate will be transported before transfer.

A comprehensive plan for follow-up of the patient after return transfer and after discharge from the hospital should be developed. This plan should outline the required services and identify the party bearing the responsibility for follow-up.

To ensure optimal care during a return transfer, the following guidelines are recommended:

- The patient's (or parents') informed consent for return transfer should be obtained.

- Return transfer should be accomplished via an adequately equipped vehicle with trained personnel so that the level of care received by the patient remains the same during transport.

- Staffing at both hospitals should be adequate to ensure a safe transition of care.

- The family should be notified of the transfer so that they may be present at the accepting facility when the transfer occurs.

- Appropriate records, including a summary of the hospital course, diagnosis, treatments, recommendations for ongoing care, and follow-up, should accompany the patient.

- The transport team should call the referring hospital and the neonate's parents to inform them of the completion of the transport and to report the neonate's condition.

- The center that provided the higher level of care should provide easily accessible consultation on current or new problems to professional staff at the return transfer facility.

Outreach Education

Critical to the appropriate use of a regional referral program is a program to educate the public and users about its capabilities. The receiving center and receiving hospitals should participate in efforts to educate the public about the kinds of services available and their accessibility.

Outreach education should reinforce cooperation between all individuals involved in the interhospital care of perinatal patients. Receiving hospitals should provide all referring hospitals with information about their response times and clinical capabilities and should ensure that providers know about the specialized resources that are available through the perinatal care network. Primary physicians should be informed as changes occur in indications for consultation and referral of perinatal patients at high risk and for the stabilization of their conditions. Each receiving hospital also should provide continuing education and information to referring physicians about current treatment modalities for high-risk situations. Effective outreach programs will improve the care capabilities of referring hospitals and may allow for some patients either to be retained or, if transferred, to be return transferred earlier in their course of care.

Program Evaluation

Ideally, the director of a regional program should coordinate program evaluation based on patient outcome data and logistic information. Program monitoring should include the following information:

- Unexpected neonatal morbidity (eg, hypothermia or tension pneumothorax) or mortality during transport
- Morbidity or mortality of patients at the receiving hospital
- Frequency of failure to transfer patients generally considered to require tertiary care (eg, newborns born at less than 32 weeks of gestation)
- Availability of all the services that may be needed by the perinatal patient
- Accessibility of services, capability to connect the patient quickly and appropriately with the services needed, and programs to promote patient and community awareness of available and appropriate regional referral programs

These data should be tracked as part of the ongoing quality improvement programs of the transport team and the receiving hospital.

Resources

American Academy of Pediatrics, Section on Transport Medicine. Guidelines for air and ground transport of neonatal and pediatric patients. 3rd ed. Elk Grove Village (IL): AAP; 2006.

American College of Obstetricians and Gynecologists. Guidelines for women's health care. 2nd ed. Washington, DC: ACOG; 2002.

Guidelines for the transfer of critically ill patients. Guidelines Committee of the American College of Critical Care Medicine; Society of Critical Care Medicine and American Association of Critical-Care Nurses Transfer Guidelines Task Force. Crit Care Med 1993;21:931–7.

March of Dimes Birth Defects Foundation. Toward improving the outcome of pregnancy: the 90s and beyond. White Plains (NY): MDBDF; 1993.

chapter 4

Antepartum Care

A comprehensive antepartum-care program involves a coordinated approach to medical care and psychosocial support that optimally begins before conception and extends throughout the antepartum period. Health care professionals should integrate the concept of family-centered care into antepartum care (see "Family-Centered Care" in Chapter 1). Care should include an assessment of the parents' attitudes toward the pregnancy, the support systems available, and the need for parenting education. Couples should be encouraged to work with their caregivers in developing a birthing plan and in making well-informed decisions about pregnancy, labor, delivery, and the postpartum period.

Preconception Care

Preconception care consists of the identification of those conditions that could affect a future pregnancy or fetus and that may be amenable to intervention. For example, adverse effects on the fetus, including spontaneous abortion or congenital anomalies, caused by maternal phenylketonuria or poorly controlled diabetes mellitus can be reduced if strict metabolic control is achieved before conception and continued throughout pregnancy. Conversely, establishing metabolic control of these conditions later in pregnancy is believed to be of lesser benefit. Alternatively, prenatal diagnosis of fetal genetic abnormalities can provide parents with options regarding the continuation of the pregnancy and permit targeted prenatal and neonatal care to optimize outcomes.

All health encounters during a woman's reproductive years, particularly those that are a part of preconception care, should include counseling on appropriate medical care and behavior to optimize pregnancy outcomes. The following maternal assessments may serve as the basis for such counseling:

- Family planning and pregnancy spacing
- Family history

- Genetic history (both maternal and paternal)
- Medical, surgical, psychiatric, and neurologic histories
- Current medications (prescription and nonprescription)
- Substance use, including alcohol, tobacco, and illicit drugs
- Domestic abuse and violence
- Nutrition
- Environmental and occupational exposures
- Immunity and immunization status
- Risk factors for sexually transmitted diseases
- Obstetric history
- Gynecologic history
- General physical examination
- Assessment of socioeconomic, educational, and cultural context

Vaccination(s) should be offered to women found to be at risk for or susceptible to rubella, varicella, and hepatitis B. Special vaccination, such as Pneumovax, may be indicated for patients who have undergone splenectomy for any reason (trauma, idiopathic thrombocytopenic purpura) or have functional asplenia caused by sickle cell disease. All pregnant women should be tested for human immunodeficiency virus (HIV) infection with patient notification as part of the routine battery of prenatal blood tests unless they decline the test (ie, opt-out approach) (see "Routine Testing" in this chapter and Chapter 9 for further discussion of viral infections). Physicians should be aware of and follow their states' prenatal HIV-screening requirements. A number of tests can be performed for specific indications:

- Screening for sexually transmitted diseases
- Testing for maternal diseases based on medical or reproductive history
- Mantoux test with purified protein derivative for tuberculosis
- Screening for genetic disorders based on racial and ethnic background:
  — Sickle hemoglobinopathies (African Americans)
  — β-thalassemia (Mediterraneans, Southeast Asians, and African Americans)
  — α-thalassemia (Southeast Asians, Mediterraneans, and African Americans)
  — Tay–Sachs disease (Ashkenazi Jews, French Canadians, and Cajuns)

—Canavan disease and familial dysautonomia (Ashkenazi Jews)

—Cystic fibrosis (CF) (while carrier frequency is higher among Caucasians of European and Ashkenazi Jewish descent, carrier screening should be made available to all couples)

- Screening for other genetic disorders on the basis of family history (eg, fragile X syndrome for family history of nonspecific, predominantly male-affected, mental retardation; Duchenne's muscular dystrophy)

Patients should be counseled regarding the benefits of the following activities:

- Exercising
- Reducing weight before pregnancy, if obese
- Increasing weight before pregnancy, if underweight
- Avoiding food faddism
- Avoiding pregnancy within one month of receiving a live attenuated viral vaccine (eg, rubella)
- Preventing HIV infection
- Determining the time of conception by an accurate menstrual history
- Abstaining from tobacco, alcohol, and illicit drug use before and during pregnancy
- Taking folic acid, 0.4 mg per day, while attempting pregnancy and during the first trimester of pregnancy for prevention of neural tube defects (NTD); women who have had a prior NTD-affected pregnancy are at high risk of having a subsequent affected pregnancy and should consume 4 mg of folic acid per day in the periconception period (see "Preconception Nutritional Counseling" later in this chapter)
- Maintaining good control of any preexisting medical conditions (eg, diabetes, hypertension, systemic lupus erythematosus, asthma, seizures, thyroid disorders, and inflammatory bowel disease)

Preconception Nutritional Counseling

Consumption of a balanced diet with the appropriate distribution of the basic food pyramid groups is especially important during pregnancy. Diet can be affected by food preferences, cultural beliefs, and eating patterns. A woman who is a vegan or food faddist or who has special dietary restrictions secondary to medical illnesses, such as phenylketonuria, diabetes mellitus, inflammatory bowel disease, or renal disease, may require special dietary measures as well as vitamin and mineral supplements. Women who frequently diet to lose weight, fast, skip meals, or have eating disorders or unusual eating habits should be identified and counseled. The patient's access to food and the ability to purchase food can be pertinent. One way to evaluate nutritional status is to calculate the woman's body mass index at the preconception visit (Table 4–1). Additional risk factors for nutritional problems include adolescence, tobacco and substance abuse, history of pica during a previous pregnancy, high parity, and mental illness.

Neural tube defects, such as anencephaly and spina bifida, have multifactorial origins, but their etiology often may involve abnormalities in homocysteine metabolism that are potentially remediable by folic acid dietary supplementation. Indeed, the first occurrence of NTDs may be reduced by as much as 36% if women of reproductive age take 0.4 mg of folic acid daily both before conception and during the first trimester of pregnancy as recommended by the Centers for Disease Control and Prevention and the U.S. Public Health Service. A woman with a history of a prior NTD-affected pregnancy (recurrence risk 2–5%) or who is being treated with anticonvulsive medication may reduce the risk of NTDs by more than 80% if she supplements her daily diet with 4 mg of folic acid for the months in which conception is attempted and for the first trimester of pregnancy. This daily dose should be achieved by adding a separate supplement to a single multivitamin tablet to provide a total of 4 mg of folate while avoiding excessive intake of fat-soluble vitamins (see "Vitamin and Mineral Toxicity" in this chapter). The U.S. Food and Drug

Table 4–1. Recommended Ranges of Total Weight Gain for Pregnant Women by Prepregnancy Body Mass Index for Singleton Gestation*

Weight-for-Height Category		Recommended Total Weight Gain	
Category	Body Mass Index	kg	lb
Low	<19.8	12.5–18	28–40
Normal	19.8–26	11.5–16	25–35
High	26–29	7–11.5	15–25
Obese	>29	At least 7	At least 15

*The range for women carrying twins is 35–45 lb (16–20 kg). Young adolescents (<2 years after menarche) and African-American women should strive for gains at the upper end of the range. Short women (<62 in or <157 cm) should strive for gains at the lower end of the range.

Reprinted and adapted with permission from Nutrition during pregnancy and lactation, an implementation guide. Copyright 1992 by the National Academy of Sciences. Courtesy of the National Academy Press, Washington, DC.

Administration has established rules under which specified grain products are required to be fortified with folic acid at levels ranging from 0.43 mg to 1.4 mg per pound of product. These amounts are designed to enable women to more easily consume 0.4 mg of folic acid daily. However, these amounts of fortified folic acid are intended to keep the daily intake of folic acid less than 1 mg. Because the amount of folic acid consumed in fortified grain products may be less than the amount recommended to prevent NTDs, supplementation still is recommended.

Routine Antepartum Care

Women who receive early and regular prenatal care are more likely to have healthier infants. The early diagnosis of pregnancy is important in establishing a management plan. This plan of care should take into consideration the medical, nutritional, psychosocial, and educational needs of the patient and her family, and it should be periodically reevaluated and revised in accordance with the progress of the pregnancy.

All pregnant women should have access in their community to readily available and regularly scheduled obstetric care, beginning in early pregnancy and continuing through the postpartum period. Pregnant women also should have access to unscheduled or emergency visits on a 24-hour basis. Timing of access varies depending on the nature of the problem.

Incarcerated Women

Generally, pregnant inmates, because of their disadvantaged background, are at a higher risk for poor pregnancy outcomes than the general population. Many facilities do not offer adequate prenatal care. Incarcerated women should receive adequate prenatal care. Applying physical restraints to pregnant women should be needed only very rarely, in extreme situations, for short periods. If restraint is needed after the first trimester, it should be performed with the individual on her side, not flat on her back or stomach. If she needs to be restrained for more than several minutes, she should be allowed to be on her side, preferably on her left side. Pressure should not be applied to the abdomen either directly or indirectly while restraining the patient.

Women With Physical Disabilities

Pregnancy and parenting for women with physical disabilities pose unique medical and social challenges but rarely are precluded by the disability itself.

Few, if any, physical disabilities directly limit fertility. Health care professionals have the responsibility to provide appropriate reproductive health services to these women or arrange adequate consultation or referral. Nonbiased preconception counseling for couples in which one partner has a physical disability may decrease subsequent psychosocial and medical complications of pregnancy. Screening and provision of disability-specific information, such as folate supplementation for women who have spina bifida, is highly desirable.

Once pregnancy occurs, the patient should have early contact with an obstetrician. Counseling about prenatal testing and options should be comprehensive and nondirective. Regular consultation or referral may be required to achieve the optimum outcome, such as in cases of spinal cord injury or multiple sclerosis. Detailed pregnancy care plans should be developed in negotiation with managed care plans and other insurers to increase access to and use of prenatal care services, ensure appropriate postpartum hospital length of stay, and arrange postpartum home care services, if necessary. Cesarean delivery should be done for obstetric indications. Community resources for childbirth, breastfeeding, and parenting education should be identified early in the pregnancy, and timely referrals should be made for the pregnant woman and her family.

General Patient Education

Patient education is an essential element of prenatal care. The physician or other providers participating in antepartum care should discuss the following information with each patient:

- Scope of care that is provided in the office (see Appendix G)
- Laboratory studies that may be performed
- Expected course of the pregnancy
- Signs and symptoms to be reported to the physician (eg, vaginal bleeding, rupture of membranes, or decreased fetal movements)
- Anticipated schedule of visits
- Physician coverage of labor and delivery
- Cost to the patient of prenatal care and delivery (eg, insurance plan participation)
- Practices to promote health maintenance (eg, use of safety restraints, including lap and shoulder belts)
- Educational programs available
- Options for intrapartum care

- Planning for hospital discharge and child care
- Encouraging breastfeeding (see Chapter 7)
- Choosing the child's physician

Specialized Counseling

Sauna and Hot Tub Exposure

There are extensive animal data to indicate that hyperthermia induced during organogenesis is teratogenic. The major malformations most commonly thought to result from human maternal febrile illnesses are NTDs. Many early studies were troubled with methodologic problems of recall bias and most could not distinguish etiologically between the fever and the infectious agent that caused it or the medications that were used to treat it. Some prospective studies now suggest that it is the fever per se that is teratogenic. Studies in the late 1970s suggested that sauna and hot tub use also might cause hyperthermia and congenital malformations. The probability of significantly increasing core body temperature depends on the temperature of the sauna or hot tub, duration of exposure, and for hot tubs, the extent of submersion. Many women will not voluntarily remain in a hyperthermic environment long enough to increase their core temperatures, but some may. Pregnant women might reasonably be advised to remain in saunas for no more than 15 minutes and hot tubs for no more than 10 minutes. As an additional precaution, there is less surface area to absorb heat and more surface area to radiate it if the head, arms, shoulders and upper chest are not submerged in a hot tub.

Nutrition in Pregnancy

Each pregnant woman should be provided with information about balanced nutrition, as well as ideal caloric intake and weight gain. Height and weight should be recorded for all women at the initial prenatal visit to allow calculation of body mass index. Maternal nutrition can contribute positively to maintaining or improving the woman's health, as well as to the delivery of a healthy, term newborn of an appropriate weight. Nutrition counseling is an integral part of perinatal care for all patients. It should focus on a well-balanced, varied, nutritional food plan that is consistent with the patient's access to food and food preferences. Nutrition consultation should be offered to all obese women, and they should be encouraged to follow an exercise program. Patient educational materials on nutrition are available from the American College of Obstetricians and Gynecologists (www.acog.org), the U.S. Public Health

Service (www.dhhs.gov/phs), and the March of Dimes Foundation (www. marchofdimes.org). Dietary counseling and intervention based on special or individual needs usually are most effectively accomplished by referral to a nutritionist or registered dietitian.

The recommended dietary allowances for most vitamins and minerals increase during pregnancy (Table 4–2). The National Academy of Sciences recommends 27 mg of iron supplementation (present in most prenatal vitamins) be given to pregnant women daily because the iron content of the standard American diet and the endogenous iron stores of many American women are not sufficient to provide for the increased iron requirements of pregnancy. The U.S. Preventive Services Task Force recommends that all pregnant women be routinely screened for iron-deficiency anemia. The treatment of frank iron-deficiency anemia requires dosages of 60–120 mg of elemental iron each day. Iron absorption is facilitated by or with vitamin C supplementation or ingestion between meals or at bedtime on an empty stomach. See Table 4–3 for examples of vitamin and mineral food sources. Women should supplement their diets with folic acid before and during pregnancy (see "Preconception Nutritional Counseling" in this chapter). Women should be cautioned to keep these supplements and any other medications out of the reach of children.

Women also should be instructed about appropriate weight gain. See Table 4–1 for the Institute of Medicine guidelines for weight gain associated with optimal outcomes by maternal prepregnancy weight. In general, caloric intake is calculated at 25–35 kcal/kg of optimal body weight. An additional 100–300 kcal per day is recommended during pregnancy. Because optimal outcome can occur over a relatively wide range of weight gain, the provider can be flexible. These recommendations can be adjusted to specific subgroups of patients, such as adolescents and women who are obese, of lower socioeconomic status, or short. Following the Institute of Medicine weight-gain guidelines for singleton gestations improves the likelihood of delivering a normal-weight newborn. Assessment of weight gain during pregnancy is important and should be documented appropriately, preferably on a form specifically designed for that purpose (see example in Appendix A). If a patient is financially unable to meet nutritional needs, she should be referred to federal food and nutrition programs, such as the Special Supplemental Food Program for Women, Infants, and Children.

Pregnant and nursing women should be reminded not to eat certain fish with high levels of mercury, including shark, swordfish, king mackerel, and tile-

Table 4-2. Recommended Daily Dietary Allowances for Adolescent and Adult Pregnant and Lactating Women

	Pregnant			Lactating		
	14–18 years	19–30 years	31–50 years	14–18 years	19–30 years	31–50 years
Fat-soluble vitamins						
Vitamin A	750 µg	770 µg	770 µg	1,200 µg	1,300 µg	1,300 µg
Vitamin D*	5 µg	5 µg	5 µg	5 µg	5 µg	5 µg
Vitamin E	15 mg	15 mg	15 mg	19 mg	19 mg	19 mg
Vitamin K	75 µg	90 µg	90 µg	75 µg	90 µg	90 µg
Water-soluble vitamins						
Vitamin C	80 mg	85 mg	85 mg	115 mg	120 mg	120 mg
Thiamin	1.4 mg	1.4 mg	1.4 mg	1.4 mg	1.4 mg	1.4 mg
Riboflavin	1.4 mg	1.4 mg	1.4 mg	1.6 mg	1.6 mg	1.6 mg
Niacin	18 mg	18 mg	18 mg	17 mg	17 mg	17 mg
Vitamin B_6	1.9 mg	1.9 mg	1.9 mg	2 mg	2 mg	2 mg
Folate	600 µg	600 µg	600 µg	500 µg	500 µg	500 µg
Vitamin B_{12}	2.6 µg	2.6 µg	2.6 µg	2.8 µg	2.8 µg	2.8 µg
Minerals						
Calcium*	1,300 mg	1,000 mg	1,000 mg	1,300 mg	1,000 mg	1,000 mg
Phosphorus	1,250 mg	700 mg	700 mg	1,250 mg	700 mg	700 mg
Iron	27 mg	27 mg	27 mg	10 mg	9 mg	9 mg
Zinc	12 mg	11 mg	11 mg	13 mg	12 mg	12 mg
Iodine	220 µg	220 µg	220 µg	290 µg	290 µg	290 µg
Selenium	60 µg	60 µg	60 µg	70 µg	70 µg	70 µg

*Recommendations measured as Adequate Intake (AI) instead of Recommended Daily Dietary Allowance (RDA). An AI is set instead of an RDA if insufficient evidence is available to determine an RDA. The AI is based on observed or experimentally determined estimates of average nutrient intake by a group (or groups) of healthy people.

Data from Institute of Medicine. Dietary reference intakes for calcium, phosphorus, magnesium, vitamin D, and fluoride. Washington, DC: National Academy Press; 1997; Institute of Medicine (US). Dietary reference intakes for thiamin, riboflavin, niacin, vitamin B6, folate, vitamin B12, pantothenic acid, biotin, and choline. Washington, DC: National Academy Press; 1998; Institute of Medicine (US). Dietary reference intakes for vitamin C, vitamin E, selenium, and carotenoids. Washington, DC: National Academy Press; 2000; and Institute of Medicine (US). Dietary reference intakes for vitamin A, vitamin K, arsenic, boron, chromium, copper, iodine, iron, manganese, molybdenum, nickel, silicon, vanadium, and zinc. Washington, DC: National Academy Press; 2002.

Table 4–3. Vitamin and Mineral Food Sources

Nutrient	Food Source
Vitamin A	Green leafy vegetables; dark yellow vegetables (eg, carrots and sweet potatoes); whole, fortified skim and low-fat milks; liver
Vitamin C	Citrus fruits (eg, oranges, lemons, grapefruit), strawberries, broccoli, tomatoes
Vitamin D	Fortified milk, fish liver oils, exposure to sunlight
Vitamin E	Vegetable oils, whole-grain cereals, wheat germ, green leafy vegetables
Folate	Green leafy vegetables, orange juice, strawberries, liver, legumes, nuts
Calcium	Milk and milk products; sardines and salmon with bones; collard, kale, mustard, and turnip greens
Iron	Meat, liver, dried beans and peas, iron-fortified cereals, prune juice

fish. The U.S. Food and Drug Administration and the U.S. Environmental Protection Agency advise pregnant and nursing women to consume no more than 12 ounces (two average meals) per week of a variety of fish and shellfish that are low in mercury content (guidance available at www.cfsan.fda.gov/~dms/admehg3.html). Five of the most commonly eaten fish that are low in mercury are shrimp, canned light tuna, salmon, pollock, and catfish. Pregnant and nursing women should consume no more than two 6-ounce cans of tuna per week (total fish consumption should not exceed 12 ounces per week). Because albacore tuna also is high in mercury, it is advisable to choose light tuna instead. Pregnant and nursing women also should check local advisories about the safety of fish caught in local lakes, rivers, and coastal areas. If no advice is available, they should consume no more than 6 ounces (one average meal) per week of fish caught in local waters and no other fish during that week.

Nausea and Vomiting of Pregnancy

Nausea and vomiting of pregnancy affects more than 70% of pregnant women and can diminish the woman's quality of life. Most mild cases of nausea and vomiting can be resolved with lifestyle and dietary changes. Effective treatments for mild cases include consuming more protein, vitamin B_6, or vitamin B_6 with doxylamine. Effective and safe treatments for more serious cases include antihistamine H1-receptor blockers and phenothiazines. The most severe form of pregnancy-associated nausea and vomiting is hyperemesis gravidarum, which occurs in less than 2% of pregnancies. This may require more intense therapy, including hospitalization, additional medications, intravenous hydration and nutrition, and if refractory, total parenteral nutrition.

Vitamin and Mineral Toxicity

Although vitamin A is essential, excessive vitamin A (more than 10,000 international units per day) may be associated with fetal malformations. The amount of vitamin A in standard prenatal vitamins (4,000–5,000 international units) is considered the maximum recommended dose before and during pregnancy and is well below the probable minimum human teratogenic dose. Dietary intake of vitamin A in the United States is adequate to meet the needs of most pregnant women throughout gestation. Therefore, additional supplementation besides a prenatal vitamin during pregnancy is not recommended except in women in whom the dietary intake of vitamin A may not be adequate, such as strict vegetarians. Vitamin tablets containing 25,000 international units or more of vitamin A are available as over-the-counter preparations; however, pregnant women or those planning to become pregnant who use high doses of vitamin A supplements (and retinol) should be cautioned about the potential teratogenicity, as excess vitamin A is associated with anomalies of bones, the urinary tract, and the central nervous system. The use of beta carotene, the precursor of vitamin A found in fruits and vegetables, has not been shown to produce vitamin A toxicity.

Excessive vitamin and mineral intake (ie, more than twice the recommended dietary allowances) should be avoided during pregnancy. For example, excess iodine is associated with congenital goiter. There also may be toxicity from excessive use of other fat-soluble vitamins (D, E, and K).

Exercise in Pregnancy

In the absence of either medical or obstetric complications, 30 minutes or more of moderate exercise per day on most if not all days of the week is recommended for pregnant women. Generally, participation in a wide range of recreational activities appears to be safe during pregnancy; however, each sport should be reviewed individually for its potential risk, and activities with a high risk of falling or those with a high risk for abdominal trauma should be avoided. Pregnant women also should avoid supine positions during exercise as much as possible.

Recreational and competitive athletes with uncomplicated pregnancies can remain active during pregnancy and should modify their usual exercise routines as medically indicated. Pregnant competitive athletes may require close obstetric supervision. Women should not take up a new strenuous sport during pregnancy, and previously inactive women and those with medical or obstetric complications should be evaluated before recommendations for physical activity participation during pregnancy are made. Additionally, a physically active woman with a history of or risk for preterm delivery or intrauterine growth restriction should be advised to reduce her activity in the second and third trimesters. Warning signs to terminate exercise while pregnant include:

- Chest pain
- Vaginal bleeding
- Dizziness
- Headache
- Decreased fetal movement
- Amniotic fluid leakage
- Muscle weakness
- Calf pain or swelling
- Preterm labor
- Regular uterine contractions

Tobacco Use

Inquiry into tobacco use and smoke exposure should be a routine part of the prenatal visit. Patients should be strongly discouraged from smoking. Multiple studies have demonstrated a clear association between maternal smoking and perinatal morbidity and mortality. Placenta previa, abruptio placentae, and preterm rupture of membranes are factors in many pregnancy losses in smokers. It is estimated that there would be a 5% reduction in perinatal mortality if smoking during pregnancy were eliminated. Infant health risks include sudden infant death syndrome, hospitalization, and neurodevelopmental abnormalities. For pregnant women who smoke fewer than 20 cigarettes per day, the provision of a 5–15-minute five-step counseling session and pregnancy-specific educational materials increases cessation rates. Physicians should use the following five smoking cessation guidelines for all patients who continue to smoke during pregnancy:

1. Ask about smoking status. Providers should ask the patient at the first prenatal visit to choose a statement that best describes her smoking status from a list of statements on smoking behavior. Using this multiple-choice method is more likely to elicit an accurate response than asking

a question that elicits a simple "yes" or "no" answer. A smoking-cessation chart, a tobacco-use sticker, or a vital-signs stamp that includes smoking status may be useful in the medical record to remind providers to ask patients about smoking status at follow-up visits.

2. Advise patients who smoke to stop by providing clear, strong advice to quit with personalized messages about the benefits of quitting and the effect of continued smoking on the woman, fetus, and newborn. Congratulate patients who report having stopped smoking and affirm their efforts with a statement about the benefits of quitting.

3. Assess the patient's willingness to attempt to quit smoking within the next 30 days. One approach to this assessment is to say, "Quitting smoking is one of the most important things you can do for your health and your baby's health. If we can give you some help, are you willing to try?" If the patient is willing, the provider can move to the next step. If the patient is unwilling to try, the provider may consider having a brief discussion with the patient to educate and reassure her about quitting. Quitting advice, assessment, and assistance should be offered at subsequent prenatal care visits.

4. Assist patients who are interested in quitting by providing pregnancy-specific, self-help smoking cessation materials. Enhance the patient's problem-solving skills by asking when and where she typically smokes and suggesting how she might avoid these situations that trigger the desire to smoke. Offer support on the importance of 1) having a smoke-free space at home, 2) seeking out a "quitting buddy," such as a former smoker or nonsmoker, both at work and at home, and 3) understanding nicotine withdrawal, such as irritability and cravings. Communicate caring and concern and encourage the patient to talk about the process of quitting. The provider also may refer the patient to a smoker's quitline. Telephone quitlines offer information, direct support, and ongoing counseling and have been very successful in helping pregnant smokers quit and remain smoke free. Great Start (1-866-66-START) is a national pregnancy-specific smoker's quitline operated by the American Legacy Foundation. Some states also have proactive, direct fax referral capability for providers to connect pregnant smokers directly to their state quitline. By dialing the national quitline network (1-800-QUIT NOW), callers are routed immediately to their state smoker's quitline.

5. Arrange follow-up visits to track the progress of the patient's attempt to quit smoking. For current and former smokers, smoking status should

be monitored throughout pregnancy, providing opportunities to congratulate and support success, reinforce steps taken toward quitting, and advise those still considering a cessation attempt.

Although nicotine-replacement products or other pharmaceuticals, such as smoking cessation aids, are effective for reducing smoking in nonpregnant women, they have not been sufficiently evaluated to determine their effectiveness and safety in pregnancy. Nicotine gum and patches should be considered in pregnant women only after nonpharmacologic treatments (eg, counseling) have failed and if the increased likelihood of smoking cessation, with its potential benefits, outweighs the unknown risk of nicotine replacement and potential concomitant smoking.

Substance Use and Abuse

All pregnant women should be questioned at their first prenatal visit about their past and present use of alcohol, nicotine, and other drugs, including the recreational use of prescription and over-the-counter medications. Use of specific screening questionnaires may improve detection rates. A woman who acknowledges the use of alcohol, nicotine, cocaine, opioids, amphetamines, or other mood-altering drugs should be counseled about the perinatal implications of their use during pregnancy and offered referral to an appropriate drug-treatment program if chemical dependence is suspected. Large numbers of women of childbearing age abuse potentially addictive and mood-altering drugs. Use of cocaine, marijuana, diazepam, opioids (including morphine, heroin, codeine, meperidine, methadone, and oxycodone), other prescription drugs, and approximately 150 other substances can lead to chemical dependency. Depending on geographic location, it is estimated that 1–40% of pregnant women have used one of these substances during pregnancy. Data suggest that approximately 1 in 10 neonates is exposed to one or more mood-altering drugs during pregnancy; the number varies only slightly for publicly versus privately insured patients.

Women should be dissuaded from alcohol consumption during pregnancy because there is no known safe threshold. Patients should be informed that prenatal alcohol consumption is a preventable cause of birth defects, including mental retardation and neurodevelopmental deficits. Fetal alcohol syndrome is characterized by three findings: 1) growth restriction, 2) facial abnormalities, and 3) central nervous system dysfunction. Although fetal alcohol syndrome is more prevalent among chronic alcoholics (prevalence 6–50%), it has been reported with lesser amounts of alcohol use.

Chemical dependency is likely to be a chronic, relapsing, and progressive disease. Many drug-dependent pregnant women do not seek early prenatal care and therefore are at increased risk for medical and obstetric complications. Drug-exposed neonates often go unrecognized and are discharged from the newborn nursery to homes where they are at increased risk for a complex of medical and social problems, including abuse and neglect.

To reinforce and encourage continued abstinence, periodic questioning or drug or metabolite testing may be desirable for a pregnant woman who reports substance use before or during pregnancy. Testing of the mother or the neonate or both also may be useful in some clinical situations, even when substance use has not been suspected previously. Such circumstances include the presence of unexplained intrauterine growth restriction, third-trimester stillbirth, unexpected preterm birth, or abruptio placentae in a woman not known to have hypertensive disease. Because positive test results have implications for patients that transcend their health, patients should give informed consent before testing. The requirements for consent to test vary from state to state, and practitioners should be familiar with the testing and the reporting requirements in their states.

Warning signs of drug abuse include noncompliance with prenatal care (eg, late entry to care, multiple missed appointments, or no prenatal care), evidence of poor nutrition, encounters with law enforcement, and marital and family disputes during the pregnancy. Screening of all patients at delivery is not recommended. Screens are likely to be negative when drugs were used early in pregnancy, and a urine screen can be negative even when women have taken certain drugs during the 48 hours before delivery. Toxicologic analysis of hair and meconium have been reported to be more sensitive methods of identifying illicit drug use, although urine remains the most frequently used specimen for screening. Because the components of urine toxicology screens vary among laboratories, physicians should verify with their laboratory which metabolites are included in its screen.

To identify drug-exposed neonates, the child's physician should obtain a thorough maternal history from all new mothers in a nonthreatening, organized manner. Practitioners also should be aware that laws in some states consider in utero drug exposure to be a form of child abuse or neglect and require reporting of positive drug test results in pregnant women or their newborns to the state's child protection agency. Although most over-the-counter medications pose no risk to pregnant women, patients also should consult with their health care providers before using nonprescription drugs or herbal remedies.

Domestic Violence

Risk assessment during pregnancy universally should include identification of women who are victims of domestic violence. Domestic violence, including intimate-partner violence, has been identified as a significant public health problem, affecting millions of American women each year. Trauma, including trauma caused by domestic violence, is one of the most frequent causes of maternal death in the United States. There is no single profile of an abused woman. Victims come from all racial, economic, educational, religious, ethnic, and social backgrounds. Victims are both adolescents and adults. In pregnant adolescents, the prevalence of abuse, particularly sexual abuse, may be greater than for adult pregnant women.

Research indicates that most abused women continue to be victimized during pregnancy. Violence against women also may begin or escalate during pregnancy and affects both maternal and fetal well-being. The prevalence of violence during pregnancy ranges from 1% to 20%, with most studies identifying rates between 4% and 8%. The presence of violence between intimate partners also affects the children in the household. Studies demonstrate that child abuse occurs in 33–77% of families in which there is abuse of adults. Among women who are being abused, 27% have demonstrated abusive behavior toward their children while living in the violent environment.

Abuse may involve threatened or actual physical, sexual, verbal, or psychologic abuse. The fundamental issues at play are power, control, and coercion. There is no clearly established set of symptoms that signal abuse. However, listed as follows are some of the obstetric presentations of abused women:

- Unwanted pregnancy
- Late entry into prenatal care or missed appointments
- Substance abuse or use
- Poor weight gain and nutrition
- Multiple, repeated somatic complaints

With the possible exception of preeclampsia, domestic violence is more prevalent than any major medical condition detected through routine prenatal screening. Detection may be possible by discussing with the patient that pregnancy sometimes places increased stress on a relationship and then by asking how the woman and her partner resolve their differences. In many cases, however, women will not disclose their abuse unless asked directly. Abused women usually are forthright when asked directly in a caring, nonjudgmental manner. The likelihood of disclosure increases with repeated inquiries.

Screening should be conducted in private with only the patient present. Translation services may be helpful in inquiring about these issues with women who have limited English proficiency. It is important to avoid using a family member or friend as an interpreter. Screening can be accomplished by prefacing the following questions with the simple statement that "because violence against women is so common, I ask all of my patients the following questions:"

- Within the past year, have you been threatened or actually hit, slapped, kicked, or otherwise physically hurt by anyone?

- Since you have been pregnant, have you been threatened or actually hit, slapped, kicked, or otherwise physically injured by anyone?

- Within the past year, has anyone forced you into sexual relations when you were not willing?

If a patient confides that she is being abused, verbatim accounts of the abuse should be recorded in the patient's medical record. The clinician should inquire about her immediate safety and the safety of her children. Clinicians should become familiar with local resources, and referrals to appropriate counseling, legal, and social-service advocacy programs should be made. Additionally, physicians should be familiar with state laws that may require reporting of domestic violence. Child abuse is always reportable. When the clinician suspects abuse, whether or not it is corroborated by the woman, supportive statements should be offered, and the need for follow-up should be addressed. It is important to encourage abused women, with the assistance of social services, to begin to create an "escape" plan, with a reliable safe haven for retreat, particularly if they believe the violence is escalating.

Antepartum Surveillance

Antepartum surveillance begins with the first prenatal visit, at which time the physician or nurse begins to compile an obstetric database. Appendix A contains a format for documenting information and the database recommended by the American College of Obstetricians and Gynecologists.

The frequency of follow-up visits is determined by the individual needs of the woman and an assessment of her risks. The frequency and regularity of scheduled prenatal visits should be sufficient to enable providers to accomplish the following activities:

- Monitor the progression of the pregnancy

- Provide education and recommended screening and interventions

- Reassure the woman

- Assess the well-being of the woman and her fetus
- Detect medical and psychosocial complications and institute indicated interventions

Generally, a woman with an uncomplicated pregnancy is examined every 4 weeks for the first 28 weeks of pregnancy, every 2–3 weeks until 36 weeks of gestation, and weekly thereafter. Women with medical or obstetric problems, as well as younger adolescents, may require closer surveillance; the appropriate intervals between scheduled visits are determined by the nature and severity of the problems (see Appendix G).

During each regularly scheduled visit, the health care provider should evaluate the woman's blood pressure, weight, urine for the presence of protein levels, uterine size for progressive growth and consistency with the estimated date of delivery, and fetal heart rate. After the patient reports quickening and at each subsequent visit, she should be asked about fetal movement. She should be queried about contractions, leakage of fluid, or vaginal bleeding at the appropriate point in pregnancy, given her potential risk factors.

Estimated Date of Delivery

Management of pregnancy requires establishing an estimated date of delivery. Problems such as intrauterine growth restriction, preterm labor, and postterm pregnancy are managed most effectively when an accurate estimated date of delivery is known. In addition, accurate gestational dating is important for the application and interpretation of certain antepartum tests (eg, maternal serum screening for trisomy 21 and NTDs or assessment of fetal maturity). If there is a size–date discrepancy or if menstrual dates are uncertain, an ultrasound examination is indicated for the purpose of dating. Such an examination is most accurate when performed before 20 weeks of gestation. Ultrasound examination results are considered to be consistent with menstrual dates if there is gestational age agreement to within 3 days by crown–rump length (CRL) measurement obtained at 6–10 weeks of gestation, within 5 days by CRL measurement obtained at 10–14 weeks of gestation, or within 7 days by the average of multiple biometric measurements obtained at 14–20 weeks of gestation. If dates are not consistent, refer to ultrasound examination results.

Routine Testing

Certain laboratory tests should be performed routinely in pregnant women. The following tests are performed early in pregnancy, as appropriate, and the results are made available to the physician responsible for care of the newborn:

- Hematocrit or hemoglobin levels
- Urinalysis, including microscopic examination
- Urine testing to detect asymptomatic bacteriuria (eg, urine culture, or urine dip for esterase and leukocytes followed by a urine culture if results are positive)
- Determination of blood group and CDE (Rh) type
- Antibody screen
- Determination of immunity to rubella virus
- Syphilis screen (Rapid plasma regain testing should be performed at first visit for populations at risk for poor prenatal care. Women at high risk or in high-prevalence areas should be rescreened in the third trimester.)
- Chlamydia screen (Women younger than 25 years or at high risk should be rescreened in the third trimester.)
- Cervical cytology (as needed)
- Hepatitis B virus surface antigen
- Human immunodeficiency virus antibody testing

Pregnant women universally should be tested for HIV infection with patient notification as part of the routine battery of prenatal blood tests unless they decline the test (ie, opt-out approach), as permitted by local and state regulations. Refusal of testing should be documented. In some states, it is necessary to obtain the woman's written authorization before disclosing her HIV status to health care providers who are not members of her health care team (see Chapter 9 for management). Women at high risk for HIV infection should be retested during the third trimester, ideally before 36 weeks of gestation. Repeat testing in high-HIV-prevalence areas and using rapid HIV testing in patients with unknown HIV status in labor and delivery also should be considered.

For couples planning pregnancy or seeking prenatal care, it is recommended that screening be offered to those at higher risk of having children with CF (Caucasians, including Ashkenazi Jews, and anyone with a family history of CF) and in whom the testing is most sensitive in identifying carriers of a CF mutation. It is further recommended that screening should be made available to couples in other racial and ethnic groups who are at lower risk and in whom the tests may be less sensitive. To ensure that they are aware of the availability of CF-carrier screening, couples in these lower-risk groups should be provided with written information about testing. For those couples to whom screening will be offered, it is recommended that this be done when they seek preconception counseling or infertility care or during the first and early second trimester of pregnancy.

Recommended intervals for additional tests that are indicated after the first prenatal visit are detailed on the ACOG Antepartum Record (see Appendix A). Additional laboratory evaluations, such as testing for sexually transmitted diseases, genetic disorders (see "Preconception Care" in this chapter), and tuberculosis, are recommended or offered on the basis of the patient's history, physical examination, parental desire, or in response to public health guidelines. Pregnancy is not a contraindication for Mantoux test with purified protein derivative for tuberculosis and may be indicated in high-risk areas or for health care workers. Tests for sexually transmitted diseases may be repeated in the third trimester if the woman has specific risk factors for these diseases. These tests may be mandated by local and state regulations. Early in the third trimester, measurement of hemoglobin or hematocrit levels should be repeated.

Fetal Imaging

Ultrasonography is the most commonly used fetal imaging tool and should be performed only by technologists or physicians who have undergone specific training and only when there is a valid medical indication for the examination. Second- and third-trimester ultrasound examinations include three types:

1. Standard—Evaluation of fetal presentation, amniotic fluid volume, cardiac activity, placental position, fetal biometry, and an anatomic survey

2. Limited—Evaluation to address a specific clinical question (eg, fetal presentation)

3. Specialized—A detailed anatomic examination performed when an anomaly is suspected on the basis of history, biochemical screening results, or the results of a limited or standard examination (eg, fetal echocardiogram, biophysical profile, Doppler ultrasound results, additional biometric study results)

Each type of ultrasound examination should be performed only when indicated and should be appropriately documented. First-trimester ultrasonography is becoming more common and can be performed abdominally or vaginally. Patients with an abnormal fetal ultrasound examination result should be referred for evaluation and management of fetal anomalies. Fetal magnetic resonance imaging does not involve radiation exposure and is being used more often. The most common use of fetal magnetic resonance imaging is to further delineate a fetal anomaly or rule out placenta accreta identified or suspected on ultrasound examination results. Although the safety of ultrasonography has been established, comparatively few studies have analyzed the safety of magnetic resonance imaging, although this technology is being used with increasing frequency in pregnant patients, and there are no known risks.

Immunizations

The risk of exposure to disease and its deleterious effects on the pregnant woman and the fetus must be balanced against the efficacy and potential risks of the vaccine. Preconception immunization is preferred when possible. Avoiding pregnancy within 1 month of receiving a live attenuated viral vaccine (eg, rubella) is recommended. No vaccine has been associated with documented risk to the fetus. Recommendations for immunization during pregnancy are available from the Centers for Disease Control and Prevention (www.cdc.gov/nip). All women who will be pregnant during the influenza season should be offered influenza vaccine, regardless of their stage of pregnancy. Pregnant women with medical conditions that increase their risk for complications from influenza should be offered the vaccine before the influenza season, regardless of the stage of pregnancy. Administration of the injectable, inactivated influenza vaccine is considered safe at any stage of pregnancy. In contrast, the intranasal influenza vaccine employs a live attenuated virus and should not be used in pregnant women. If indicated, other vaccines that are safe in pregnancy include tetanus, hepatitis B, and pneumococcus (recommended for pregnant patients with prior splenectomy or functional asplenia). In studies of meningococcal vaccination with MPSV4 during pregnancy, adverse effects have not been documented among either pregnant women or newborns. On the basis of these data, the Centers for Disease Control and Prevention states that pregnancy should not preclude vaccination with meningococcal polysaccharide vaccine, if indicated. No data are available on the safety of meningococcal conjugate vaccines during pregnancy. Both rubella and varicella vaccinations are not recommended during pregnancy.

Ongoing Risk Assessment and Management

Identification of risk factors for poor outcomes is critical to minimize maternal and neonatal morbidity and mortality. Appendixes B and C provide essential data important for early and ongoing risk assessment. Although a correlation can be seen between antenatal risk factors and the development of problems, a significant percentage of intrapartum and neonatal problems occur among patients without identified antenatal risk factors. In many instances, special obstetric problems require a multidisciplinary approach to antepartum care. Some conditions may require the involvement of a maternal–fetal medicine subspecialist, geneticist, pediatrician, neonatologist, anesthesiologist, or other medical specialist in the evaluation, counseling, and care of the patient.

Antibody Testing

Antibody tests should be repeated in unsensitized, D-negative patients at 28–29 weeks of gestation (see also "Isoimmunization in Pregnancy" in this chapter). These patients also should receive anti-D immune globulin at a dose of 300 µg prophylactically at that time. In addition, any patient who is unsensitized and D-negative should receive anti-D immune globulin if she has had one of the following conditions or procedures:

- Ectopic gestation
- Abortion (either threatened, spontaneous, or induced)
- Procedures associated with possible fetal-to-maternal bleeding, such as chorionic villus sampling (CVS) or amniocentesis
- Conditions associated with fetal–maternal hemorrhage (eg, abdominal trauma, abruptio placentae)
- Unexplained vaginal bleeding during pregnancy
- Delivery of a newborn who is D-positive

Diabetes Mellitus Screening

All pregnant patients should be screened for gestational diabetes mellitus (GDM), whether by patient history, clinical risk factors, or a laboratory screening test to determine blood glucose levels. Although universal glucose challenge screening for GDM is the most sensitive approach, there may be pregnant women at low risk who are less likely to benefit from testing. Such low-risk women should have all of the following characteristics:

- Age younger than 25 years
- Not a member of a racial or ethnic group with a high prevalence of diabetes mellitus (ie, not of Hispanic, African, Native American, South or East Asian, or Pacific Islands ancestry)
- Body mass index of 25 or less

- No history of abnormal glucose tolerance
- No history of adverse pregnancy outcomes usually associated with GDM
- No known diabetes mellitus in first-degree relative

Teratogens

Major birth defects are apparent at birth in 2–3% of the general population, and their possible occurrence is a frequent cause of anxiety among pregnant women. Many patient inquiries concern the teratogenic potential of environmental exposures. Unfortunately, there often is little scientifically valid information on which a risk estimate in human pregnancy can be based. Patients should be counseled that relatively few agents have been identified that are known to cause malformations in exposed pregnancies. Relatively few patients are exposed to agents that are known to be associated with increased risk for fetal malformations or mental retardation. The health care provider may wish to consult with or refer such patients to health care professionals with special knowledge or experience in teratology and birth defects. The Organization of Teratology Information Services provides information on teratology issues and exposures in pregnancy (www.otispregnancy.org).

Many patients raise questions about the methods of detecting birth defects related to drug exposure. Amniocentesis or CVS for chromosome analysis is not helpful for the diagnosis of birth defects caused by teratogens. Although obstetric ultrasonography has been the mainstay of surveillance for teratogen-induced congenital anomalies, its sensitivity varies with the experience and skill of the imager as well as the specific anatomic abnormality. However, even in expert hands, the overall sensitivity of ultrasonography in the detection of fetal anatomic anomalies is in the range of 50–70%.

Concerns frequently are expressed over the teratogenic potential of diagnostic imaging modalities used during pregnancy, including X-ray, nuclear imaging, contrast agents, and magnetic resonance imaging. The imaging modality that causes the most anxiety for both obstetrician and patient is X-ray or ionizing radiation. Much of this anxiety is secondary to a general misperception that any radiation exposure is harmful and may result in injury to or anomaly of the fetus. This anxiety may lead to inappropriate therapeutic abortion. In fact, most diagnostic X-ray procedures are associated with few, if any, risks to the fetus. Exposure to less than 5 rads has not been associated with an increase in fetal anomalies or pregnancy loss. Moreover, according to the American College of Radiology, no single diagnostic X-ray procedure results in radiation exposure to a degree that would threaten the well-being of a developing preembryo, embryo, or fetus.

Concern about radiation exposure during pregnancy should not prevent medically indicated diagnostic X-ray studies when these are important for the care of the woman. When such a study is indicated, the minimal dose of radiation should be used. Because magnetic resonance imaging does not use ionizing radiation, it may be the preferred test. Both spiral computed tomography and ventilation–perfusion scanning expose the fetus to only small amounts of radiation. However, most centers avoid the use of iodinated contrast agents in pregnancy because of the risk of neonatal hypothyroidism. Patients concerned about previously performed or planned diagnostic studies should have counseling to allay these concerns.

Most diagnostic studies in which radioisotopes are used are not hazardous to the fetus and result in low levels of radiation exposure. A typical technetium Tc 99m scan results in a fetal dose of less than 0.5 rads, and a thallium 201 scan also results in a low dose. Many of these isotopes are excreted in the urine. Therefore, women should be advised to drink plenty of fluids and to void frequently after a radionuclide study.

One important exception is the use of iodine 131 for the treatment of Graves' disease. The fetal thyroid gland begins to incorporate iodine actively by the end of the first trimester. Administration of iodine 131 after this time can result in concentration of the radiation within, and destruction of, the fetal thyroid gland. Therefore, Iodine 131 is contraindicated for therapeutic use during pregnancy. By comparison, there are few reports on the safety of radioisotope imaging of the maternal thyroid during pregnancy, and such studies should be undertaken only after careful consideration of the risks and benefits of the procedure.

Maternal Serum Screening

There are now several screening options for trisomy 21 and 18, including first-trimester combined serum screening (pregnancy associated plasma protein-A and free β-hCG) with ultrasound assessment of fetal nuchal translucency (10–13 weeks of gestation) and second-trimester triple (alpha-fetoprotein (AFP), estriol, β-hCG) or quadruple (AFP, estriol, β-hCG, inhibin-A) marker serum screening (15–20 weeks of gestation). In addition, there are several combined first- and second-trimester fetal aneuploidy screening approaches, including integrated and contingent testing. Only the second-trimester screening includes a serum screen for NTDs with elevated maternal serum AFP (MSAFP), so women who opt for the first-trimester screening also should be offered second-trimester MSAFP testing or ultrasound screening for NTDs. All women presenting for prenatal care before 20 weeks of gestation should be offered screening for aneuploidy. The first-trimester combined screening has similar detection rates to the second-trimester quadruple screen for women younger than 35 years at the time of delivery. All women, regardless of age, should have the option of invasive prenatal diagnosis (ie, CVS or amniocentesis) for fetal aneuploidy. All serum samples should be submitted to a clinical laboratory that has a quality improvement program, normative data specific to each week of gestational age, and interpretations and risk assessment that take into account maternal weight, race, diabetic status, and, for trisomy 21 screening, maternal age. The laboratory should be able to confirm that the specific combination of tests and the particular assays performed will yield a minimum detection rate for trisomy 21 of approximately 70% and a positive rate of screening of 5% or less after ultrasound examination correction of gestational age. Specific training, standardization, use of appropriate ultrasound equipment, and ongoing quality assessment are required to achieve optimal Down syndrome diagnostic accuracy for nuchal translucency measurement, and this procedure should be limited to centers and individuals meeting these criteria.

Trisomy 21

All women should be provided with their specific fetal risk for trisomy 21. A serum marker screening result typically is considered positive if it indicates a midtrimester risk of trisomy 21 that is equal to or greater than that of a 35-year-old woman bearing a fetus with trisomy 21 (ie, 1:270 midtrimester risk). If ultrasound examination results do not reveal an error in gestational dating or diagnose a fetal disorder, amniocentesis should be offered to analyze fetal karyotype. If first-trimester or contingent screening is employed, patients with a positive screen may be offered CVS at 11–12 weeks of gestation.

Neural Tube Defects

The results of second-trimester MSAFP testing may be used to screen for NTDs. The use of a standard screening cutoff (2.5 multiples of the median) will detect approximately 80% of cases of open spina bifida and 90% of cases of anencephaly. Patients with elevated MSAFP levels are evaluated by ultrasonography to detect identifiable causes of false–positive results (eg, fetal death, multiple gestation, underestimation of gestational age) and for targeted study of fetal anatomy for NTDs and other defects associated with elevated MSAFP values (eg, omphalocele, gastroschisis, cystic hygroma). Amniocentesis may be recommended to confirm the presence of open defects and to obtain a fetal karyotype. Amniocentesis may be offered even when ultrasound examination results do not reveal an identifiable defect or cause for the elevated MSAFP level, particularly if the ultrasound examination was suboptimal because of maternal obesity or abdominal scarring. It is important to remember that periconceptional supplementation with folic acid (0.4 mg/d) significantly decreases the first occurrence of NTDs. Periconceptional supplementation with 4 mg/d of folic acid decreases repeat occurrences of NTDs as well (see "Preconception Nutritional Counseling" in this chapter).

Prenatal Diagnosis of Genetic Disorders in Patients at Increased Risk

Prenatal genetic diagnosis should be offered in circumstances in which there is a definable increased risk for a fetal genetic disorder that may be diagnosed by one or more methods. Prenatal genetic screening or diagnosis should be voluntary and informed. In most circumstances, test results are normal and provide patients with a high degree of reassurance that a particular disorder does not affect a fetus, although there is no guarantee that it is normal and with no abnormalities. Early prenatal genetic diagnosis also affords patients the option to terminate affected pregnancies. Alternatively, a diagnosis of a genetic disorder may allow a patient to prepare for the birth of an affected child and, in some circumstances, may be important in establishing a plan for care during pregnancy, labor, delivery, and the immediate neonatal period.

Genetic Risk Assessment and Counseling

Many couples at increased risk for having children with genetic disorders can benefit from genetic counseling (see "Preconception Care" in this chapter). An example of current screening criteria is listed in the ACOG Antepartum Record in Appendix A. Health care providers should be aware that many single-gene disorders are discovered each year and may be tracked using Internet databases, such as "Online Mendelian Inheritance in Man" (www.ncbi.nlm.nih.gov/entrez/query.fcgi?db=OMIM).

Sometimes the problem is relatively straightforward. For example, the health care provider can readily explain the well-known relationship between advanced maternal age and autosomal trisomies. The maternal age-adjusted risks for chromosome abnormalities are shown in Table 4–4. Increasing paternal age, particularly after age 50 years, predisposes the fetus to an increase in gene mutations that can affect X-linked recessive and autosomal dominant

Table 4–4. Chromosome Abnormalities in Term, Liveborn Neonates*

Maternal Age	Risk of Trisomy 21 at Delivery	Risk of Chromosomal Abnormalities[†]
20	1/1,667	1/526
21	1/1,667	1/526
22	1/1,667	1/526
23	1/1,429	1/500
24	1/1,250	1/476
25	1/1,250	1/476
26	1/1,176	1/476
27	1/1,111	1/455
28	1/1,053	1/435
29	1/1,000	1/417
30	1/952	1/385
31	1/909	1/385
32	1/769	1/322
33	1/602	1/286
34	1/485	1/238
35	1/378	1/192
36	1/289	1/156
37	1/224	1/127
38	1/173	1/102
39	1/136	1/83
40	1/106	1/66
41	1/82	1/53
42	1/63	1/42
43	1/49	1/33
44	1/38	1/26
45	1/30	1/21
46	1/23	1/16
47	1/18	1/13
48	1/14	1/10
49	1/11	1/8

*Because sample sizes for some intervals are relatively small, 95% confidence limits are sometimes relatively large. Nonetheless, these figures are suitable for genetic counseling.

[†]47,XXX excluded for ages 20–32 years (data not available).

Modified from Hook EB, Cross PK, Schreinemachers DM. Chromosomal abnormality rates at amniocentesis and in live-born infants. JAMA 1983;249:2034–2038. Copyrighted 1983, American Medical Association and Hook EB. Rates of chromosome abnormalities at different maternal ages. Obstet Gynecol 1981;58:282–85.

disorders, such as neurofibromatosis, achondroplasia, Apert's syndrome, and Marfan syndrome. Currently, it is not possible to screen prenatally for all autosomal dominant and X-linked diseases in the presence of advanced paternal age. Fetal ultrasonography may detect some autosomal dominant disorders, but this technique cannot be relied on as a screening modality. Chromosomal analysis cannot be used to detect these disorders. Only genetic counseling on an individual basis is recommended for couples to address their specific concerns if advancing paternal age is an issue.

In other cases, referral to a geneticist may be necessitated by the complexities of determining risks, evaluating a family history of such abnormalities, interpreting laboratory test results, or providing counseling. Regardless of the indication, counseling is essential before genetic screening or antenatal diagnostic tests are performed.

Prenatal genetic counseling addresses the risk of occurrence of a genetic disorder in a family. In this process, the primary health care provider, a medical geneticist, or other trained professional attempts to help the individual or family in the following areas:

- Comprehending the medical facts, including the diagnosis, probable course of the disorder, and available management
- Appreciating the way in which heredity contributes to the disorder and the risk of occurrence or recurrence in specific relatives
- Understanding the options for dealing with the risk of recurrence, including prenatal genetic diagnosis
- Choosing the course of action that seems appropriate in view of the risk and the family's goals and act in accordance with that decision
- Making the best possible adjustment to the disorder in an affected family member and to the risk of recurrence in another family member

The key elements in genetic counseling are accurate diagnosis, communication, and nondirective presentation of options. The counselor's function is not to dictate a particular course of action but to provide information that will allow couples to make informed decisions.

Diagnostic Testing

Amniocentesis

Transabdominal amniocentesis is the technique most commonly used for obtaining fetal cells for genetic studies. This well-established, safe, and reliable procedure usually is performed at approximately 16 weeks of gestation. The cells obtained via amniocentesis can be used for blood typing or cytogenetic, metabolic, or other DNA testing. Alpha-fetoprotein and acetylcholinesterase levels can be measured in the supernatant amniotic fluid to detect open fetal NTDs. Significant maternal injury from amniocentesis is rare, and the estimated risk of spontaneous abortion caused by amniocentesis at 15 weeks of gestation or later is less than 1%. Increased loss rates are associated with more than three needle insertions. Amniocenteses performed at 11–13 weeks of gestation have been associated with relatively high postprocedure loss rates of 2–5%, an increased occurrence (1.4%) of talipes equinovarus (clubfoot), and increased cell culture failure rates.

Chorionic Villus Sampling

Chorionic villus sampling is a technique for removing a small sample (5–40 mg) of placental tissue (chorionic villi) for performing chromosomal, metabolic, or DNA studies. It generally is performed between 10 weeks and 12 weeks of gestation, either by a transabdominal or a transcervical approach. Chorionic villi, however, cannot be used for the prenatal diagnosis of NTDs. Therefore, women who have undergone cytogenetic testing by CVS should be offered MSAFP, or detailed ultrasound examinations, or both for NTD detection. Most prospective studies have shown that the procedure-related risk of pregnancy loss following CVS is not significantly different from the loss rate following amniocentesis. The possibility that CVS performed before 10 weeks of gestation may cause limb reduction defects remains controversial but should be discussed in counseling. Until further information is available, CVS should not be performed before 10 weeks of gestation.

Invasive Diagnostic Testing in Women Who Are Rh D Negative

Because both amniocentesis and CVS can result in fetal-to-maternal bleeding, the administration of anti-D immune globulin is indicated for women who are D negative and unsensitized and undergo either of these procedures. Chorionic villus sampling should not be performed in women who are red cell antibody sensitized because it may worsen the antibody response.

Tests of Fetal Well-Being

The goals of antepartum fetal surveillance are as follows:

- Identifying patients at increased risk for stillbirth

- Reducing the risk of fetal demise after 24 weeks of gestation
- Avoiding unnecessary intervention

Although there have been no randomized clinical trials that clearly demonstrate improved perinatal outcome with the use of antepartum testing or that determine the optimal time to initiate testing, these tests have become an integral part of clinical care of pregnancies suspected to be at increased risk of fetal demise. Indications for initiating such testing typically include the following conditions:

- Maternal conditions
    — Antiphospholipid syndrome
    — Hyperthyroidism (poorly controlled)
    — Hemoglobinopathies (hemoglobin SS, SC, or S-thalassemia)
    — Significant heart disease
    — Systemic lupus erythematosus
    — Chronic renal disease
    — Insulin-treated diabetes mellitus
    — Hypertensive disorders
- Pregnancy-related conditions
    — Pregnancy-induced hypertension
    — Decreased fetal movement
    — Oligohydramnios
    — Polyhydramnios
    — Intrauterine growth restriction
    — Postterm pregnancy
    — Isoimmunization (moderate to severe)
    — Previous fetal demise (unexplained or recurrent risk)
    — Multiple gestation (with significant growth discrepancy)

There are several tests used in clinical practice to assess fetal status. Commonly available tests (which are described in more detail in the following section) include the following procedures:

- Assessment of fetal movement (eg, kick counts)
- Nonstress test (NST)

- Biophysical profile (BPP)
- Modified biophysical profile (NST plus amniotic fluid index [AFI])
- Contraction stress test (CST) or oxytocin challenge test (OCT)
- Doppler ultrasonography of umbilical artery blood flow velocity

An important consideration in deciding when to begin antepartum testing is the prognosis for neonatal survival if intervention is undertaken for abnormal test results. Initiating testing at 32–34 weeks of gestation is appropriate for most pregnancies at increased risk of stillbirth, although in pregnancies with multiple or particularly worrisome high-risk conditions, testing may be initiated as early as 26–28 weeks of gestation. However, because the potential for iatrogenic harm to pregnancies is highest in preterm gestations, the low specificity of these tests needs to be considered. The implications of a nonreassuring fetal heart rate tracing at these early gestational ages still are unclear.

When the clinical condition that has prompted testing persists, a reassuring test (reactive NST, negative CST, or normal BPP) should be repeated periodically (either weekly or, depending on the test used and the presence of certain high-risk conditions, twice weekly) until delivery to monitor continued fetal well-being. In most clinical situations, a normal test result indicates that intrauterine fetal death is highly unlikely in the next 7 days. The risk of fetal death within 7 days of a reactive NST is approximately 3 per 1,000 fetuses. The risk of fetal death within 7 days of a BPP of 8–10 or a negative OCT or CST result is 0.6–0.8 per 1,000 fetuses. In contrast, an abnormal test result or nonreassuring fetal assessment frequently (50–90%) is falsely positive (ie, worrisome) and, therefore, should be corroborated whenever possible before potentially harmful interventions are undertaken. In the presence of certain high-risk conditions, such as prolonged pregnancy, insulin-treated diabetes mellitus beyond 36 weeks of gestation, intrauterine growth restriction, or pregnancy-induced hypertension, twice-weekly testing may be appropriate.

The sequence of tests to determine fetal well-being may vary by practice and protocol. Each test has advantages and disadvantages, and no single test has been shown to be superior to the others in any specific clinical situation. The NST is the most commonly used screening test for antepartum fetal evaluation. It is easily performed in an outpatient setting with minimal staffing, and it can be easily archived for review. The BPP requires a trained ultrasonographer and ultrasound equipment. However, unless the study is videotaped, it cannot be reviewed. The BPP does have a lower false–positive rate (20%) than NST alone (75–90%) and is supplanting the CST as a supplemental test following a nonreactive NST because of its ease of performance. Regardless of which antepartum surveillance test is used, the results and interpretation should be noted in the patient's medical record.

Assessment of Fetal Movement

A decrease in the maternal perception of fetal movement may, but does not invariably, precede fetal death, in some cases by several days. This observation provides the rationale for fetal movement assessment by the mother (kick counts) as a means of antepartum fetal surveillance. Whether programs of fetal movement assessment actually can reduce the risk of stillbirth is unclear. Neither the ideal number of kicks nor the ideal duration of daily movement count assessment has been defined. Perhaps more important than any single quantitative guideline is the mother's perception of a decrease in fetal activity in relation to a previous level. One approach to assessing fetal movement is to have the woman count distinct fetal movements on a daily basis after 28 weeks of gestation. The perception of 10 distinct movements in a period of up to 2 hours is considered reassuring. After 10 movements have been perceived, the count can be discontinued for that day. In the absence of a reassuring count, a biophysical means of fetal assessment (NST and AFI, BPP, or CST) should be used.

Nonstress Test

For the NST, the fetal heart rate is monitored with an external transducer for at least 20 minutes. The tracing is observed for fetal heart rate accelerations peaking at least 15 beats per minute higher than the baseline and acceleration lasting 15 seconds from baseline to baseline. The testing can be continued for an additional 40 minutes or longer to take into account the typical fetal sleep–wake cycle. Because fetal heart rate reactivity is a function of fetal maturity, more than 15% of NSTs performed before 32 weeks of gestation may be nonreactive in the absence of fetal compromise. Before 32 weeks of gestation, accelerations usually peak at 10 beats per minute and persist for 10 seconds. The results of an NST are considered reactive (reassuring) if two or more fetal heart rate accelerations are detected within a 20-minute period, with or without fetal movement discernible by the mother. A nonreactive tracing is one without sufficient fetal heart rate accelerations in a 40-minute period. Vibroacoustic stimulation (lasting 1 second) of a fetus that elicits fetal heart rate accelerations also is reassuring. The use of such stimulation can safely reduce overall testing time.

Contraction Stress Test

For a CST, the fetal heart rate is obtained using an external transducer, and uterine contraction activity is monitored with a tocodynamometer. A baseline tracing is obtained for 10–20 minutes. If at least three contractions of 40 seconds or more are present in a 10-minute period, uterine stimulation is not necessary. If the contractions are not present, they are induced with either nipple stimulation or intravenously administered oxytocin. With nipple stimulation, the patient is instructed to rub one nipple gently through her clothing for 2 minutes or until a contraction begins. Stimulation is then stopped and restarted after 5 minutes if an adequate contraction frequency has not been attained. The cycle is repeated until an adequate contraction pattern is obtained. If the use of oxytocin is preferred by the patient or if nipple stimulation is unsuccessful, an intravenous infusion of low-dose oxytocin can be initiated, usually at a rate of 0.5–1 mU/min, and increased every 15–20 minutes until an adequate contraction pattern occurs (ie, three contractions in 10 minutes). The results of the CST can be categorized as follows:

- Negative—No late or significant variable decelerations

- Positive—Late decelerations following 50% or more of contractions, even if the frequency of contractions is less than three in 10 minutes

- Equivocal-suspicious—Intermittent late or significant variable decelerations

- Equivocal-hyperstimulatory—Fetal heart rate decelerations that occur in the presence of contractions more frequent than every 2 minutes or lasting longer than 90 seconds

- Unsatisfactory—Fewer than three contractions within 10 minutes or a tracing that cannot be interpreted

Both oxytocin and nipple stimulation can produce tachysystole (contractions that occur more frequently than every 2 minutes or exceed 90 seconds in duration). If fetal heart rate decelerations occur in the presence of hyperstimulation, retesting is appropriate to ensure correct interpretation. Relative contraindications to inducing contractions for CSTs generally include the following conditions:

- Preterm labor or certain patients at high risk for preterm delivery

- Preterm rupture of membranes

- Classic uterine incision scar or history of extensive uterine surgery

- Known placenta previa

Biophysical Profile

Biophysical profile testing consists of an NST with the addition of four observations using real-time ultrasonography. The five components of a reassuring BPP are:

1. Nonstress test, if result is reactive—Because the probability of fetal well-being is identical with scores of 10 out of 10 and 8 out of 10, the NST may be excluded if all other parameters of the BPP are reassuring in more than 97% of cases without adverse consequences.

2. Fetal breathing movements—One or more episodes of rhythmic fetal breathing movements of 30 seconds or more within 30 minutes

3. Fetal movement—Three or more discrete body or limb movements within 30 minutes

4. Fetal tone—One or more episodes of fetal extremity extension with return to flexion, or opening or closing of a hand within 30 minutes

5. Quantification of amniotic fluid volume—A pocket of amniotic fluid that measures at least 2 cm in two planes perpendicular to each other

With BPP testing, a score of 2 (present) or 0 (absent) is assigned to each of the five observations. A score of 8 or 10 is reassuring. A score of 6 is equivocal and generally should lead to delivery if the patient is at term, whereas retesting within 12–24 hours may be appropriate for a preterm fetus. A score of 4 or less is nonreassuring and warrants further evaluation and consideration of delivery. Irrespective of the score, more frequent BPP testing or consideration of delivery may be warranted when oligohydramnios is present.

Modified Biophysical Profile

As another approach to fetal surveillance, the modified BPP combines the use of an NST as a short-term indicator of fetal status with the assessment of AFI as an indicator of long-term placental function. The AFI is a semiquantitative, four-quadrant assessment of amniotic fluid depth. A value of less than or equal to five is considered indicative of oligohydramnios. The modified BPP is less cumbersome than complete BPP assessment and appears to be as predictive of fetal well-being as other approaches of biophysical fetal surveillance. Indeed, the rate of stillbirth within one week of a normal modified BPP is the same as that with the full BPP.

Doppler Ultrasonography of Umbilical Artery

Umbilical artery Doppler flow ultrasonography is a noninvasive technique to assess resistance to blood flow in the placenta. It is not a screening test for detecting fetal compromise in the general population, but it can be used in conjunction with other biophysical tests in high-risk pregnancies associated with suspected intrauterine growth restriction. Umbilical artery Doppler flow velocimetry is based on the characteristics of the systolic blood flow and the diastolic blood flow. The most commonly used index to quantify the flow velocity waveform is the systolic/diastolic ratio. As peripheral resistance increases, diastolic flow decreases and may become absent or reversed, and the systolic/diastolic ratio increases. Reversed end-diastolic flow can be seen with severe cases of intrauterine growth restriction secondary to uteroplacental insufficiency and may suggest impending fetal demise.

Assessment of Fetal Pulmonary Maturation

Fetal pulmonary maturity always should be taken into consideration when delivering a fetus electively or preterm in high-risk pregnancies. Fetal lung maturity should be confirmed before all elective deliveries at less than 39 weeks of gestation for patients who are not infected with HIV. All efforts should be made to administer a course of antenatal corticosteroids to women whose pregnancies are at high risk for preterm delivery between 24–34 weeks of gestation to promote fetal lung maturation (see Chapter 6). The following fetal maturity tests are available:

- Surfactant/albumen ratio (fetal lung maturity index)
- Lecithin/sphingomyelin ratio
- Phosphatidylglycerol
- Foam stability index
- Fluorescence polarization
- Optical density at 650 nm
- Lamellar body counts
- Saturated phosphatidylcholine

Although the lecithin/sphingomyelin ratio as first used is the industry standard for determining fetal lung maturity, the other tests rapidly are replacing the lecithin/sphingomyelin ratio in clinical practice because of their technical ease. Regardless of the test used, the probability of respiratory distress syndrome after a mature test result beyond 34 weeks of gestation is less than 5%. In contrast, all available tests that show immature results are relatively poor in predicting respiratory distress syndrome. However, because no test indicating maturity can completely eliminate the risk of respiratory distress syndrome or other neonatal complications, the risk of adverse neonatal outcome following delivery must be weighed against the potential risk of allowing the pregnancy to remain in utero.

Issues to Discuss With Patients Before Delivery

Working

A woman with an uncomplicated pregnancy usually can continue to work until the onset of labor. Women with medical or obstetric complications of pregnancy may need to make adjustments based on the nature of their activities, occupations, and specific complications. It also has been reported that pregnant women whose occupations require standing or repetitive, strenuous, physical lifting have a tendency to give birth earlier and have smaller-for-gestational-age infants. Although a period of 4–6 weeks generally is required for a woman's physiologic condition to return to normal, the patient's individual circumstances should be considered when recommending resumption of full activity. It also is important for the development of children and the family unit that adequate family leave be available for parents to be able to participate in early childrearing. The federal Family and Medical Leave Act and state laws should be consulted to determine the family and medical leave that is available.

Air Travel During Pregnancy

In the absence of obstetric or medical complications, pregnant women can observe the same general precautions for air travel as the general population and can fly safely up to 36 weeks of gestation. However, most airlines provide liberal maternity leave policies allowing flight attendants to stop flying with confirmation of pregnancy. Some restrict the working air travel of flight attendants after 20–24 weeks of gestation and restrict commercial airline pilots from flying once pregnancy is diagnosed. Air travel is not recommended at any time during pregnancy for women who have medical or obstetric complications for which likely emergencies cannot be predicted. Such complications may include increased risks for or evidence of preterm delivery, pregnancy-induced hypertension, poorly controlled diabetes mellitus, or sickle cell disease, which may be exacerbated by high altitude.

In-craft environmental conditions, such as low cabin humidity and changes in cabin pressure, coupled with the physiologic changes of pregnancy, do result in maternal adaptations that could have transient effects on the fetus. These changes should not affect normal pregnant women; however, pregnant women with medical problems that may be exacerbated by a hypoxic environment who must travel by air should be prescribed supplemental oxygen during air travel.

The risks of lower extremity edema and venous thrombotic events are increased by long hours of air travel immobilization and may be minimized by the use of support stockings, periodic movement of the lower extremities and staying well hydrated. Pregnant air travelers may help minimize in-flight discomfort by avoiding gas-producing foods and drinks before and during flight. Additionally, preventive antiemetic medication should be considered for pregnant women with increased nausea. Because air turbulence cannot be predicted and the risk for trauma is significant, pregnant women, as well as all air travelers, should be instructed to continuously use their seat belts while seated. The seatbelt should be belted low on the hipbones, between the protuberant abdomen and pelvis.

Childbirth Education Classes and Choosing a Newborn Care Provider

Couples should be referred to appropriate educational literature and urged to attend childbirth education classes. Studies have shown that prepared childbirth education programs can have a beneficial effect on performance in labor and delivery. The prenatal period should be used to expose the prospective parents to information about labor and delivery, pain relief, obstetric complications and procedures, breastfeeding, normal newborn care, and postpartum adjustment. Other family members also should be encouraged to participate in childbirth education programs. Adequate preparation of family members may benefit the mother, the neonate, and, ultimately, the family unit. Many hospitals, community agencies, and other groups offer such educational programs. The participation of physicians, certified nurse midwives, and hospital obstetric nurses in educational programs is desirable to ensure continuity of care and consistency of instruction. National organizations, such as the Childbirth Education Association, are available for assistance as well. Integration of parenting education in prenatal education is beneficial in facilitating transition to parenthood. If a patient has a birth plan, she should be encouraged to review it with her provider before labor. Sometime in the third trimester, it should be determined if the patient has a newborn care provider. If she does not have one, she should be referred to the appropriate resources to identify her newborn care provider before delivery, if possible.

Anticipating Labor

As pregnancy progresses into the third trimester, all women should be informed of what to do if contractions become regular, if membrane rupture is suspected, or if vaginal bleeding occurs. Patients should be given a telephone number to call where assistance is available 24 hours per day. Patients should be encouraged to refrain from consumption of solid food when active labor ensues. Pregnant women are at highest risk of aspiration pneumonitis when stomach contents are greater than 25 mL and when the pH of those contents is less than 2.5. Pregnancy slows gastric emptying, and labor can delay it further. The type of aspiration pneumonitis that produces the most severe physiologic and histologic alteration is partially digested food. A detailed discussion of the analgesic and anesthetic options available for labor and delivery should be held during the third trimester.

Breech Presentation at Term

If the fetus persists in a breech presentation at 36–38 weeks of gestation, women should be offered an external cephalic version. Contraindications to the procedure include multifetal gestation, nonreassuring fetal testing, müllerian duct anomalies, and suspected placental abruption or previa. Relative contraindications include intrauterine growth restriction and oligohydramnios. The success rate of external cephalic version ranges from 35–86%, with an average success rate of approximately 58%. Planned cesarean delivery is the most common and safest route of delivery for fetuses at term in breech presentations. However, planned vaginal delivery of a term singleton breech may be reasonable under hospital-specific protocol guidelines for both eligibility and labor management if the care provider is experienced in vaginal breech deliveries. Before embarking on a plan for a vaginal breech delivery, women should be informed that the risk of perinatal or neonatal mortality or short-term serious neonatal morbidity might be somewhat higher than if a cesarean delivery is planned. Informed consent for vaginal delivery should be obtained and documented. In those instances in which breech vaginal deliveries are pursued, great caution should be used.

Vaginal Birth After Cesarean Delivery

If the patient has had a prior cesarean delivery, the risks and benefits of a trial of labor versus repeat cesarean delivery should be discussed with the patient.

Advantages of a successful vaginal delivery include decreased risks for hemorrhage and infection, a shorter postpartum hospital stay, and a less painful, more rapid recovery. The patient should be informed of contraindications to a trial of labor (eg, prior classic or T-shaped cesarean incision, previous uterine rupture, lack of resources to perform emergency cesarean delivery during labor) as well as relative contraindications (eg, two prior uterine surgeries with no previous vaginal delivery). The patient also should be informed that although uterine rupture occurs more often in women undergoing a trial of labor than in women who elect repeat cesarean delivery, rupture rates during attempted vaginal birth after cesarean delivery generally are less than 1%. Uterine rupture has been associated with fetal death as well as severe neonatal neurologic injury and may occur no matter what resources are available to manage it. Risk of uterine rupture increases with multiple uterine surgeries, uterine tachysystole, use of cervical ripening agents, or induction of labor with oxytocin. Hospitals that offer vaginal trial of labor in women with prior cesarean delivery should have the personnel necessary to monitor labor and to perform a cesarean delivery—including the obstetrician and operating room and anesthesia staff—immediately available during active labor. No woman should be mandated to undergo a trial of labor. The ultimate decision to attempt vaginal delivery after cesarean delivery or to undergo a repeat cesarean delivery should be made by the informed patient and her physician.

Childbearing for Women Older Than 50 Years

Because of advances in assisted reproductive technology, it is now possible for women aged 50 years and older to become pregnant and to have successful obstetric outcomes. Nonetheless, pregnancy in this age group is rare, and because of the small number of patients, recommendations for pregnancy management are based on retrospective studies, case series, and expert opinion. Before starting fertility treatment, these women should be counseled about the complications associated with pregnancy in this age group. Risks include multiple gestation, preeclampsia, gestational diabetes, abnormal placentation, stillbirth, cesarean delivery, and, possibly, cardiac complications. These risks also are associated with women aged 40 years and older. These women also should have a medical workup before undergoing fertility treatment to determine that they are healthy. Once these women are pregnant, their blood pressure should be monitored frequently. Most often, these pregnancies are secondary to egg donation, and the risk of fetal aneuploidy is that of the egg donor. First-trimester screening, chorionic villus sampling, and amniocenteses are all options for these women. Invasive testing may not be as critical for egg-donor recipients because the egg donors are usually young. An anatomical survey should be performed at approximately 18–20 weeks gestation. Also, glucose-tolerance testing in the early third trimester is suggested. Cesarean delivery can be reserved for obstetric indications. Long-term outcomes regarding parenting that affect pediatric and maternal outcomes of childbearing by women older than 50 years are unknown.

Umbilical Cord Blood Banking

Prospective parents may seek information regarding umbilical cord blood banking. Balanced and accurate information regarding the advantages and disadvantages of public versus private banking should be provided. Health care providers should dispense the following information:

- There is clinical potential of hematopoietic stem cells found in cord blood.
- The indications for autologous transplantation are limited.
- Banking should be considered if there is a family member with a current or potential need to undergo stem cell transplantation.
- Where logistically possible, collection and support of umbilical cord blood for public banking is encouraged.

Support of Breastfeeding

During prenatal visits, the patient should be counseled regarding the nutritional advantages of human breast milk. Human milk is the most appropriate nutrient for newborns and provides significant immunologic protection against infection. Newborns who are breastfed have a decreased incidence of infection and require fewer hospitalizations than formula-fed neonates. Women should be provided with information regarding available lactation consultation services and organizations (see "Breastfeeding" in Chapter 7). Maternal benefits start in the immediate postpartum period with the release of oxytocin during milk letdown. This results in increased uterine contractions, aiding with uterine involution, and a decrease in maternal blood loss.

Circumcision

The topic of newborn male circumcision should be discussed. Newborn circumcision is an elective procedure to be performed, at the request of the parents, on newborn boys who are physiologically and clinically stable. The American Academy of Pediatrics 1999 Task Force suggests that existing scientific evidence demonstrates potential medical benefits of newborn male circumcision (eg, reduced incidences of phimosis, urinary tract infection, and penile cancer). However, the data are not sufficient to recommend routine neonatal circumcision. Appropriate anesthesia must be provided for the procedure (see "Circumcision" in Chapter 7).

Newborn Screening

Newborn screening is a public health issue that has moved into the spotlight because of advances in genetic medicine. Although newborn screening tests are designed to detect infants with specific metabolic disorders who would benefit from early diagnosis and treatment, they also may identify couples who are carriers of disorders. Because of advances in genetics and technology, newborn screening programs are capable of testing for approximately 30 disorders, including infections, genetic diseases, and inherited and metabolic disorders.

Newborn hearing screening can detect possible hearing loss in the first days of a baby's life. If a possible hearing loss is found, further tests will be done to confirm the results. If a hearing loss is confirmed, treatment and early intervention can start promptly. Early intervention helps babies with hearing loss and their families learn important communication skills. For more specific information on this screening, see "Hearing Screening" in Chapter 7.

Newborn screening programs are designed for maximal sensitivity and specificity; the false-negative rate must be kept at an absolute minimum so that no cases will be missed. However, this results in significant false–positive rates. Therefore, confirmatory testing is essential. A false-positive test result can cause parental anxiety. Counseling by the obstetric provider can be of great value. Prenatal education about newborn screening not only provides parents with an understanding of the reasons for obtaining their newborn's blood specimen but also informs them that an initial positive test result does not necessarily mean that their child will be affected. For more information, see "Newborn Screening" in Chapter 7.

Dental Care in Pregnancy

Caries, poor dentition, and periodontal disease may be associated with an increased risk for preterm delivery. It is very important that pregnant women continue usual dental care in pregnancy. This dental care includes routine brushing and flossing, scheduled cleanings, and any medically needed dental work. Many dentists will require a note from the obstetrician stating that dental care requiring local anesthesia, antibiotics, or narcotic analgesia is not contraindicated in pregnancy. The dentist should be aware that pregnant women's gums do bleed more easily.

Preparation for Discharge

Prospective parents should be aware of the timing of hospital discharge after delivery. The couple should be encouraged to prepare for discharge by setting up required resources for home health services and acquiring a newborn car seat, newborn clothing, and a crib that meets standard safety guidelines. The prospective parents should be apprised of proper newborn positioning during sleep. Reports have shown a significant reduction in the incidence of sudden infant death syndrome among newborns that are placed on their backs (as opposed to the prone position) during sleep (see Chapter 7, "Care of the Neonate" for more information). The patient should be informed of the various options of pregnancy prevention and birth control. This may be done by individual instruction, reading material, or a variety of films or videotapes.

Psychosocial Services

Confronting psychosocial issues, such as providing appropriate childcare, the need for simultaneous employment, guilt associated with unintended pregnancy, and other family conflicts, may be the most distressing aspect of a woman's pregnancy and postpartum recovery. A woman with ambivalent feelings about her pregnancy may benefit from additional support from the health care team. Patients should be informed that postpartum "blues" are a normal phenomenon that occur in more than 70% of women. Women may manifest a wide range of symptoms, including weeping, depression, restlessness, mood lability, and negative feelings toward their newborns. The blues are transient (lasting less than 2 weeks) and mild, not interfering with the patient's ability to care for herself or her child. All patients should be followed for the development of more severe postpartum depression and offered culturally appropriate treatment or referral to community resources (see also "Follow-up Care" in Chapter 5). Women with a history of depression or a family history of depression are at increased risk for postpartum depression.

A woman with negative feelings about her pregnancy should receive additional support from the health care team, and she may need professional advice on the alternatives to completing the pregnancy and keeping the newborn. Family members and their interactions with the pregnant woman should be considered in whatever recommendations are made to the woman. Physicians should be aware of individuals and community agencies to which patients can be referred for additional counseling and assistance when necessary. More information is available at the American Psychiatric Association web site (www.psych.org).

Conditions of Special Concern

Adolescent Pregnancy

Pregnancy, birth, and abortion rates in teenagers have declined 30–40% since 1990 and are now at record lows. In the 2003 *National Vital Statistics Report*, only 6,471 births occurred in minors younger than 15 years. Approximately 82% of women younger than 20 years who give birth are unmarried. Approximately 2–4% of unmarried adolescents relinquish their newborns for adoption.

The status of laws requiring mandatory parental involvement in a minor's abortion decision currently is in flux. Most states have statutes addressing this issue, although the content and degree of enforcement of these laws vary considerably. Minors typically have legal rights protecting their privacy regarding the diagnosis and treatment of pregnancy. The clinician should assess the adolescent's ability to understand the implications of the diagnosis of pregnancy and the options available. The duration of the pregnancy should be determined and documented. The following three options are available:

1. Continuation of the pregnancy with the intent of raising the child
2. Continuation of the pregnancy with the intent of relinquishing the newborn for adoption
3. Termination of the pregnancy

The patient should be informed about the options available, return for visits as needed, and understand the importance of a timely decision. She should be encouraged to include her parents (or a surrogate parent) and the father of the fetus. The patient's right to decide the outcome of the pregnancy and who should be involved should be respected. Many states have laws regarding adolescent rights, and the physician should be aware of these state laws when making health care decisions.

If the adolescent chooses to continue the pregnancy, she should be referred for psychosocial support. There is an increased incidence of delivery of low birth weight neonates, neonatal death, preterm delivery, preeclampsia, anemia, and sexually transmitted diseases (STD) among pregnant adolescents, necessitating increased monitoring and appropriate medical management. Pregnant adolescents should be counseled about the effects of STDs on themselves and their fetuses. They should receive repetitive reinforcement that condoms should be used during pregnancy for STD protection.

Postterm Gestation

Approximately 10% (3–14%) of pregnancies extend beyond 42 weeks of gestation (294 days or more from the first day of the last menstrual period) and are considered postterm. Although some apparent cases of postterm pregnancy are the result of an inability to define the time of conception accurately, some patients clearly progress to excessively long gestations that can represent a significant risk to the fetus. Accurate assessment of gestational age will minimize the misdiagnosis of postterm gestation.

Antepartum assessments by cervical examination, fetal heart rate testing (NST or CST), ultrasound evaluation of amniotic fluid volume, BPP, or a combination of these tests may be initiated between 41 weeks and 42 weeks of gestation. Although no firm recommendation can be made on the basis of published research regarding the frequency of antenatal surveillance among postterm patients, many practitioners use twice-weekly testing. If fetal testing is not reassuring, delivery is indicated. Even when fetal testing is reassuring but reliable dating establishes a gestational age of 41–42 weeks, induction of labor is an acceptable management strategy.

Antepartum Hospitalization

Pregnant patients with complications who require hospitalization before the onset of labor should be admitted to a designated antepartum area, either inside or near the labor and delivery area. Obstetric patients with serious and acute complications should be assigned to an area where more intensive care and surveillance are available, such as the labor and delivery area or an intensive care unit. An obstetrician–gynecologist or a specialist in maternal–fetal medicine should be involved, either as the primary or the consulting physician, in the care of an obstetric patient with complications. When sufficiently recovered, the pregnant patient should be returned to the obstetric service, provided that her return does not jeopardize her care.

Acutely ill obstetric patients who are likely to give birth to neonates requiring intensive care should be cared for in specialty or subspecialty perinatal care centers, depending on the medical needs of the maternal–fetal dyad. When feasible, antepartum transfer to specialty or subspecialty perinatal care centers should be encouraged for these women.

Written policies and procedures for the management of pregnant patients seen in the emergency department or admitted to nonobstetric services should be established and approved by the medical staff and must comply with the requirements of federal and state transfer laws. When warranted by patient volume, a high-risk antepartum care unit should be developed to provide specialized nursing care and facilities for the mother and the fetus at risk. When this is not feasible, written policies are recommended that specify how the care and transfer of pregnant patients with obstetric, medical, or surgical complications will be handled and where these patients will be assigned.

Whether an obstetric patient is admitted to the antepartum unit or to a nonobstetric unit, her condition should be evaluated soon thereafter by the primary physician or appropriate consultants. The evaluation should encompass a complete review of current illnesses as well as a medical, family, and social history. The condition of the patient and the reason for admission should determine the extent of the physical examination performed and the laboratory studies obtained. A copy of the patient's current prenatal record should become part of the hospital medical record as soon as possible after admission. These policies also must comply with the requirements of federal and state transfer laws.

Isoimmunization in Pregnancy

The pathogenesis of blood group isoimmunization resulting in hemolytic disease of the newborn has been well described. Rational methods of assessing the extent of the disease, including amniocentesis, umbilical cord blood sampling, and middle cerebral artery Doppler ultrasound measurements and of treating the fetus have been developed. Since 1967, preventive therapy has been available for Rh D isoimmunization in the form of anti-D immune globulin (RhoGAM), which has been associated with a decrease in the incidence of Rh D isoimmunization. However, despite the decreased incidence, Rh D isoimmunization remains the most common cause of serious hemolytic disease of the fetus and newborn. Among the etiologies of residual Rh D isoimmunization cases are failure to accurately type the patient's blood, transfusion of mismatched blood, early or severe fetal-to-maternal hemorrhage, and failure to administer a sufficient amount of anti-D immune globulin at delivery. Other RBC antigens associated with hemolytic disease of the fetus and newborn include c, Kell, E, e, C^w, C, Ce, Kp^a, Kp^b, cE, k, Jk^a, s, Wr^a, and Fy^a.

If isoimmunization is noted during routine prenatal testing, the genotype of the father can be determined, or in the case of anti-D, estimated. In the case of paternal heterozygosity for the offending antigen, the fetal blood type often can be determined by DNA analysis of fetal cells obtained at amniocentesis. Should such a study reveal the absence of the target gene, the fetus has a 98.5% probability of not being at risk. Discordance between the apparent fetal amniocyte genotype and RBC phenotype can result from rearrangement of the paternal Rh (D) gene locus (2% of patients). If the fetus is affected, the patient should be referred for consultation with a maternal–fetal medicine specialist with experience in the management of such cases (see also "Antibody Testing" in this chapter).

Pregnancy Outcomes in Women Older Than 35 Years as of the Estimated Delivery Date

In 2003, birth rates for women in their 30s were the highest in more than three decades (95.2 per 1,000 for ages 30–34; 43.8 per 1,000 for ages 35–39) and continue to increase. The birth rate for women aged 40–44 years increased to 8.7 per 1,000 births in 2003, a greater than 200% increase since 1981. In 2003, more than 100,000 births occurred in women older than 39 years. Several factors have contributed to this increase in older pregnant women, including delayed childbearing because of career, aging of the "baby boom" generation, and assisted reproductive technologies (ART). With increasing maternal age, there is an increase in the presence of underlying medical conditions. It is important to review the potential additional risks that advanced maternal age may pose and counsel the patient accordingly:

- Cesarean delivery—In nearly all studies, an increase in the prevalence of cesarean delivery in older pregnant women has been noted. This increase persists despite similar labor management of older nulliparous women compared with nulliparous women aged 20–29 years.

- Stillbirth and growth restriction—After correcting for the higher prevalence of aneuploidy in older pregnant women, results from the preponderance of published reports fail to demonstrate an increase in perinatal morbidity or mortality in previously healthy women.

- Assisted reproductive technology and multiple gestation—Women older than 35 years are more likely to conceive via some form of ART than women younger than 35 years. With ART, there is a well-reported increase in multiple gestations.

- Aneuploidy—The incidence of fetal aneuploidy increases with increasing maternal age. This increased risk has been well reported. Advanced paternal age, particularly after age 50 years, is implicated in an increase in gene mutations that can affect X-linked recessive and autosomal dominant disorders, such as neurofibromatosis, achondroplasia, Apert's syndrome, and Marfan syndrome.

- Medical conditions—There is no consensus in the literature as to whether older patients without preexisting medical conditions have a higher prevalence of preeclampsia, placenta previa, breech presentation, preterm delivery, or operative vaginal delivery. In general, increases in perinatal and maternal morbidity are likely because of the increased risk of developing medical disorders with advancing age.

Nonobstetric Surgery in Pregnancy

Nonobstetric surgery is sometimes necessary during pregnancy, and there are no data to support specific recommendations. However, obstetric consultation to confirm gestational age and make recommendations about fetal monitoring is highly recommended. The decision to use fetal monitoring should be individualized and depends on fetal age and type of surgery. Pregnant patients who undergo nonobstetric surgery are best managed with communication between involved services, including obstetrics, anesthesia, surgery, and nursing.

Multifetal Gestations

The incidence of twin and higher-order multiple gestations has increased significantly over the past 20 years primarily because of the availability and increased use of ovulation-inducing drugs and ART, such as in vitro fertilization. Between 1971 and 2002, the number of triplet births increased more than fourfold, from 1,034 to 6,898. In addition, there were 434 quadruplet births in the United States in 2002. There is increased fetal, neonatal, and maternal morbidity and mortality associated with multifetal gestations. The practicing obstetrician managing these high-risk patients should be familiar with their special antepartum and intrapartum problems, but consultation with maternal–fetal medicine specialists may be necessary. Methods to limit high-order multiple pregnancies include monitoring hormone levels and follicle numbers during superovulation and limiting transfer to two embryos during in vitro fertilization cycles. Transferring two embryos can limit the occurrence of triplets in younger candidates who have a good prognosis without significantly decreasing the overall pregnancy rate. The American Society for Reproductive

Medicine and the Society for Assisted Reproductive Technology have developed updated recommendations on the number of embryos per transfer to reduce the risk of multiple gestation.

Antepartum Management

Counseling. Ideal antepartum care requires recognition of the following four issues in management and a frank discussion with the patient regarding how these issues may affect her pregnancy:

1. Nutritional considerations—It is recommended that maternal dietary intake in a multiple gestation be increased by approximately 300 kcal per day more than that for a singleton pregnancy. Supplementation should include iron and folic acid. Although optimal weight gain for women with multiple gestations has not been determined, it has been suggested that women with twin gestations gain 35–45 lb.

2. Prenatal diagnosis—The usual indications for prenatal diagnosis and counseling in a singleton pregnancy apply to twin and higher-order gestations. Because the incidence of twin gestation increases with maternal age, women with multiple gestations often are candidates for prenatal genetic diagnosis. Genetic counseling should make clear to the patient the need to obtain a sample from each fetus, the risk of chromosomal abnormalities, potential complications of the procedure, the possibility of discordant results, and the ethical and technical concerns when the chromosomes of one fetus are found to be abnormal. There is evidence that the combined risk of fetal chromosome abnormality is higher in dizygotic twin gestations than a singleton gestation.

   Maternal serum alpha-fetoprotein screening programs contribute to the early detection of multiple gestations. Depending on the laboratory, a value greater than 4.5 multiples of the median in an uncomplicated twin gestation is abnormal, requiring further comprehensive ultrasound evaluation by an experienced ultrasonographer and possible amniocentesis for the detection of amniotic fluid AFP and acetylcholinesterase. Although maternal serum screening with MSAFP for NTDs can be useful in twin pregnancies, the effectiveness of serum screening with other analytes for trisomy 21 or trisomy 18 is less well established in multiple gestations.

   There is no clear evidence of an increased risk of amniocentesis in twin versus singleton gestations, except that the patient may have the risk of at least two procedures. Chorionic villus sampling is an appropriate method of first-trimester prenatal diagnosis in multiple gestations. Difficulties that can arise with CVS in twin gestations include the inability to obtain an adequate sample and contamination of one sample with tissue from the second. In approximately 1% of patients, tissue can be obtained from only one placenta. When CVS is performed at centers with experienced operators, twin–twin contamination occurs in approximately 4–6% of samples, leading to possible prenatal diagnostic errors.

3. Multifetal reduction—The greater the number of fetuses within the uterus, the greater the risk of preterm delivery and adverse perinatal outcome. Multifetal pregnancy reduction may be performed to decrease the risk of serious perinatal morbidity and mortality associated with preterm delivery by reducing the number of fetuses. Unintended pregnancy loss is the main risk of multifetal pregnancy reduction, varying with both the number of starting fetuses and the number of "finishing" viable fetuses from 2.5% to nearly 17%. Most studies have concluded that the risks associated with continuation of a quadruplet or higher pregnancy clearly outweigh the risks associated with fetal reduction. Multifetal pregnancy reduction of triplet gestations to twin gestations results in outcomes comparable to those seen in unreduced twin gestations.

4. Management of other complications—The patient carrying a multiple gestation should be informed that she is at risk for a number of other potential complications including, but not limited to, preterm labor, preterm premature rupture of membranes, discordant fetal growth and intrauterine growth restriction, abnormal fluid volumes, preeclampsia, death of one fetus, and discordancy for fetal anomalies. Twin–twin transfusion syndrome, monoamniotic twinning, conjoined twins, and acardia (or twin reversed arterial perfusion sequence) are complications of monochorionic gestations. The most significant, common, and likely unpreventable complication of multiple pregnancy is preterm delivery. Women pregnant with multiple gestations are at a higher risk for complications of tocolysis, such as the development of pulmonary edema, because of higher blood volume, lower colloid osmotic pressure, and anemia. No benefit has been shown from the use of oral tocolysis in multiple gestations to prevent the onset of preterm labor or preterm birth. Antenatal corticosteroids should be administered for induction of fetal lung maturation to women with multiple pregnancies who experience preterm labor or preterm membrane rupture at less than 34 weeks of gestation.

Antepartum Surveillance. When intrauterine growth restriction, abnormal fluid volumes, growth discordance, pregnancy-induced hypertension, fetal anomalies, monoamnionicity, or other pregnancy complications occur, fetal surveillance, including NSTs or the modified or standard BPP, is indicated. The BPP is as reliable in multiple gestations as in singleton gestations. Although some patients may find it difficult to distinguish fetal movements between twins, fetal movement counting can be an adjunct to these antepartum surveillance techniques. Umbilical cord velocimetry may be helpful in evaluating the severely growth-restricted fetus, but its role in antepartum fetal surveillance of the singleton or multiple gestation is yet to be determined.

Ultrasonography. Ultrasonography can be useful in both prenatal diagnosis and surveillance of multiple gestations. Ultrasonography has a role in evaluating fetal growth and amniotic fluid volume once the diagnosis is established. Beginning at viability, serial estimations of fetal growth by ultrasonography (every 4–6 weeks after viability) are a prudent measure because physical examination is less reliable.

Controversies in Management

There are many diagnostic or therapeutic modalities used in the care of multiple gestations that are of unclear or unproven benefit. Some examples of these modalities are listed as follows:

- Vaginal ultrasonography—This procedure has been used to measure cervical width, length, and funneling and to examine the relationship of these measurements to the risk of preterm birth. Although this is a promising technique, further evaluation of transvaginal ultrasonography by a prospective randomized study is necessary to determine its role in the prevention of preterm birth.

- Prophylactic cerclage—This procedure is not recommended as a routine prophylactic measure in multiple gestations because in prospective trials in twins it has not been associated with any benefit and has been associated with increased risk of preterm labor.

- Bed rest—Not only is hospital bed rest costly, stressful, and disruptive, there is no clear consensus that it is of any benefit. Numerous studies have failed to show that bed rest in hospital decreases the incidence of preterm delivery, lengthens gestation, or reduces neonatal morbidity in multiple gestations.

- Home uterine activity monitoring—Home uterine activity monitoring has been shown in a large randomized controlled trial not to improve perinatal outcome in multiple gestations.

- Maintenance or prophylactic tocolysis—There are no consistent data to support efficacy of maintenance or prophylactic tocolysis for prolonged gestation or improving neonatal outcome.

Resources

Adashek JA, Peaceman AM, Lopez-Zeno JA, Minogue JP, Socol ML. Factors contributing to the increased cesarean birth rate in older parturient women. Am J Obstet Gynecol 1993;169:936–40.

The adolescent's right to confidential care when considering abortion. American Academy of Pediatrics. Committee on Adolescence. Pediatrics 1996;97:746–51.

Air travel during pregnancy. ACOG Committee Opinion No. 264. American College of Obstetricians and Gynecologists. Obstet Gynecol 2001;98:1187–8.

Alfirevic Z, Neilson JP. Biophysical profile for fetal assessment in high-risk pregnancies. Cochrane Database of Systematic Reviews 1996, Issue 1. Art. No.: CD000038. DOI: 10.1002/14651858.CD000038.

American College of Medical Genetics, American College of Obstetricians and Gynecologists. Preconception and prenatal carrier screening for cystic fibrosis. Clinical and laboratory guidelines. Bethesda (MD): ACMG; Washington, DC: ACOG; 2001.

American College of Obstetricians and Gynecologists. Access to reproductive health care for women with disabilities. In: Special issues in women's health. Washington DC: ACOG; 2005. p. 39–59.

American College of Obstetricians and Gynecologists. Antepartum fetal surveillance. ACOG Practice Bulletin 9. Washington, DC: ACOG; 1999.

American College of Obstetricians and Gynecologists. Assessment of fetal lung maturity. ACOG Educational Bulletin 230. Washington, DC: ACOG; 1996.

American College of Obstetricians and Gynecologists. External cephalic version. ACOG Practice Bulletin 13. Washington, DC: ACOG; 2000.

American College of Obstetricians and Gynecologists. Health and health care of incarcerated adult and adolescent females. In: Special issues in women's health. Washington, DC: ACOG; 2005. p. 89–101.

American College of Obstetricians and Gynecologists. Intimate partner violence and domestic violence. In: Special issues in women's health. Washington, DC: ACOG; 2005. p. 169–88.

American College of Obstetricians and Gynecologists. Prevention of Rh D alloimmunization. ACOG Practice Bulletin 4. Washington, DC: ACOG; 1999.

American College of Obstetricians and Gynecologists. Smoking and women's health. In: Special issues in women's health. Washington, DC: ACOG; 2005. p. 151–67.

American College of Obstetricians and Gynecologists. Substance use: obstetric and gynecologic implications. In: Special issues in women's health. Washington, DC: ACOG; 2005. p. 105–50.

American Medical Association. H-420.960 Effects of work on pregnancy. Chicago (IL): AMA; 1999; Available at: http://www.ama-assn.org/apps/pf_new/pf_online? f_n=browse&doc=policyfiles/HnE/H-420.960.HTM&&s_t=&st_p= &nth=1&prev_pol=policyfiles/HnE/H-415.999.HTM&nxt_pol=policyfiles/HnE/H-420.959.HTM&. Retrieved January 3, 2007.

Bianco A, Stone J, Lynch L, Lapinski R, Berkowitz G, Berkowitz RL. Pregnancy outcome at age 40 and older. Obstet Gynecol 1996;87:917–22.

Breastfeeding: maternal and infant aspects. American College of Obstetricians and Gynecologists. ACOG Clin Rev 2007;12(suppl):1S–16S.

Breastfeeding: maternal and infant aspects. ACOG Committee Opinion No. 361. American College of Obstetricians and Gynecologists. Obstet Gynecol 2007;109: 479–80.

Briggs GG, Freeman RK, Yaffe SJ. Drugs in pregnancy and lactation: a reference guide to fetal and neonatal risk. 7th ed. Philadelphia (PA): Lippincott Williams & Wilkins; 2005.

Chasnoff IJ, Landress HJ, Barrett ME. The prevalence of illicit-drug or alcohol use during pregnancy and discrepancies in mandatory reporting in Pinellas County, Florida. N Engl J Med 1990;322:1202–6.

Chiarotti M, Strano-Rossi S, Offidani C, Fiori A. Evaluation of cocaine use during pregnancy though toxicological analysis of hair. J Anal Toxicol 1996;20:555–8.

Circumcision. ACOG Committee Opinion No. 260. American College of Obstetricians and Gynecologists. Obstet Gynecol 2001;98:707–8.

Counseling the adolescent about pregnancy options. American Academy of Pediatrics. Committee on Adolescence. Pediatrics 1998;101:938–40.

Cuniff C. Prenatal screening and diagnosis for pediatricians. American Academy of Pediatrics Committee on Genetics. Pediatrics 2004;114:889–94.

Dildy GA, Jackson GM, Fowers GK, Oshiro BT, Varner MW, Clark SL. Very advanced maternal age: pregnancy after age 45. Am J Obstet Gynecol 1996;175:668–74.

Drug-exposed infants. American Academy of Pediatrics. Committee on Substance Abuse. Pediatrics 1995;96:364–7.

Exercise during pregnancy and the postpartum period. ACOG Committee Opinion No. 267. American College of Obstetricians and Gynecologists. Obstet Gynecol 2002; 98:171–3.

Gestational diabetes. ACOG Practice Bulletin No. 30. American College of Obstetricians and Gynecologists. Obstet Gynecol 2001;98:525–38.

Graham JM Jr, Edwards MJ, Edwards MJ. Teratogen update: gestational effects of maternal hyperthermia due to febrile illnesses and resultant patterns of defects in humans. Teratology 1998;58:209–21.

Hemoglobinopathies in pregnancy. ACOG Practice Bulletin No. 78. American College of Obstetricians and Gynecologists. Obstet Gynecol 2007;109:229–37.

Immunization during pregnancy. ACOG Committee Opinion No. 282. American College of Obstetricians and Gynecologists. Obstet Gynecol 2003;101:207–12.

Influenza vaccination and treatment during pregnancy. ACOG Committee Opinion No. 305. American College of Obstetricians and Gynecologists. Obstet Gynecol 2004;104:1125–6.

Joint Commission on Accreditation of Healthcare Organizations. Comprehensive accreditation manual for hospitals: the official handbook. Oakbrook Terrace (IL): JCAHO; 2007.

Klein JD. Adolescent pregnancy: current trends and issues. American Academy of Pediatrics Committee on Adolescence. Pediatrics 2005;116:281–6.

Landry SH, Whitney JA. The impact of prenatal cocaine exposure: studies of the developing infant. Semin Perinatol 1996;20:99–106.

Management of alloimmunization during pregnancy. ACOG Practice Bulletin No. 75. American College of Obstetricians and Gynecologists. Obstet Gynecol 2006;108:457–64.

Management of postterm pregnancy. ACOG Practice Bulletin No. 55. American College of Obstetricians and Gynecologists. Obstet Gynecol 2004;104:639–46.

March of Dimes Birth Defects Foundation. Toward improving the outcome of pregnancy: the 90s and beyond. White Plains (NY): MDBDF; 1993.

Martin JA, MacDorman MF, Mathews TJ. Triplet births: trends and outcomes, 1971–94. Vital Health Stat 21 1997;(55):1–20.

Meningococcal vaccination for adolescents. ACOG Committee Opinion No. 314. American College of Obstetricians and Gynecologists. Obstet Gynecol 2005;106:667–9.

Metzger BE, Coustan DR. Summary and recommendations of the Fourth International Workshop-Conference on Gestational Diabetes Mellitus. The Organizing Committee. Diabetes Care 1998;21(suppl 2):B161–7.

Mode of term singleton breech delivery. ACOG Committee Opinion No. 340. American College of Obstetricians and Gynecologists. Obstet Gynecol 2006;108:235–7.

Multiple gestation: complicated twin, triplet, and high-order multifetal pregnancy. ACOG Practice Bulletin No. 56. American College of Obstetricians and Gynecologists. Obstet Gynecol 2004;104:869–83.

National Institutes of Health (US). National Center for Complementary and Alternative Medicine. Available at: http://nccam.nih.gov/. Retrieved December 18, 2006.

Nausea and vomiting of pregnancy. ACOG Practice Bulletin No. 52. American College of Obstetricians and Gynecologists. Obstet Gynecol 2004;103:803–14.

Newborn screening. ACOG Committee Opinion No. 287. American College of Obstetricians and Gynecologists. Obstet Gynecol 2003;102:887–9.

Nonobstetric surgery in pregnancy. ACOG Committee Opinion No. 284. American College of Obstetricians and Gynecologists. Obstet Gynecol 2003;102:431.

Obesity in pregnancy. ACOG Committee Opinion No. 315. American College of Obstetricians and Gynecologists. Obstet Gynecol 2005;106:671–5.

Obstetric management of patients with spinal cord injuries. ACOG Committee Opinion No. 275. American College of Obstetricians and Gynecologists. Obstet Gynecol 2002; 100:625–7.

Peipert JF, Bracken MB. Maternal age: an independent risk factor for cesarean delivery. Obstet Gynecol 1993;81:200–5.

Prenatal and perinatal human immunodeficiency virus testing: expanded recommendations. ACOG Committee Opinion No. 304. American College of Obstetricians and Gynecologists. Obstet Gynecol 2004;104:1119–24.

Prenatal and preconceptional carrier screening for genetic diseases in individuals of Eastern European Jewish descent. ACOG Committee Opinion No. 298. American College of Obstetricians and Gynecologists. Obstet Gynecol 2004;104:425–8.

Psychosocial risk factors: perinatal screening and intervention. ACOG Committee Opinion No. 343. American College of Obstetricians and Gynecologists. Obstet Gynecol 2006;108:469–77.

Recommendations to prevent and control iron deficiency in the United States. Centers for Disease Control and Prevention. MMWR Recomm Rep 1998;47(RR-3):1–29.

Rodis JF, Egan JF, Craffey A, Ciarleglio L, Greenstein RM, Scorza WE. Calculated risk of chromosomal abnormalities in twin gestations. Obstet Gynecol 1990;76:1037–41.

Screening for fetal chromosomal abnormalities. ACOG Practice Bulletin No. 77. American College of Obstetricians and Gynecologists. Obstet Gynecol 2007;109: 217–27.

Smoking cessation during pregnancy. ACOG Committee Opinion No. 316. American College of Obstetricians and Gynecologists. Obstet Gynecol 2005;106:883–8.

Spohr HL, Willms J, Steinhausen HC. Prenatal alcohol exposure and long-term developmental consequences. Lancet 1993;341:907–10.

Tan KH, Smyth R. Fetal vibroacoustic stimulation for facilitation of tests of fetal wellbeing. Cochrane Database of Systematic Reviews 2001, Issue 1. Art. No.: CD002963. DOI: 10.1002/14651858.CD002963.

Update on carrier screening for cystic fibrosis. ACOG Committee Opinion No. 325. American College of Obstetricians and Gynecologists. Obstet Gynecol 2005;106: 1465–8.

Vaginal birth after previous cesarean delivery. ACOG Practice Bulletin No. 54. American College of Obstetricians and Gynecologists. Obstet Gynecol 2004;104:203–12.

Wald N, Cuckle H, Wu TS, George L. Maternal serum unconjugated oestriol and human chorionic gonadotrophin levels in twin pregnancies: implications for screening for Down's syndrome. Br J Obstet Gynaecol 1991;98:905–8.

Wald NJ, Law MR, Morris JK, Wald DS. Quantifying the effect of folic acid [published erratum appears in Lancet 2002;359:630]. Lancet 2001;358:2069–73.

Wapner R, Thom E, Simpson JL, Pergament E, Silver R, Filkins K, et al. First-trimester screening for trisomies 21 and 18. First Trimester Maternal Serum Biochemistry and Fetal Nuchal Translucency Screening (BUN) Study Group. N Eng J Med 2003;349:1405–13.

chapter 5

Intrapartum and Postpartum Care of the Mother

The goal of all labor and delivery units is a safe birth for mothers and their newborns. At the same time, staff should attempt to make the patient feel welcome, comfortable, and informed throughout the labor and delivery process. Ongoing risk assessment should determine appropriate care for the woman. The father, partner, or other primary support person should be made to feel welcome and should be encouraged to participate throughout the labor and delivery experience.

Labor and delivery is a normal physiologic process that most women experience without complications. Obstetric staff can greatly enhance this experience for the woman and her family by exhibiting a caring attitude and helping them understand the process. Efforts to promote healthy behaviors can be as effective during labor and delivery as they are during antepartum care. Physical contact between the newborn and the parents in the delivery room should be encouraged. Every effort should be made to foster family interaction and to support the desire of the family to be together.

Because intrapartum complications can arise, sometimes quickly and without warning, ongoing risk assessment and surveillance of the mother and the fetus are essential. The hospital, including a birthing center within a hospital complex, or freestanding birthing centers that meet the standards of the Accreditation Association for Ambulatory Health Care or the Joint Commission or the American Association of Birth Centers provide the safest setting for labor, delivery, and the postpartum period. This setting ensures accepted standards of safety that cannot be matched in a home-birthing situation. The collection and analysis of data on the safety and outcome of deliveries in other settings have been problematic. The development of approved, well-designed research protocols, prepared in consultation with obstetric departments and their related institutional review boards, is appropriate to assess safety, feasibility, and birth outcomes in such settings. Until such data are available, home births are not encouraged. There may be exceptional situations, however, such as in geographically isolated areas, in which special programs are required.

Admission

Pregnant women may come to a hospital's labor and delivery area not only for obstetric care but also for evaluation and treatment of nonobstetric illnesses. However, a nonobstetric condition, such as highly transmissible infectious diseases (eg, varicella), is best treated in another area of the hospital. The obstetric department should establish policies in consultation with other hospital units or personnel, such as the emergency department or infectious disease director, for coordinated care of pregnant women. Departments should agree on the conditions that are best treated in the labor and delivery area and those that should be treated in other hospital-care units. Patients with medical or surgical conditions that could reasonably be expected to result in obstetric consequences should be evaluated by qualified obstetric-care providers. The priority of that evaluation and the site where it is best performed should be determined by the patient's needs (including gestational age of the fetus) and the care unit's ability to provide for those needs. The obstetric department also should establish policies for the admission of nonobstetric patients according to state regulations (see "Nonobstetric Patients" in Chapter 2). Federal and state regulations address the management and treatment of patients in hospital acute-care areas, including labor and delivery (see Appendix F).

Written departmental policies regarding triage of patients who come to a labor and delivery area should be reviewed periodically for compliance with appropriate regulations. A pregnant woman who comes to the labor and delivery area should be evaluated in a timely fashion. Obstetric nursing staff may perform this initial evaluation, which should minimally include assessment of:

- Maternal vital signs
- Fetal heart rate
- Uterine contractions

The responsible obstetric provider should be informed promptly if any of the following findings are present or suspected:

- Vaginal bleeding
- Acute abdominal pain

- Temperature of (100.4°F) or higher
- Preterm labor
- Preterm rupture of membranes (PROM)
- Hypertension
- Nonreassuring fetal heart rate pattern

Any patient who is suspected to be in labor or who has rupture of the membranes or vaginal bleeding should be evaluated promptly in an obstetric service area. Whenever a pregnant woman is evaluated for labor, the following factors should be assessed and recorded in the patient's permanent medical record:

- Maternal vital signs
- Frequency and duration of uterine contractions
- Documentation of fetal well-being
- Urinary protein concentration
- Cervical dilatation and effacement, unless contraindicated (eg, placenta previa, preterm PROM) or cervical length as ascertained by transvaginal ultrasonography
- Fetal presentation and station of the presenting part
- Status of the membranes
- Date and time of the patient's arrival and of notification of the provider
- Estimation of fetal weight and assessment of maternal pelvis

If the patient is in prodromal or early labor and has no complications, admission to the labor and delivery area may be deferred after initial evaluation and documentation of fetal well-being (see Appendix F). A patient with a transmissible infection should be admitted to a site where isolation techniques may be followed according to hospital policy.

If a woman has received prenatal care and a recent examination has confirmed the normal progress of pregnancy, her admission evaluation may be limited to an interval history and physical examination directed at the presenting condition. Previously identified risk factors should be recorded in the medical record. If no new risk factors are found, attention may be focused on the following historic factors:

- Time of onset and frequency of contractions
- Status of the membranes

- Presence or absence of bleeding
- Fetal movement
- History of allergies
- Time, content, and amount of the most recent food or fluid ingestion
- Use of any medication

Serologic testing for hepatitis B virus surface antigen may be necessary as described in Chapter 9. Women who have not received prenatal care or who received care late in pregnancy are more likely to have sexually transmitted diseases and substance abuse problems. Social problems, such as poverty and family conflict, also may affect patients' health. A shortened obstetric hospital stay poses even greater problems for patients who have had no prenatal care. Routine obstetric screening tests (eg, hemoglobin, type and Rh), social intervention, and additional education may be needed within this limited period.

If no complications are detected during initial assessment in the labor and delivery area and if contraindications have been ruled out, qualified nursing personnel may perform the initial pelvic examination. Once the results of the examination have been obtained and documented, the provider responsible for the woman's care in the labor and delivery area should be informed of her status. The provider can make a decision regarding her management. The timing of the provider's arrival in the labor area should be based on this information and hospital policy. If epidural, spinal, or general anesthesia is anticipated, or if conditions exist that place the patient at risk for requiring rapid institution of an anesthetic, anesthesia personnel should be informed of the patient's presence soon after her admission. If a preterm delivery, infected or depressed newborn, or newborn with a prenatally diagnosed congenital anomaly is expected, the provider who will assume responsibility for the newborn's care should be informed. When the patient has been examined and instructions regarding her management have been given and noted on her medical record, all necessary consent forms should be signed and incorporated into the medical record.

By 36 weeks of gestation, preregistration for labor and delivery at the hospital should be confirmed. By 36 weeks of gestation, a copy of the prenatal medical record (see "ACOG Antepartum Record" in Appendix A) should be on file in the hospital's labor registration area, including information pertaining to the patient's antepartum course, or equivalent electronic medical record should be accessible. Consideration should be given to providing periodic updates to the prenatal medical record on file.

At the time of a patient's admission to the labor and delivery area, pertinent information from the prenatal record should be noted in the admission records. Because labor and delivery is a dynamic process, all entries into a patient's medical record should include the date and time of occurrence. Blood typing and screening tests need not be repeated if they were performed during the antepartum period and no antibodies were present, provided that the report is in the hospital records. If results of the woman's antenatal laboratory evaluation are not known and cannot be obtained, blood typing, Rh D type determination, hepatitis B virus antigen testing, and serologic testing for syphilis should be performed before the woman is discharged. State laws governing testing of umbilical cord blood may vary. Serologic testing for human immunodeficiency virus (HIV) infection and other tests should be encouraged and performed according to state law. Rapid HIV testing can be done in labor if the mother's HIV status is unknown (see additional information on rapid HIV testing in Chapter 4 under "Routine Testing" and Chapter 9 under "Human Immunodeficiency Virus"). Collection of umbilical cord blood may be useful for subsequent evaluation of ABO incompatibility if the mother is type O. Policies should be developed to ensure expeditious preparation of blood products for transfusion if the patient is at increased risk of hemorrhage or if the need arises.

At all times in the hospital labor and delivery area, the safety and well-being of the mother and the fetus are the primary concern and responsibility of the obstetric staff. This concern, however, should not unnecessarily restrict the activity of women with uncomplicated labor and delivery or exclude people who are supportive of her. The woman should have the option to stay out of bed during the early stages of labor, to ambulate, and to rest in a comfortable chair as long as the fetal status is reassuring. Concerns such as showers during labor, placement of intravenous lines, use of fetal heart rate monitoring, and restrictions on ambulation should be reviewed in departmental policies, taking into consideration physicians' preferences as well as patients' desires, comfort, privacy, and sense of participation. Likewise, the use of drugs for relief of pain during labor and delivery should depend on the needs and desires of the woman. The development of a birth plan that has been discussed previously with a woman's provider and placed in her medical record may promote her participation in and satisfaction with her care.

The woman's health care team should communicate regarding all factors that may pose a risk to her, her fetus, or her newborn. Obstetric departmental policies should include recommendations for transmitting to the nursery those maternal and fetal historical and laboratory data that may affect the care of the newborn. Information on conditions that may influence neonatal care also should be communicated. The lack of such data, perhaps because of a lack of prenatal care, also should be made known to the nursery personnel. The physician who will care for the newborn should be identified on the maternal medical record (see Appendix A). Health care professionals who provide anesthesia should be notified of women who may be at significant risk of complications from anesthetic procedures (eg, women with hypertension or who are morbidly obese).

Labor

The onset of true labor is established by observing progressive change in a woman's cervix in the setting of regular, phasic, uterine contractions. This may require two or more cervical examinations that are separated by an adequate period to observe change. Even a well-prepared woman may arrive at the hospital labor and delivery area before true labor has begun. A policy that allows for adequate evaluation of patients for labor and that prevents unnecessary admissions to the labor and delivery unit is advisable (see Appendix F).

False Labor at Term

Uterine contractions in the absence of cervical change commonly are called false labor. Treatment for this condition should be based on individual circumstances. Patients who are having uterine contractions and are not yet in active labor may be observed for evidence of cervical change in a casual, comfortable area. After observation and evaluation by appropriate hospital-designated personnel and assurance of fetal well-being, the patient may be discharged (see Appendix F).

Premature Rupture of Membranes at Term

Premature rupture of membranes is considered to be present when there is leakage of amniotic fluid before the onset of labor. Preparations for labor and delivery should begin when PROM occurs, whether at or before term, because labor frequently ensues. Management of PROM is not uniform, and several acceptable strategies exist for the care of patients with PROM. These strategies should address methods of diagnosis, induction of labor, and timing and use of antibiotics for both prophylaxis and treatment of the mother and the fetus.

The diagnosis of PROM is established by history, physical examination, and laboratory test result confirmation. Diagnosis based on history alone is correct in more than 90% of patients. Nevertheless, all patients reporting symptoms that suggest ruptured membranes should be examined with a sterile speculum as soon as possible to confirm this diagnosis. In any labor occurring after rupture of membranes, vaginal examinations should be limited in number and attention paid to clean technique. Gross pooling of amniotic fluid in the vagina is nearly 100% diagnostic of PROM. Supportive laboratory testing includes vaginal pH, fern testing, and ultrasound estimation of amniotic fluid volume. The obstetric providers who perform the examination to confirm or rule out PROM should be aware of the causes of false-positive and false-negative test results that occur with the use of pH and fern testing. These causes include leakage of alkaline urine, cervical mucus, bacterial vaginosis, and blood. Given equivocal findings, exclusion of PROM remote from term may require an amniocentesis with instillation of indigo carmine dye.

Management is determined by the presence or absence of PROM and gestational age. For women with PROM at term, labor should be induced at the time of presentation to reduce the risk of maternal and neonatal complications. Delivery is recommended when PROM occurs at or beyond 34 weeks of gestation. With PROM at 32–33 completed weeks of gestation, labor induction may be considered if fetal pulmonary maturity has been documented. Patients with PROM before 32 weeks of gestation should be managed expectantly until 33 completed weeks of gestation if no maternal or fetal contraindications exist. A 48-hour course of intravenous ampicillin and erythromycin followed by 5 days of amoxicillin and erythromycin is recommended during expectant management of preterm PROM remote from term to prolong pregnancy and to reduce infectious- and gestational age-dependent neonatal morbidity. For a woman with preterm PROM and a viable fetus, the safety of expectant management at home has not been established.

If intraamniotic infection is diagnosed at any gestational age, antibiotics should be initiated and labor should be induced. The diagnosis of intraamniotic infection alone is not an indication for cesarean delivery, which should be reserved for obstetric indications only. In the presence of chorioamnionitis, the duration of PROM does not correlate with the risk of neonatal sepsis.

Management of Labor

Ideally, every woman admitted to the labor and delivery area should know who her principal, designated health care provider will be. Members of the obstetric team should observe the patient to follow the progress of labor, record her vital signs and the fetal heart rate in her medical record at regular intervals, and make an effort to ensure her understanding of the events taking place. The provider principally responsible for the patient's care should be kept informed of her progress and notified promptly of any abnormality. When the patient is in active labor, that provider should be readily available (see "Preface," and "Cesarean Delivery" in this chapter).

Patients in active labor should avoid oral ingestion of anything except sips of clear liquids, occasional ice chips, or preparations for moistening the mouth and lips. Ideally, intravenous access should be secured when the active phase of labor begins. The progress of labor should be evaluated by periodic vaginal examinations, and her provider should be notified of labor progress. Sterile, water-soluble lubricants may be used to reduce discomfort during vaginal examinations. Antiseptics, such as povidone-iodine and hexachlorophene, have not been shown to decrease infections acquired during the intrapartum period. Furthermore, these agents may produce local irritation and are absorbed through maternal mucous membranes.

For women who are at no increased risk of complications, evaluation of the quality of the uterine contractions and pelvic examinations should be sufficient to detect abnormalities in the progress of labor. Vital signs should be recorded at regular intervals of at least every 4 hours. This frequency may be increased, particularly as active labor progresses, according to clinical signs and symptoms. Documentation of the course of a woman's labor may include, but need not be limited to, the presence of physicians, midwives, or nurses, position changes, cervical status, oxygen and drug administration, blood pressure levels, temperature, amniotomy or spontaneous rupture of membranes, color of amniotic fluid, and Valsalva maneuver.

Fetal Heart Rate Monitoring

Either electronic fetal heart rate monitoring or intermittent auscultation may be used to determine fetal status during labor. Obstetric unit guidelines should clearly delineate the procedures to be followed for using these techniques according to the phase and stage of labor.

The method of fetal heart rate monitoring for fetal surveillance during labor may vary depending on the risk assessment at admission, the preferences of the patient and obstetric staff, and departmental policy. If no risk factors are present at the time of the patient's admission, a standard approach to fetal surveillance is to determine, evaluate, and record the fetal heart rate every 30 minutes in the active phase of the first stage of labor and at least every 15 minutes in the second stage of labor.

If risk factors are present at admission or appear during labor, there is no difference in perinatal outcome between intermittent auscultation and continuous fetal monitoring if one of the following methods for fetal heart rate monitoring is used:

- During the active phase of the first stage of labor, the fetal heart rate should be determined, evaluated, and recorded at least every 15 minutes, preferably before, during, and after a uterine contraction, when intermittent auscultation is used. If continuous electronic fetal heart rate monitoring is used, the heart rate tracing should be evaluated at least every 15 minutes.

- During the second stage of labor, the fetal heart rate should be determined, evaluated, and recorded at least every 5 minutes if auscultation is used. If continuous electronic fetal heart rate monitoring is used, the tracing should be evaluated at least every 5 minutes.

The appropriate use of electronic fetal heart rate monitoring includes recording and interpreting the tracings. Nonreassuring findings should be noted and communicated to the physician or certified nurse midwife so that the appropriate intervention can occur. When a change in the rate or pattern has been noted, it also is important to document a subsequent return to reassuring findings. Terms that describe the fetal heart rate patterns (eg, early, late, variable, or prolonged decelerations; tachycardia and bradycardia; accelerations; and variability) should be used in both medical record entries and verbal communication among obstetric personnel.

Internal fetal heart rate monitoring and internal uterine pressure monitoring may be used to gain further information about fetal status and uterine contractility, respectively. Relative contraindications to internal fetal monitoring include maternal HIV infection and other high-risk factors for fetal infection, including herpes simplex virus and hepatitis B or hepatitis C virus. However, if there are indications for fetal scalp monitoring, it is reasonable in a woman who has a history of recurrent herpes simplex virus and no active lesions.

Fetal scalp or acoustic stimulation that results in acceleration of the fetal heart rate is reassuring when the fetal heart rate pattern is difficult to interpret. If electronic fetal monitoring is used, all fetal heart rate tracings should be identified with the patient's name, hospital number, and the date and time of admission. All fetal heart rate tracings should be easily retrievable from storage so that the events of labor can be studied in proper relationship to the tracings.

Induction and Augmentation of Labor

Each hospital's department of obstetrics and gynecology should develop written protocols for preparing and administering oxytocin solution or other agents for labor induction or stimulation. Indications for induction and augmentation of labor should be stated. The qualifications of personnel authorized to administer oxytocic agents for this purpose should be described. The methods for assessment of the woman and the fetus before and during administration of these agents should be specified. Fetal heart rate monitoring should be performed as delineated for high-risk patients in active labor (see "Fetal Heart Rate Monitoring" in this chapter).

Labor is induced when the benefits to either the woman or the fetus outweigh those of continuing the pregnancy. If oxytocin is used, the infusion should be administered by a device that permits precise control of the flow rate to ensure accurate, minute-to-minute control. Oxytocin also is used to augment labor and enhance inadequate uterine contractions in women in whom an assessment of the relationship between the maternal pelvis and fetal size is otherwise normal. Buccal, intranasal, or intramuscular administration of oxytocin should not be used to induce or augment labor.

Various regimens exist for the administration of varying techniques and agents to stimulate uterine contractions. These regimens vary in initial dose, amount of incremental dose increase, and interval between dose increases. Each hospital's department of obstetrics and gynecology should determine which regimens will be standard for that hospital so that obstetric staff in the labor and delivery area may develop further guidelines for their application to individual patients. Regimens described as low dose and with a less-frequent dosage increase are associated with a lower incidence of uterine hyperstimulation. Higher and more frequent dosage increases are credited with shortening time in labor and reducing the incidence of chorioamnionitis and the number of cesarean deliveries performed for dystocia but increased rates of uterine hyperstimulation.

Cervical Ripening

Cervical ripening may be beneficial if the cervix is unfavorable for induction. Acceptable interventions for preparing an unfavorable cervix for induction include mechanical dilation with laminaria or a 30 mL Foley catheter placed in the cervical canal, use of misoprostol (as detailed in the following paragraphs), and intravaginal or intracervical administration of prostaglandin E_2 (PGE_2) in doses appropriate for cervical ripening. If the fetus' estimated gestational age is near term, routine intravenous oxytocin induction or misoprostol administration usually is effective. High-dose PGE_2 suppositories and more concentrated intravenous oxytocin regimens both are effective for terminating a pregnancy complicated by fetal death, especially at a gestational age of 28 weeks or less. Because of the risk of uterine rupture, the use of prostaglandins after 28 weeks of gestation should be discouraged if the woman has had prior transfundal uterine surgery.

Misoprostol, a prostaglandin E_1 analog, has been demonstrated to be an effective agent for cervical ripening and the induction of labor. When compared with placebo, misoprostol use may decrease overall cesarean delivery rates, decrease oxytocin requirements, and achieve higher rates of vaginal delivery within 24 hours of induction. Misoprostol use also compares favorably with the use of intracervical and intravaginal PGE_2 preparations, with many studies demonstrating shorter times to delivery and reduced oxytocin requirements. Misoprostol should not be used for cervical ripening or induction of labor in patients with prior cesarean delivery or previous major uterine surgery.

When given vaginally in doses of 50 µg or more, misoprostol use has been associated with an increased rate of uterine hyperstimulation, uterine tachysystole, and meconium passage. These problems are less common with a dose of 25 µg of misoprostol administered intravaginally every 3–6 hours.

Misoprostol currently is available in 100-µg and 200-µg tablets, and the 100-µg tablet is not scored. If misoprostol is used for cervical ripening and induction, one quarter of a 100-µg tablet (ie, approximately 25 µg) should be considered for the initial dose. Doses should not be administered more frequently than every 3–6 hours. Both fetal heart rate and uterine activity should be monitored carefully in these patients. Doses should be held in the presence of a nonreassuring fetal heart rate or regular and frequent uterine contractions of moderate intensity. Oxytocin should not be administered less than 4 hours after the last misoprostol dose.

When a patient is admitted for labor induction, a physician who has privileges to perform cesarean deliveries should be readily available (see "Preface" and "Cesarean Delivery" in this chapter). The patient's medical record should document who is the responsible physician. A qualified member of the obstetric team should perform a vaginal examination for evaluation of the cervix before the induction is initiated. Personnel who are familiar with the effects of the agents used and who are able to identify both maternal and fetal complications should be in attendance during administration of the agent(s).

Hyperstimulation can occur with any of the available chemical techniques of cervical ripening or labor induction or augmentation. When the continuous administration of PGE_2 via vaginal insert is the technique used, the fetal heart rate and uterine activity should be monitored continuously as long as the device is in place and for at least 15 minutes after it is removed.

Induction of labor by "stripping" or "sweeping" the amniotic membranes is a relatively common practice. Risks associated with this procedure include infection, bleeding from an undiagnosed placenta previa or low-lying placenta, and accidental rupture of membranes. Membrane stripping may be associated with a higher frequency of spontaneous labor and with a decreased incidence of postterm gestation.

Artificial rupture of membranes is another method of labor induction that may be used, particularly when the cervix is favorable. Routine early amniotomy results in a modest reduction in the duration of labor but may result in an increased rate of intraamniotic infection and cesarean delivery for fetal heart rate abnormalities, although not overall cesarean delivery rates. Moreover, it would seem reasonable to delay amniotomy in an uncomplicated intrapartum patient with normal fluid unless the cervix is significantly dilated (see "Amnioinfusion" as follows). Care should be taken to palpate for an umbilical cord and to avoid dislodging the fetal head when artificially rupturing membranes. The fetal heart rate should be evaluated and recorded before and immediately after the procedure.

Amnioinfusion

The transcervical infusion of sterile, balanced salt solutions during labor (amnioinfusion) may be used to ameliorate severe, variable decelerations in the fetal heart rate tracing that are suspected to be caused by umbilical cord compression. Meta-analysis confirms that amnioinfusion lowers caesarean delivery rates in the setting of oligohydramnios with repetitive variable fetal heart rate decelerations. There is no proven benefit of amnioinfusion for other fetal heart rate abnormalities, such as late decelerations, and the resultant increase in uterine tone may exacerbate underlying uteroplacental vascular insufficiency. Because it is possible to introduce fluid into the uterus at too rapid a rate, each obstetric unit should establish a protocol for intrauterine pressure monitoring during amnioinfusion or limitations of the volume and infusion rate when the technique is used. Based on the totality of published data, routine prophylactic amnioinfusion for meconium-stained amniotic fluid is not indicated. Prophylactic use of amnioinfusion in this setting should be done only in the setting of additional clinical trials. Data are not available on whether amnioinfusion for fetal heart rate variable decelerations in the presence of meconium-stained fluid decreases meconium aspiration syndrome or other meconium-related morbidities. However, amnioinfusion is a reasonable approach to treatment of repetitive, variable decelerations irrespective of amniotic fluid meconium status.

Analgesia and Anesthesia

Management of discomfort and pain during labor and delivery is an essential part of good obstetric practice. It is the responsibility of the obstetrician or certified nurse midwife, in consultation with the anesthesiologist, if appropriate, to develop the most appropriate response to the woman's request for analgesia or anesthesia. In the absence of a medical contraindication, maternal request is a sufficient medical indication for pain relief during labor.

Some patients tolerate the pain of labor by using techniques learned in childbirth preparation programs. Although specific techniques vary, classes usually seek to relieve pain through the general principles of education, support, relaxation, paced breathing, focusing, and touch. The staff at the bedside should be knowledgeable about these pain management techniques and should be supportive of the patient's decision to use them.

Unless contraindicated, pharmacologic analgesics to ameliorate the pain of contractions should be made available on request to women in labor. The choice and availability of analgesic and anesthetic techniques depend on the experience and judgment of the obstetrician and anesthesiologist, the physical condition of the patient, the circumstances of labor and delivery, and the personal preferences of the patient. Parenteral pain medications for labor pain decrease fetal heart rate variability and may limit the obstetrician's ability to interpret the fetal heart rate tracing. Considerations should be given to other agents in the setting of minimal or absent fetal heart rate variability. High doses of narcotics potentially are depressing to both the woman and the fetus, and both patients should be monitored. Barbiturates, tranquilizers, and narcotics can be administered during prodromal and early labor to allow the patient to rest.

Epidural analgesia offers the most effective form of intrapartum pain relief and is used by most women in the United States. A catheter is placed in the epidural space, allowing for a continuous infusion of pain medication during labor. The advantage of this method of analgesia is that the medication may be titrated over the course of labor as needed. In addition, epidural catheters placed for labor may be dosed and used for cesarean delivery, postpartum tubal ligation, postcesarean pain control, or for repair of obstetric lacerations following vaginal delivery, if needed.

Spinal anesthesia is performed by giving a single injection of anesthesia. This provides excellent pain relief for procedures of limited duration, such as cesarean delivery, postpartum tubal ligation, or for vaginal delivery in a patient who is rapidly progressing in labor.

Combined spinal–epidural analgesia offers the advantages of the rapid onset of spinal analgesia along with the ability to use the indwelling epidural catheter to titrate medication throughout labor. It also may be used and dosed to provide anesthesia for a cesarean delivery and dosed for postcesarean pain control before being removed.

It also should be noted that a low-grade maternal fever might be associated with a normally functioning epidural in the absence of infection. If the temperature is greater than (100.4°F), it may be difficult to differentiate this "epidural temperature" from the temperature associated with chorioamnionitis. In this group of patients, neonatal surveillance blood cultures do not reveal occult infection.

Depending on the technique used, the experience of the anesthesiologist, and the patient's response, ambulation to some extent may be possible during regional analgesia.

In the past, reports regarding the timing of epidural anesthesia and its effect on the labor course have offered conflicting results. More recent data now indicate that low-dose neuraxial analgesia in early labor does not increase the rate of cesarean delivery and may result in a shorter duration of labor. Thus, there seems to be little justification to withhold this form of pain relief in women in early labor at less than 4 cm cervical dilation.

Paracervical block, when used for pain relief during labor, may result in fetal bradycardia. The fetal heart rate should be monitored closely before, during, and after the administration of paracervical block. Bupivacaine is contraindicated for use in paracervical block. At the time of delivery, local anesthetics may be injected into the tissues of the perineum and the vagina to provide anesthesia for episiotomy and repair of vaginal and perineal lacerations. Local anesthetics also may be injected to perform a pudendal block in patients who did not receive regional anesthesia during labor. This regional block may provide adequate anesthesia for outlet operative deliveries and performance of any necessary episiotomy or repair.

Spinal analgesia using low-dose dilute concentrations of local anesthetics with opioids may provide excellent analgesia with rapid onset for the second stage of labor. Spinal anesthesia with higher-dose local anesthetics can provide profound sensory and motor blockade if needed for maternal indications or to facilitate instrumented vaginal delivery. Although spinal anesthesia can provide adequate pain relief and muscle relaxation for nearly all vaginal deliveries, it typically results in profound sensory and motor blockade, which impairs maternal expulsive efforts. Therefore, spinal anesthesia typically is not administered until delivery is imminent or the physician has made a decision to perform an operative delivery. General anesthesia rarely is necessary for vaginal delivery and should be used only for specific indications.

For most cesarean deliveries, properly administered regional or general anesthesia is effective and has little adverse effect on the newborn. Because of the maternal risks associated with intubation and the possibility of aspiration during induction of general anesthesia, regional anesthesia is the preferred technique and should be available in all hospitals that provide obstetric care. The advantages and disadvantages of both techniques should be discussed with the patient as completely as possible. Examples of circumstances in which rapid induction of general anesthesia may be indicated include a prolapsed umbilical cord with severe fetal bradycardia and ominous fetal heart rate patterns from other or unknown causes.

Analgesia or anesthesia during labor and delivery has little or no lasting effect on the physiologic status of the neonate. No evidence exists that suggests that the administration of analgesia or anesthesia during childbirth per se has a significant effect on the child's later mental and neurologic development.

Regional anesthesia in obstetrics should be initiated and maintained only by health care providers who are approved through the institutional credentialing process to administer or supervise the administration of obstetric anesthesia. These individuals must be qualified to manage anesthetic complications. An obstetrician may administer the anesthesia if granted privileges for these procedures. However, having an anesthesiologist or anesthetist provide this care permits the obstetrician to give undivided attention to the delivery.

It is the responsibility of the director of anesthesia services to make recommendations regarding the clinical privileges of all anesthesia service personnel. If obstetric analgesia (other than pudendal or local techniques) is provided by obstetricians, the director of anesthesia services should participate with a representative of the obstetric department in the formulation of procedures designed to ensure the uniform quality of anesthesia services throughout the hospital.

Specific recommendations regarding these procedures are provided in the *Accreditation Manual for Hospitals* published by the Joint Commission. The directors of departments providing anesthesia services are responsible for implementing processes to monitor and evaluate the quality and appropriateness of these services in their respective departments.

Regional anesthesia should be administered only after the patient has been examined and the fetal status and progress of labor have been evaluated by a qualified individual. A physician with obstetric privileges who has knowledge of the maternal and fetal status and the progress of labor and who approves initiation of labor anesthesia should be readily available (see "Preface" and "Cesarean Delivery" in this chapter) to deal with any obstetric complications that may arise. When regional anesthesia is administered during labor, the patient's vital signs should be monitored at regular intervals by a qualified member of the health care team.

When any of the following risk factors are present, anesthetic consultation in advance of delivery may be considered to permit formulation of a management plan:

- Marked obesity
- Severe edema or anatomic abnormalities of the face, neck, or spine, including trauma or surgery
- Abnormal dentition, small mandible, or difficulty opening the mouth
- Extremely short stature, short neck, or arthritis of the neck
- Goiter
- Serious maternal medical problems, such as cardiac, pulmonary, or neurologic diseases
- Bleeding disorders
- Severe preeclampsia
- Previous history of anesthetic complications
- Obstetric complications likely to lead to operative delivery (eg, placenta previa or high-order multiple gestation)

When such risk factors are identified, a physician who is credentialed to provide general and regional anesthesia should be consulted in the antepartum period to allow for joint development of a plan of management, including optimal location for delivery. Strategies thereby can be developed to minimize the need for emergency induction or general anesthesia in women for whom this would be especially hazardous. For those women at risk, consideration should be given to the planned placement in early labor of an intravenous line and an epidural or spinal catheter with confirmation that the catheter is functional. If a woman at unusual risk of complications from anesthesia is identified (eg, prior failed intubation), strong consideration should be given to antepartum referral of the patient to allow for delivery at a hospital that can manage such anesthesia on a 24-hour basis.

Aspiration is a significant cause of anesthetic-related maternal morbidity and mortality, and the more acidic the aspirate, the greater the harm done. Therefore, prophylactic administration of an antacid before induction of a major regional or general anesthesia is appropriate. Particulate antacids may be harmful if aspirated; a clear antacid, such as a solution of 0.3 mol/L of sodium citrate or a similar preparation, may be a safer choice.

On rare occasions, it may be impossible to intubate an obstetric patient after the induction of general anesthesia. Equipment for emergency airway management, such as the laryngeal mask airway, combi tube, and fiberoptic laryngoscope, should be available whenever general anesthesia is administered.

Delivery

Vaginal Delivery

Vaginal delivery is associated with less risk of maternal operative and postoperative complications than nonelective cesarean delivery and results in shorter hospital stays. Vaginal delivery requires consideration of:

- The availability of professionals with special skills in neonatal resuscitation
- The availability of anesthesia personnel
- Obstetric attendants for the delivery
- The potential need to move a patient from a LDR room to an operative suite

The risk assessment performed on the patient's admission, the course of the patient's labor, the fetal presentation, any abnormalities encountered during the labor process, and the anesthetic technique in use or anticipated for delivery will all have an effect on the need for other professionals. At least one obstetric nurse, preferably the woman's designated primary nurse for the labor, should be present in the delivery room throughout the delivery. Under no circumstances should an attempt be made to delay birth by physical restraint or anesthetic means.

Episiotomy may be used to aid in the management of delivery in some situations. The routine use of episiotomy is not necessary and may lead to an increase in the risk of third- and fourth-degree perineal lacerations and a delay in the patient's resumption of sexual activity. Episiotomy always should be done for specific medical indication. Median episiotomy is associated with higher rates of injury to the anal sphincter and rectum, and mediolateral episiotomy may be preferable to median episiotomy in selected cases.

Vaginal Birth After Cesarean Delivery

Despite extensive data regarding the risks and success rates of vaginal birth after cesarean delivery (VBAC), there is relatively little information regarding how labor should be conducted (see "Vaginal Birth After Cesarean Delivery" in Chapter 4). Examples of the information that is available are listed as follows:

- Limited data suggest that external cephalic version for breech presentation may be as successful for VBAC candidates as for women who have not undergone previous cesarean delivery.

- The use of prostaglandins for cervical ripening or labor induction in VBAC candidates is discouraged, as noted previously (see "Cervical Ripening" in this chapter). If induction of labor is necessary for a clear and compelling clinical indication, the potential increased risk of uterine rupture with the use of prostaglandins should be discussed with the patient and documented in the medical record.

- Oxytocin may be used for both labor induction and augmentation with close patient monitoring in VBAC candidates, although such inductions are associated with a nearly 50% increased risk of uterine rupture compared with candidates having spontaneous labor.

- Once labor has begun, the patient should be evaluated promptly. Continuous electronic monitoring of both fetal heart rate and uterine contractions is recommended. The most common sign of uterine rupture is a nonreassuring fetal heart rate pattern with variable decelerations that may evolve into late decelerations, bradycardia, and undetectable fetal heart rate. Personnel familiar with the potential complications of VBAC should be vigilant for nonreassuring fetal heart rate patterns and inadequate progress in labor. Because uterine rupture may be catastrophic and evolve rapidly, VBAC should be attempted in institutions equipped to respond to emergencies with physicians immediately available to provide emergency care, including emergent cesarean delivery.

- Epidural analgesia and anesthesia may be used safely during a trial of labor and planned VBAC. Assurance of adequate pain relief during labor may encourage more women to choose a trial of labor. Success rates for VBAC are similar in women who do and those who do not receive epidural analgesia, as well as in those women who receive other types of pain relief. Epidural analgesia rarely masks the signs or symptoms of uterine rupture. The anesthesia service should be available whenever there is a patient attempting VBAC in active labor on the labor floor.

The need to explore the uterus after a successful VBAC is controversial. Most asymptomatic scar dehiscences heal well, and there is no data to suggest that future pregnancy outcome is improved if the dehiscence is surgically repaired versus spontaneous healing. Excessive vaginal bleeding or signs of hypovolemia at delivery require prompt and complete assessment of the previous scar and the entire genital tract.

Operative Vaginal Delivery

Forceps and vacuum extraction are valuable tools to perform operative vaginal delivery. Operator experience and preference should determine which instrument is used in a particular situation. The vacuum extractor is associated with an increased incidence of neonatal cephalohematomata, retinal hemorrhages, and jaundice when compared with forceps delivery. Forceps delivery, on the other hand, is associated with a higher rate of maternal perineal injuries. Neonatal care providers should be made aware of the mode of delivery to observe for potential complications associated with operative vaginal delivery. The following definitions and indications relate to both techniques.

Station. Station refers to the relationship of the estimated distances, in centimeters, between the leading bony portion of the fetal head and the level of the maternal ischial spines. In classifying forceps and vacuum extraction procedures, the station of the fetal head should be noted. Engagement of the head occurs when the biparietal diameter has passed through the pelvic inlet. It is clinically diagnosed when the leading bony portion of the fetal head is at or below the level of the ischial spines (station 0 or more). The preferred method to describe station beyond the level of the ischial spines is to estimate centimeters (+1 to +5 cm) below the spines.

Outlet Operative Vaginal Delivery. Outlet operative vaginal delivery is the application of forceps or vacuum when 1) the fetal scalp is visible at the introitus without separating the labia, 2) the fetal skull has reached the pelvic floor, 3) the fetal sagittal suture is in the anterior–posterior diameter or in the right or left occiput anterior or posterior position, and 4) the fetal head is at or on the perineum. According to this definition, rotation cannot exceed 45 degrees. There is no difference in perinatal outcome when deliveries involving the use of outlet operative vaginal deliveries are compared with similar spontaneous deliveries, and no data support the concept that rotating the head on the pelvic floor 45 degrees or less increases the rate of morbidity.

Low Operative Vaginal Delivery. Low operative vaginal delivery is the application of forceps or vacuum when the leading point of the fetal skull is at station +2 or more and is not on the pelvic floor. Low operative vaginal delivery applications have two subdivisions: 1) rotation 45 degrees or less (eg, left or right to occiput anterior, or left or right occipitoposterior to occiput posterior) and 2) rotation more than 45 degrees. Although rotation of the fetal head often accompanies the use of the vacuum extractor, the vacuum never should be used to provide a direct rotational force to the fetal scalp.

Midpelvis Operative Vaginal Delivery. Midpelvis operative vaginal delivery is the application of forceps or vacuum when the fetal head is engaged but the leading point of the skull is above station +2. Under very unusual circumstances, such as the sudden onset of severe fetal or maternal compromise, application of forceps or vacuum above station +2 may be attempted while simultaneously initiating preparations for a cesarean delivery in the event that the operative vaginal delivery maneuver is unsuccessful. Neither forceps nor vacuum should be applied to an unengaged fetal presenting part or when the cervix is not completely dilated.

Indications for a forceps or vacuum extraction operation and the position and station of the vertex at the time of application of the forceps or vacuum apparatus should be identified in a detailed operative description in the patient's medical record. These indications include the following items:

- Shortening the second stage of labor—Outlet forceps or vacuum extraction may be used to shorten the second stage of labor in the best interests of the woman or the fetus.
- Ending a prolonged second stage—The following periods are approximate; when these intervals are exceeded without continuing progress,

the risks and benefits of allowing labor to continue should be assessed and documented:

— Nulliparous patients: more than 3 hours with a regional anesthetic or more than 2 hours without a regional anesthetic

— Parous patients: more than 2 hours with a regional anesthetic or more than 1 hour without a regional anesthetic

- Nonreassuring fetal heart rate
- Maternal indications (eg, cardiac disease, exhaustion)

The following conditions are required for forceps or vacuum extraction operations:

- A person with privileges for such procedures
- Assessment of maternal pelvis–fetal size relationship, including clinical pelvimetry, and an estimation of fetal weight, and the position and station of the fetal calvarium
- Adequate anesthesia
- Willingness to abandon attempted operative vaginal delivery
- Ability to perform emergency cesarean delivery (see "readily available" in the "Preface" and in "Cesarean Delivery" in this chapter)

Cesarean Delivery

All hospitals offering labor and delivery services should be equipped to perform emergency cesarean delivery. The required personnel, including nurses, anesthesia personnel, neonatal resuscitation team members, and obstetric attendants, should be in the hospital or readily available (also see "Preface"). Any hospital providing an obstetric service should have the capability of responding to an obstetric emergency. No data correlate the timing of intervention with outcome, and there is little likelihood that any will be obtained. However, in general, the consensus has been that hospitals should have the capability of beginning a cesarean delivery within 30 minutes of the decision to operate. Some indications for cesarean delivery can be appropriately accommodated in longer than 30 minutes. Conversely, examples of indications that may mandate more expeditious delivery include hemorrhage from placenta previa, abruptio placentae, prolapse of the umbilical cord, and uterine rupture. Sterile materials and supplies needed for emergency cesarean delivery should be kept sealed but properly arranged so that the instrument table can be made ready at once for an obstetric emergency.

In-house obstetric and anesthesia coverage should be available in subspecialty-care units. The anesthesia and pediatric staff responsible for covering the labor and delivery unit should be informed in advance when a complicated delivery is anticipated and when a patient with risk factors requiring a high-acuity level of care is admitted.

Before elective, repeat cesarean delivery, the maturity of the fetus should be established. For patients with an indication for an elective repeat cesarean delivery, fetal maturity may be assumed if one of the following criteria is met:

- Fetal heart tones have been documented for 20 weeks by nonelectronic fetoscope or for 30 weeks by Doppler ultrasonography.

- Thirty-six weeks have elapsed since positive results were obtained from a serum or urine human chorionic gonadotropin pregnancy test performed by a reliable laboratory.

- An ultrasound measurement of the crown–rump length obtained at 6–11 weeks of gestation supports a current gestational age of 39 weeks or more.

- Clinical history and physical and ultrasound examinations performed at 12–20 weeks of gestation support a current gestational age of 39 weeks or more.

These criteria are not intended to preclude the use of menstrual dating. If any one criterion confirms gestational age assessment in a patient who has normal menstrual cycles and no immediate antecedent use of oral contraceptives, it is appropriate to schedule delivery at 39 weeks of gestation or later on the basis of menstrual dates. Another option is to await the onset of spontaneous labor. If delivery before 39 weeks of gestation or if the above criteria are not met, an amniocentesis to confirm the presence of indices of fetal pulmonary maturity is required before performing an elective cesarean delivery.

In women requiring cesarean delivery, fetal surveillance should continue until abdominal sterile preparation has begun. If internal fetal heart rate monitoring is in use, it should be continued until the abdominal sterile preparation is complete. Consideration should be given to the use of antiembolic elastic stockings or pneumatic compression boots in women considered at high risk for venous thromboembolism. When the cesarean delivery is performed for fetal indications, consideration should be given to sending the placenta for pathologic evaluation.

Multiple Gestation

The following factors should be considered in the delivery of multiple gestations:

- Labor and delivery—Confirmation of fetal presentations by ultrasound examination is indicated on admission. Each fetus should be monitored continuously during labor. Pediatric and anesthesia personnel should be immediately available, as well as blood bank services.

- Route of delivery—Controversy surrounds the preferred route of delivery for some multiple gestations, especially twins. Although cesarean delivery frequently is used for three or more fetuses, there are reports suggesting that vaginal delivery of triplet gestations, in appropriately monitored patients, is safe. Delivery should be based on individual needs and may depend on the clinician's practice and experience. In general, twins presenting as vertex–vertex should be anticipated to deliver vaginally. If the presenting twin is nonvertex, cesarean delivery is preferred by most physicians. In vertex–nonvertex presentations, cesarean delivery is not always necessary; vaginal delivery of twin B in the nonvertex presentation is a reasonable option for a neonate with an estimated weight greater than 1,500 g.

- Interval between deliveries—In the absence of other complications, such as bleeding or fetal heart rate abnormalities, the interval between deliveries for twins is not critical in determining the outcome of twin B. Following the delivery of twin A, the fetal heart rate of twin B should be monitored.

- A physician capable of carrying out an emergent cesarean delivery should manage the labor and delivery of patients with multiple gestations.

Support Persons in the Delivery Room

Childbirth is a momentous family experience. Obstetric providers willingly should provide opportunities for those accompanying and supporting the woman giving birth to participate in the process. These support persons must be informed about requirements for safety and must be willing to follow the directions of the obstetric staff concerning behavior in the delivery room. They also should understand the normal events and procedures in the labor and delivery area. They must conform to the dress code required of personnel in attendance in a delivery room. Both the obstetrician and the patient should consent to the presence of fathers, partners, or other support persons in the delivery room. Support persons should realize that their major function is to provide psychologic support to the mother during labor and delivery. Continuous support during labor from physicians, midwives, nurses, doulas, or lay individuals may have a number of benefits for women. Continuous presence of a support person appears to reduce the likelihood of medication for pain relief, operative vaginal delivery, cesarean delivery, and 5-minute Apgar scores less than 7.

The judgment of the obstetric staff, the individual obstetrician, the anesthesiologist, and the pediatric support personnel, as well as the policies of the hospital, determines whether support persons may be present at a cesarean delivery. A written policy developed by all involved hospital staff is recommended.

Postpartum Maternal Care

Immediate Postpartum Maternal Care

Monitoring of maternal status postpartum is dictated in part by the events of the delivery process, the type of anesthesia or analgesia used, and the complications identified. Postanesthesia pain management should be guided by protocols established by the anesthesiologists and obstetricians in concert. Blood pressure levels and pulse should be monitored at least every 15 minutes for 2 hours and more frequently and of longer duration if complications are encountered. The woman's temperature should be taken at least every 4 hours for 8 hours after delivery, then at least every 8 hours.

Nursing staff assigned to the delivery and immediate recovery of a woman should have no other obligations. Discharge from the delivery room, which may involve recovery from an anesthetic, should be at the discretion of the physician or certified nurse midwife or the anesthesiologist in charge.

When regional or general anesthesia has been used for either vaginal or cesarean delivery, the woman should be observed in an appropriately equipped LDR room or LDRP room or in an appropriately staffed and equipped postanesthesia care unit or equivalent area until she has recovered from the anesthetic. After cesarean delivery, policies for postanesthesia care should not differ from those applied to nonobstetric surgical patients receiving major anesthesia. Policy should ensure that a physician is available in the facility, or at least is nearby, to manage anesthetic complications and provide cardiopulmonary resuscitation for patients in the postanesthesia care unit. The patient should be discharged from the recovery area only at the discretion of, and after communication between, the attending physician or a certified nurse midwife, anesthesiologist, or certified registered nurse anesthetist in charge. Vital signs and additional signs or events should be monitored and recorded as they occur.

Postpartum Tubal Sterilization

In evaluating the feasibility and safety or advisability of immediate postpartum sterilization, consideration must be given to the advent of maternal or neonatal problems and other demands on obstetric and anesthesia staff. If postpartum tubal ligation is planned, the vaginal delivery has been uncomplicated, and the anesthetic can be continued safely, there is no contraindication to proceeding directly to the sterilization procedure. Preoperative care and evaluation, therefore, become part of delivery room care, especially if the delivery has taken place in a room designed and equipped for abdominal surgery. The obstetrician and anesthesiologist or certified registered nurse anesthetist should exercise medical judgment regarding the risks, benefits, and safety of the procedure.

When a woman has had prior or concurrent psychologic difficulties, the risks and benefits of early postpartum sterilization must be carefully considered and alternative contraceptive options reviewed. In patients who have had medical or obstetric complications during their pregnancy or who have cardiovascular, respiratory, infectious, or metabolic abnormalities during the peripartum period (such as serious anemia, hypovolemia, upper respiratory infections, or hypertension), the procedure should be deferred unless there are overriding medical indications for proceeding. Major physiologic changes occur at delivery in all patients. In particular, cardiovascular stability of the patient should be ensured.

In addition to such maternal considerations, special attention also must be paid to situations in which neonatal outcome is in doubt. Both infant survival and long-term well-being may ultimately influence a decision with respect to desire for a subsequent pregnancy.

Furthermore, consideration of the overall number of patients in relationship to available staffing of the labor–delivery suite also is relevant. An elective procedure, such as tubal ligation, should not be attempted at a time when it might compromise other aspects of patient care. Therefore, the decision to proceed with anesthesia and surgery should not only be a joint one between anesthesiologist and obstetrician but also one that appropriately involves the patient and nursing and pediatric personnel.

Subsequent Postpartum Care

The medical and nursing staff should cooperatively establish specific postpartum policies and procedures. In the postpartum period, staff should help the woman learn how to care for the general needs of herself and her neonate and should identify potential problems related to her general health.

The obstetric caregiver should note postpartum orders on the patient's medical record (see "ACOG Postpartum Form in Appendix A). If routine postpartum orders are used, they should be printed or written in the medical record, reviewed and modified as necessary for the particular patient, and signed by the obstetric caregiver before the patient is transferred to the postpartum unit. When an LDR or LDRP room is used, the same guidelines should apply.

Bed Rest, Ambulation, and Diet

It is important for the new mother to sleep, regain her strength, and recover from the effects of any analgesic or anesthetic agents that she may have received during labor. In the absence of complications, she may have a regular diet as soon as she wishes. Because early ambulation has been shown to decrease the incidence of subsequent thrombophlebitis, the mother should be encouraged to walk as soon as she feels able to do so. She should not attempt to get out of bed for the first time without assistance. She may shower as soon as she wishes. It may be necessary to administer fluids intravenously for hydration. If the patient has an intravenous line in place, her fluid and hemodynamic status should be evaluated before it is removed. If blood loss is greater than usual, the patient's hematocrit also should be assessed before discontinuing intravenous access.

Care of the Vulva

Traditional teaching includes that the patient should be taught to cleanse the vulva from anterior vulva to perineum and anus rather than in the reverse direction. Application of an ice bag to the perineum during the first 24 hours after delivery may help reduce pain and swelling that have resulted from pressure of the neonate's head. Orally administered analgesics often are required and usually are sufficient for relief of discomfort from episiotomy or repaired lacerations. Pain that is not relieved by such medication suggests hematoma formation and mandates a careful examination of the vulva, vagina, and rectum. Beginning 24 hours after delivery, moist heat in the form of a warm sitz bath may reduce local discomfort and promote healing.

Care of the Bladder

Women should be encouraged to void as soon as possible after delivery. Often women have difficulty voiding immediately after delivery, possibly because of trauma to the bladder during labor and delivery, regional anesthesia, or vulvar–perineal pain and swelling. In addition, the diuresis that often follows delivery can distend the bladder before the patient is aware of a sensation of a full bladder. To ensure adequate emptying of the bladder, the patient should be checked frequently during the first 24 hours after delivery, with particular attention to displacement of the uterine fundus and any indication of the presence of a fluid-filled bladder above the symphysis. Although every effort should be made to help the patient void spontaneously, catheterization may be necessary. If the patient continues to find voiding difficult, use of an indwelling catheter is preferable to repeated catheterization.

Care of the Breasts

The woman's decision about breastfeeding determines the appropriate care of the breasts. Breast care for a woman who chooses to breastfeed is outlined in Chapter 7. The woman who chooses not to breastfeed should be reassured that milk production will abate over the first few days after delivery if she does not breastfeed. During the stage of engorgement, the breasts may become painful and should be supported with a well-fitting brassiere. Ice packs and analgesics can help relieve discomfort during this period. Medications for lactation cessation are discouraged. Women who do not wish to breastfeed should be encouraged to avoid nipple stimulation and should be cautioned against continued manual expression of milk.

Temperature Elevation

The condition of a postpartum patient with an elevated temperature (38°C or higher [100.4°F or higher] on two occasions, 6 hours apart) should be evaluated (see "Endometritis" in Chapter 6). The nursery should be notified if the mother develops a fever at any time during the postpartum period, especially after the first 24 hours. Under most circumstances, the neonate need not be separated from the woman for infection control (see "Endometritis" in Chapter 6).

Postpartum Analgesia

After vaginal delivery, analgesic medication (including topical lidocaine cream) may be necessary to relieve perineal and episiotomy pain and facilitate maternal mobility. This is best addressed by administering the drug on an as-needed basis according to postpartum orders. Most mothers experience considerable pain in the first 24 hours after cesarean delivery. Although at one time pain most often was treated by intramuscular injections of narcotics, newer techniques, such as spinal or epidural opiates, patient-controlled epidural or intravenous analgesia, and potent oral analgesics provide better pain relief and greater patient satisfaction. Regardless of the route of administration, opioids potentially can cause respiratory depression and decrease intestinal motility. Therefore, adequate supervision and monitoring should be ensured for all postpartum patients receiving these drugs.

Immunization—Anti-D Immune Globulin, Tetanus–Diphtheria Acellular Pertussis, and Rubella

A woman who is unsensitized and D-negative and who gives birth to a neonate who is D-positive or Du-positive (ie, weak Rh positive) should receive 300 µg of anti-D immune globulin postpartum, ideally within 72 hours, even when anti-D immune globulin has been administered in the antepartum period. This dose may be inadequate in circumstances in which there is a potential for greater-than-average fetal-to-maternal hemorrhage, such as abruptio placentae, placenta previa, intrauterine manipulation, and manual removal of the placenta. In these cases, laboratory analysis should be performed to detect excessive maternal-to-fetal hemorrhage (eg, Kleihauer–Betke test) and determine the proper dose. If indicated, additional anti-D immune globulin should be given.

If a patient has not already received the tetanus–diphtheria acellular pertussis vaccine, and if it has been at least 2 years since her last tetanus–diphtheria booster, she should be given a dose before hospital discharge.

A patient who is identified as susceptible to rubella virus infection should receive the rubella vaccine in the postpartum period. The rubella vaccine can be administered before discharge, even if the patient is breastfeeding. Patients should be informed of the possibility of transient arthralgia and low-grade fever after rubella immunization.

Length of Hospital Stay

When no complications are present, the postpartum hospital stay ranges from 48 hours for vaginal delivery to 96 hours for cesarean delivery, excluding the day of delivery. When the physician and the mother want a shortened hospital stay, certain minimal criteria should be met:

- The mother is afebrile, with pulse and respirations of normal rate and quality.

- Her blood pressure level is within the normal range.
- The amount and color of lochia are appropriate for the duration of recovery.
- The uterine fundus is firm.
- Urinary output is adequate.
- Any surgical repair or wound has minimal edema and no evidence of infection and appears to be healing without complication.
- The mother is able to ambulate with ease and has adequate pain control.
- There are no abnormal physical or emotional findings.
- The mother is able to eat and drink without difficulty.
- Arrangements have been made for postpartum follow-up care.
- The mother has been instructed in caring for herself and the neonate at home, is aware of deviations from normal, and is prepared to recognize and respond to danger signs and symptoms.
- The mother demonstrates readiness to care for herself and her newborn.
- Pertinent laboratory results are available, including a postpartum measurement of hemoglobin or hematocrit, if indicated by excessive intrapartum or postpartum blood loss.
- ABO blood group and Rh D type are known, and, if indicated, the appropriate amount of anti-D immune globulin has been administered.
- The mother has received instructions on postpartum activity and exercises and common postpartum discomforts and relief measures.
- Family members or other support persons are available to the mother for the first few days following discharge.

The medical and nursing staff should be sensitive to potential problems associated with shortened hospital stays and should develop mechanisms to address patient questions that arise after discharge. With a shortened hospital stay, a home visit or follow-up telephone conference by a health care provider, such as a lactation nurse, within 48 hours of discharge is encouraged.

When a pregnancy, labor, or delivery is complicated by medical or obstetric disorders, the mother's readiness for discharge may be based on the aforementioned criteria, as modified by the individual judgment of the obstetric care provider. The stability of the woman's medical condition, the need for continued inpatient observation, and treatment and risks of complications should be taken into consideration.

Postpartum Nutritional Guidelines

Postnatal dietary guidelines are similar to those established during pregnancy (see Table 4-2 in Chapter 4). The minimal caloric requirement for adequate milk production in a woman of average size is 1,800 kcal per day. In general, an additional 500 kcal of energy daily is recommended throughout lactation. A balanced, nutritious diet will ensure both the quality and the quantity of the milk produced without depletion of maternal stores. Fluid intake by the mother is governed by thirst.

A vitamin–mineral supplement is not needed routinely. Mothers at nutritional risk should be given a multivitamin supplement with particular emphasis on calcium and vitamins B_{12} and D. Iron should be administered only if the mother herself needs it.

Maternal postpartum weight loss can occur at a rate of 2 lb per month without affecting lactation. On average, a woman will retain 2 lb more than her prepregnancy weight at 1 year postpartum. There is no relationship between body mass index or total weight gain and weight retention. Aging, rather than parity, is the major determinant of increases in a woman's weight over time.

Residual postpartum retention of weight gained during pregnancy that results in obesity is a concern. Special attention to lifestyle, including exercise and eating habits, will help these women return to a normal body mass index.

Postpartum Considerations

Before discharge, the mother should receive information about the following normal postpartum events:

- Changes in lochia pattern expected in the first few weeks
- Range of activities that she may reasonably undertake
- Care of the breasts, perineum, and bladder
- Dietary needs, particularly if she is breastfeeding
- Recommended amount of exercise
- Emotional responses
- Signs of complications (eg, temperature elevation, chills, leg pains, episiotomy or wound drainage, or increased vaginal bleeding)

The length of convalescence that the patient can expect, based on the type of delivery, also should be discussed. For women who have had cesarean delivery, additional precautions may be appropriate, such as wound care and temporary abstinence from lifting objects heavier than the newborn and from driving motor vehicles. It is helpful to reinforce oral discussions with written information.

The earliest time at which coitus may be resumed safely after childbirth is unknown. Resumption of coitus should be discussed with the couple. Risks of hemorrhage and infection are minimal approximately by 2 weeks postpartum. By this time, the uterus has involuted markedly and the endometrium and cervix have begun to reepithelialize. Thereafter, coitus can be resumed, depending on the patient's desire and comfort and on resolution of contraceptive issues.

Sexual difficulties that are common in the early months after childbirth should be discussed. Healing at the episiotomy site can cause the woman some discomfort during intercourse within the first year following delivery. In the lactating woman, the vagina often is atrophic and dry. Natural lubrication during sexual excitement may be unsatisfactory. Furthermore, the demands of the newborn's care alter the couple's ability to find time for physical intimacy.

Methods of contraception should be fully reviewed and implemented. In women who breastfeed exclusively, a return to fertility is delayed. When carefully defined criteria are met (see ACOG/AAP Breastfeeding Handbook for Physicians), the Lactational Amenorrhea Method can be used as a reliable form of contraception temporarily. Nonnursing mothers should begin using a contraceptive soon after delivery if they wish to avoid becoming pregnant. Combined oral contraceptives may be prescribed if there is no personal or family history of venous thrombosis and no known significant thrombophilia is present. Nonnursing women may receive depot medroxyprogesterone acetate within 5 days after delivery.

Progesterone-only contraceptives do not appear to have adverse effects on lactation. Women may consider initiating progesterone-only contraceptives at 6 weeks if breastfeeding exclusively, at 3 weeks if not exclusively. However, in certain situations, such as concern about patient follow-up, an earlier start may be appropriate. An intrauterine device that contains copper also is an option that does not interfere with breast milk. However, intrauterine devices generally are not inserted until 4–6 weeks postpartum. While progestin-only preparations remain the oral contraception of choice for breastfeeding women, they may begin using oral combined estrogen–progestin contraceptives at 6 weeks after delivery if breastfeeding is well established and the infant's nutritional status is monitored. If follow-up concerns are strong enough to consider an earlier start, that should be only after the period of hypercoagulability associated with pregnancy has resolved (ie, 2–4 weeks).

Patients for whom the use of oral contraceptives is contraindicated or who prefer other methods of contraception, such as foam or condoms, should be offered instruction in their use. Spermicides and barrier methods have no effect on breastfeeding. Lubricated condoms may offset vaginal dryness secondary to breastfeeding. A diaphragm or a cervical cap cannot be fitted adequately during the immediate postpartum period and should be delayed until the 4- to 6-week examination. Fertility awareness methods, such as the rhythm method, are difficult to practice accurately before the resumption of menses and, therefore, are not recommended.

At the time of discharge, the family should be given the name of the person to contact if questions or problems arise for either the mother or the newborn. Arrangements should be made for a follow-up examination and specific instructions conveyed to the woman, including when contact is advisable.

In general, the following points should be reviewed with the mother or, preferably, with both parents; specific information to be conveyed is discussed within this section:

- Condition of the newborn
- Immediate needs of the newborn (eg, feeding methods and environmental supports)
- Feeding techniques; skin care, including umbilical cord care; temperature assessment and measurement with a thermometer; and assessment of neonatal well-being and recognition of illness
- Roles of the obstetrician, pediatrician, and other members of the health care team concerned with the continuous medical care of the mother and the newborn
- Availability of support systems, including psychosocial support
- Instructions to follow in the event of a complication or emergency
- Importance of maintaining newborn immunization, beginning with an initial dose of hepatitis B virus vaccine. (For more information, see "Discharge" in Chapter 7.)

Follow-up Care

The physical and psychosocial status of the mother and the newborn should be subject to ongoing assessment after discharge. The new mother needs personalized care during the postpartum period to hasten the development of a healthy mother–infant relationship and a sense of maternal confidence. Support and reassurance should be provided as the woman masters newborn-care tasks and adapts to her maternal role. Involving the father and encouraging him to participate in the newborn's care not only can provide additional support to the woman but also can enhance the father–infant relationship.

For many women, the postpartum period can be a stressful time and may lead to the onset of mood disorders. Some patients experience postpartum "blues," which normally occur within 2–4 days postpartum. The patient's mood usually is labile, and she may feel happy or excited, only to be sad, depressed, anxious, and irritable hours later. Symptoms generally are mild and self-limited. Supportive care and reassurance are helpful in ensuring that symptoms are time-limited. However, all women with postpartum blues should be monitored for the onset of continuing or worsening symptoms because women with the blues are at high risk for the onset of a more serious condition (see also "Psychosocial Services" in Chapter 4). The incidence of postpartum major or minor depressive disorders varies from 10% to 15%, and treatment with an antidepressant drug generally is recommended for a major depressive disorder. It should be noted that recurrent depression might occur following discontinuation of psychotropic medication. Postpartum psychosis is the most severe form of mental derangement and is most common in women with preexisting disorders, such as manic–depressive illness or, less commonly, schizophrenia. Women with postpartum psychosis show severe symptoms, such as an inability to sleep and strange notions about their neonate as well as other significant individuals in their lives. This should be considered a psychiatric emergency and the patient should be referred for immediate, often inpatient, treatment.

The postpartum period is a time of developmental adjustment for the whole family. Family members have new roles and relationships, and an effort should be made to assess the progress of the family's adaptation. If a family member—parent or sibling—finds it difficult to assume the new role, the health care team should arrange for sensitive, supportive assistance. This is particularly important for adolescent mothers, for whom it may be necessary to mobilize multiple resources within the community.

Postpartum Visits

Approximately 4–6 weeks after delivery, the mother should visit her physician for a postpartum review and examination (see Appendix G). This interval may be modified according to the needs of the patient with medical, obstetric, or intercurrent complications. A visit within 7–14 days of delivery may be advisable after a cesarean delivery or a complicated gestation, such as a patient requiring antihypertensives for after-treatment of severe preeclampsia or severe hypertension.

The review at the first postpartum visit should include obtaining an interval history and performing a physical examination to evaluate the patient's current status and her adaptation to the newborn. Specific inquiries regarding breastfeeding should be made. The examination should include an evaluation of weight, blood pressure levels, breasts (if not lactating or if there are specific complaints in lactating women), and abdomen as well as a pelvic examination. Episiotomy repair and uterine involution should be evaluated and a Pap test performed, if needed. Methods of birth control should be reviewed or initiated.

As noted above, many women experience some degree of emotional lability in the postpartum period. If this persists or develops into clinically significant depression, intervention may be needed. The emotional status of a woman whose pregnancy had an abnormal outcome also should be reviewed. Counseling should address specific issues regarding her future health and pregnancies. For example, it may be advantageous to discuss VBAC or the implications of diabetes mellitus, intrauterine growth restriction, preterm birth, hypertension, fetal anomalies, or other conditions that may recur in any future pregnancy. Laboratory data should be obtained as indicated. This is a good time to review immunizations, including rubella vaccination for women who are susceptible and did not receive the vaccine immediately postpartum, and to discuss any special problems. The patient should be encouraged to return for subsequent periodic examinations.

The postpartum visit is an excellent time to begin preconception counseling for patients who may wish to have future pregnancies (see also "Preconception Care" in Chapter 4). This counseling includes risk assessment to facilitate the planning, spacing, and timing of the next pregnancy; health promotion measures; and timely intervention to reduce medical and psychosocial risks. Such intervention may include treatment of infections; counseling regarding behaviors, such as those related to sexually transmitted infections; nutrition counseling and supplementation; and appropriate referrals for follow-up care. Although physiologic considerations indicate that a woman can return to a normal work schedule 4–6 weeks after delivery, attention also should be given to maternal–infant bonding.

Resources

A multicentre randomised trial of amniotomy in spontaneous first labour at term. The UK Amniotomy Group. Br J Obstet Gynaecol 1994;101:307–9.

American Academy of Pediatrics, American College of Obstetricians and Gynecologists. Neonatal encephalopathy and cerebral palsy: defining the pathogenesis and pathophysiology. Elk Grove Village (IL): AAP; Washington, DC: ACOG; 2003.

American Academy of Pediatrics, American Heart Association. Neonatal resuscitation textbook. 5th ed. Elk Grove Village (IL): AAP; Dallas (TX): AHA; 2006.

American College of Obstetricians and Gynecologists. Assessment of fetal lung maturity. ACOG Educational Bulletin 230. Washington, DC: ACOG; 1996.

American College of Obstetricians and Gynecologists. Evaluation of cesarean delivery. Washington, DC: ACOG; 2000.

American College of Obstetricians and Gynecologists. Induction of labor. ACOG Practice Bulletin 10. Washington, DC: ACOG; 1999.

American College of Obstetricians and Gynecologists. Induction of labor with misoprostol. ACOG Committee Opinion 228. Washington, DC: ACOG; 1999.

American College of Obstetricians and Gynecologists. Operative vaginal delivery. ACOG Practice Bulletin 17. Washington, DC: ACOG; 2000.

American College of Obstetricians and Gynecologists. Response to Searle's drug warning on misoprostol. Committee Opinion 248. Washington, DC: ACOG; 2000.

American College of Obstetricians and Gynecologists, American Society of Anesthesiologists. Optimal goals for anesthesia care in obstetrics. ACOG Committee Opinion 256. Washington, DC: ACOG; Park Ridge (IL): ASA; 2001.

Analgesia and cesarean delivery rates. ACOG Committee Opinion No. 339. American College of Obstetricians and Gynecologists. Obstet Gynecol 2006;107:1487–8.

The Apgar score. ACOG Committee Opinion No. 333. American College of Obstetricians and Gynecologists, American Academy of Pediatrics. Obstet Gynecol 2006;107:1209–12.

Dystocia and augmentation of labor. ACOG Practice Bulletin No. 49. American College of Obstetricians and Gynecologists. Obstet Gynecol 2003;102:1445–54.

Episiotomy. ACOG Practice Bulletin No. 71. American College of Obstetricians and Gynecologists. Obstet Gynecol 2006;107:957–62.

Intrapartum fetal heart rate monitoring. ACOG Practice Bulletin No. 70. American College of Obstetricians and Gynecologists. Obstet Gynecol 2005;106:1453–60.

Inappropriate use of the terms fetal distress and birth asphyxia. ACOG Committee Opinion No. 326. American College of Obstetricians and Gynecologists. Obstet Gynecol 2005;106:1469–70.

Induction of labor for vaginal birth after cesarean delivery. ACOG Committee Opinion No. 342. American College of Obstetricians and Gynecologists. Obstet Gynecol 2006; 108:465–67.

Influenza vaccination and treatment during pregnancy. ACOG Committee Opinion No. 305. American College of Obstetricians and Gynecologists. Obstet Gynecol 2004;104:1125–6.

Intrapartum fetal heart rate monitoring. ACOG Practice Bulletin No. 70. American College of Obstetricians and Gynecologists. Obstet Gynecol 2005;106:1453–60.

Management of postterm pregnancy. ACOG Practice Bulletin No. 55. American College of Obstetricians and Gynecologists. Obstet Gynecol 2004;104:639–46.

Mode of term singleton breech delivery. ACOG Committee Opinion No. 340. American College of Obstetricians and Gynecologists. Obstet Gynecol 2006;108:235–7.

Multiple gestation: complicated twin, triplet, and high-order multifetal pregnancy. ACOG Practice Bulletin No. 56. American College of Obstetricians and Gynecologists. Obstet Gynecol 2004;104:869–83.

National Institute of Child Health and Human Development. Report of the workshop on acute perinatal asphyxia in term infants. NIH publication 96-3823. Washington, DC: NICHHD; 1996.

Neurological and Psychiatric Disorders. Cunningham FG, Leveno KJ, Bloom SL, Hauth JC, Gilstrap LC, Wenstrom KD. In: Williams Obstetrics. 22nd ed. New York (NY): McGraw-Hill; 2005; p. 1229–48.

New U.S. Food and Drug Administration labeling on Cytotec (misoprostol) use and pregnancy. ACOG Committee Opinion No. 283. American College of Obstetricians and Gynecologists. Obstet Gynecol 2003;101:1049–50.

Obstetric analgesia and anesthesia. ACOG Practice Bulletin No. 36. American College of Obstetricians and Gynecologists. Obstet Gynecol 2002;100:177–91.

Pain relief during labor. ACOG Committee Opinion No. 295. American College of Obstetricians and Gynecologists, American Society of Anesthesiologists. Obstet Gynecol 2004;104:213.

Pierce J, Gaudier FL, Sanchez-Ramos L Intrapartum amnioinfusion for meconium-stained fluid: meta-analysis of prospective clinical trials. Obstet Gynecol 2000;95:1051–6.

Pitt C, Sanchez-Ramos L, Kaunitz AM, Gaudier F. Prophylactic amnioinfusion for intrapartum oligohydramnios: a meta-analysis of randomized controlled trials. Obstet Gynecol 2000;96:861–6.

Premature rupture of membranes. ACOG Practice Bulletin No. 80. American College of Obstetricians and Gynecologists. Obstet Gynecol 2007;109:1007–19.

Prophylactic antibiotics in labor and delivery. ACOG Practice Bulletin No. 47. American College of Obstetricians and Gynecologists. Obstet Gynecol 2003;102:975–82.

Vaginal birth after previous cesarean delivery. ACOG Practice Bulletin No. 54. American College of Obstetricians and Gynecologists. Obstet Gynecol 2004;104:203–12.

Wong CA, Scavone BM, Peaceman AM, McCarthy RJ, Sullivan JT, Diaz NT, et al. The risk of cesarean delivery with neuraxial analgesia given early versus late in labor. N Engl J Med 2005;352:655–65.

chapter 6

Obstetric and Medical Complications

Certain complications of pregnancy, labor, or delivery may require more intensive surveillance, monitoring, and special care of the obstetric patient. Often, complications can arise without warning. In some cases, early detection and timely intervention can improve outcome. When there is a high risk of complications, it may be advisable to make arrangements for such care in advance. The pediatric and anesthesia services should be made aware of such patients so that appropriate medical care can be planned in advance of the delivery.

Management of Preterm Birth

Preterm delivery is the leading cause of neonatal mortality in the United States and accounts for 35% of all U.S. health care spending for infants and 10% of all such spending for children. Preterm birth is defined as delivery before 37 weeks of gestation; it occurs in approximately 12.5% of all live births. Although significant complications of premature delivery are most evident in delivery before 34 weeks of gestation, improvement in outcome should be sought for all infants before 37 weeks of gestation.

Of all preterm births, 40–50% result from preterm labor with intact fetal membranes, approximately 25–40% from preterm premature rupture of membranes (PROM), and 20–30% from maternal medical or obstetric complications that require early delivery. Ideally, preterm birth should occur in a hospital setting with personnel and equipment appropriate for the stage of gestation. Very low birth weight neonates (weighing less than 1,500 g) should be delivered in a subspecialty care facility whenever possible. No effective method of preventing most preterm births has been discovered; however, weekly intramuscular administration of 17 α-hydroxyprogesterone caproate (250 mg), beginning at 16–20 weeks of gestation and continuing until 36 weeks of gestation, appears to reduce spontaneous preterm births in a select group of women at very high risk who have a documented history of previous spontaneous birth at less than 37 weeks of gestation. The use of tocolytic drugs may prolong gestation for 2–7 days, which can provide time for administration of steroids and maternal transport to a facility with a neonatal intensive care unit. Corticosteroids are effective in enhancing fetal maturity when a woman is at risk of preterm birth (see "Antenatal Corticosteroid Administration" in this chapter).

Preterm Labor

Preterm labor is defined as regular contractions that occur before 37 weeks of gestation and are associated with changes in the cervix. Strategies for reducing the incidence of preterm birth in the United States have failed. Included among them have been enhanced physician and patient education about the risks for preterm labor, early detection via uterine activity monitoring, and prophylactic treatments, such as antibiotics. The goal continues to be early detection of preterm labor to allow administration of corticosteroids and delivery at a site capable of providing the needed care for the neonate. Ultrasound measurement of cervical length and fetal fibronectin testing each have good negative predictive value; thus, either approach or both combined may be helpful in determining which patients do not need tocolysis or steroids.

Diagnosis

Patients with suspected preterm labor should be examined and observed for 1–2 hours and should have their uterine activity monitored to confirm whether it is significant and whether the cervix has changed since the most recent examination. After observation, the cervical examination should be repeated, preferably by the same examiner, to determine whether cervical dilation or effacement is taking place. Alternatively, cervical length can be assessed by transvaginal ultrasound examination or vaginal fetal fibronectin assessment or both. Because preterm labor often is associated with urinary tract infections, a dipstick or a microscopic examination of urine and urine culture may be helpful. Based on the test results, antibiotic treatment can be instituted. Ultrasound examination also may be considered to confirm gestational age and to assess the presence of any congenital anomalies.

Once preterm labor is diagnosed on the basis of these evaluations, consideration should be given to initiating interventions, such as tocolysis, corticosteroid therapy, and chemoprophylaxis for group B streptococcal infection (see

"Tocolysis" and "Antenatal Corticosteroid Administration" in this chapter and "Group B Streptococci" in Chapter 9). Women diagnosed as having false labor may be discharged with outpatient follow-up.

Occult Infection

Because infections have been implicated as both a cause and a consequence of ruptured membranes, the diagnosis of infection is an important component of the evaluation of preterm labor. This diagnosis may be difficult to establish because clinical signs of infection may be absent at the initial evaluation. A variety of organisms, including group B streptococci, *Neisseria gonorrhoeae*, *Listeria monocytogenes*, *Mycoplasma* species, *Bacteroides* species, and *Ureaplasma* species, have been identified in amniotic fluid. Although the threshold at which colonization is significant enough to result in preterm labor has not been defined and the exact proportion of preterm labor that is attributable to infection is unknown, the incidence of infection is highest with ruptured membranes. In the presence of infection, the time from the onset of preterm labor to delivery is shorter, and preterm PROM is more likely. Treating women in preterm labor with antibiotics for the sole purpose of preventing preterm delivery is not recommended. While protocols for antibiotic prophylaxis against early-onset group B streptococcal sepsis should be followed, there is little evidence that this will prolong the pregnancy.

Intraamniotic Infection

Preterm labor may be the first sign of intraamniotic infection in the absence of rupture of the membranes. Organisms may be recovered from the chorioamnion in as much as 60% of women in preterm labor with intact membranes and from the amniotic fluid in 10–15% of women who are not in labor and have intact membranes. Preterm labor at early gestational ages is more likely to be associated with occult intraamniotic infection. Women with poor nutrition or of a low socioeconomic status may be at higher risk for this complication. Intraamniotic infection also may follow cervical cerclage. Diagnosis of occult infection may require amniocentesis.

All patients in preterm labor should be evaluated for evidence of intraamniotic infection. Maternal temperature and white blood cell count should be documented, and the uterus should be palpated for tenderness. Maternal or fetal tachycardia could indicate intraamniotic infection. Amniocentesis may be appropriate to detect the presence of occult intraamniotic infection by revealing a low amniotic fluid glucose concentration, the presence of white blood cells, or a positive culture.

When intraamniotic infection is diagnosed during pregnancy, broad-spectrum antibiotic therapy should be initiated and delivery effected. Vaginal delivery should be anticipated, and cesarean delivery should be reserved for standard obstetric indications. The choice of antibiotics should take into consideration the polymicrobial nature of most uterine infections that reflect endogenous vaginal flora. The combination of ampicillin or penicillin, plus an aminoglycoside, provides appropriate coverage of most organisms. If a cesarean delivery is required, anaerobes play a prominent role in postpartum endomyometritis, and clindamycin or metronidazole should be added to the regimen. Extended spectrum cephalosporins also provide appropriate coverage if a cesarean delivery is needed. Antibiotics should be given intravenously to minimize serious complications of infection in the woman and to prevent or treat transplacental infection of the fetus.

Tocolysis

Tocolytic agents do not appear to markedly prolong the length of gestation, but they may delay delivery in some women for at least 48 hours and provide a window of opportunity for transporting the patient to a regional subspecialty obstetric center and administering antenatal corticosteroid therapy. Many agents have been used, including magnesium sulfate, calcium channel blockers, oxytocin antagonists, nonsteroidal antiinflammatory drugs, and β-mimetic agonists. There is no evidence that prolonged, subcutaneous β-adrenergic pump therapy prolongs gestation beyond 48 hours, and this treatment may pose risks to the mother.

Antenatal corticosteroid therapy should be given to enhance fetal maturation at less than 34 weeks of gestation or when fetal lung immaturity has been documented (see "Antenatal Corticosteroid Administration" in this chapter).

Preterm Premature Rupture of Membranes

Preterm PROM is a major risk factor for obstetric complications because of its association with perinatal infection, preterm delivery, fetal deformation, pulmonary hypoplasia, and resultant complications. Preterm PROM is responsible for 25–35% of all preterm deliveries, depending on racial and socioeconomic considerations.

The status of the fetus should be assessed by fetal heart rate monitoring, with particular attention to variable decelerations that are suggestive of umbilical cord compression. Determining whether the woman is in labor may be difficult because repetitive digital examination of the cervix should be avoided until active labor occurs or until the decision has been made to induce labor.

When preterm PROM occurs, expectant management usually is attempted. Patients with PROM before 32 weeks of gestation should be managed expectantly until 33 completed weeks of gestation if no maternal or fetal contraindications exist. Delivery is recommended when PROM occurs at or beyond 34 weeks of gestation based on some data that the risks of fetal complications outweigh the risks of preterm delivery at this point. With PROM at 32–33 completed weeks of gestation, labor induction may be considered if fetal pulmonary maturity has been documented. The hospital's departments of obstetrics and gynecology and pediatrics should develop guidelines for the management of preterm PROM, recognizing the need to individualize patient care. If expectant management is chosen in a woman with preterm PROM, bed rest is indicated. For a woman with preterm PROM and a viable fetus, the safety of expectant management at home has not been established. Ongoing evaluations of maternal and fetal status should be performed.

The prophylactic use of antibiotics can prolong gestation in women with preterm PROM and may improve perinatal outcome. A 48-hour course of intravenous ampicillin and erythromycin followed by 5 days of amoxicillin and erythromycin is recommended during expectant management of preterm PROM remote from term to prolong pregnancy and to reduce infectious and gestational age-dependent neonatal morbidity. All women with PROM and a viable fetus, including those known to be group B streptococcus carriers and those who give birth before carrier status can be delineated, should receive intrapartum chemoprophylaxis to prevent vertical transmission of group B streptococcus regardless of prior treatments.

A single course of antenatal corticosteroids should be administered to women with PROM before 32 weeks of gestation to reduce the risks of respiratory distress syndrome, perinatal mortality, and composite morbidities. The efficacy of corticosteroid use at 32–33 completed weeks of gestation is unclear based on available evidence, but treatment may be beneficial, particularly if pulmonary immaturity is documented. Tocolytic agents may be useful to permit administration of corticosteroids and antibiotics and to facilitate transfer to a subspecialty care center.

When preterm PROM occurs before a viable gestational age, conservative management is unlikely to result in the delivery of a healthy neonate and entails significant risk of maternal morbidity. Such management may produce very preterm neonates, resulting in mortality or significant short- and long-term morbidity (see "Births at the Threshold of Viability"). Some women may elect induction of labor with no expectation of neonatal survival or resuscitation. If the woman elects to continue the pregnancy, management at home may be considered. It is strongly suggested that women who have preterm PROM at a previable gestational age be counseled by both an obstetrician and a pediatrician. A woman should participate fully in the decision regarding her pregnancy, and adequate time should be allowed for her to make an informed decision. In the presence of intraamniotic infection, delivery is indicated.

Antenatal Corticosteroid Administration

Antenatal corticosteroid therapy to induce fetal maturation is effective in reducing respiratory distress syndrome, intraventricular hemorrhage, and mortality in preterm neonates. These benefits accrue at less than 34 weeks of gestation and are not limited by sex or race. Optimal benefits begin 24 hours after the initiation of therapy and last 7 days, although treatment of less than 24 hours duration also may improve outcomes. Antenatal corticosteroid therapy also may complement the benefit of postnatal surfactant therapy and should be considered an urgent drug to be given as soon as possible.

Following a 2000 consensus conference, the National Institutes of Health affirmed their 1994 recommendation of giving a single course of corticosteroids to all pregnant women between 24 weeks and 34 weeks of gestation who are at risk of preterm delivery within 7 days. Repeated corticosteroid courses should not be used routinely because clinical trials show decreased brain size, decreased birth weight, and adrenal insufficiency in neonates exposed to repeated doses. Treatment should consist of two doses of 12 mg of betamethasone given intramuscularly 24 hours apart or four doses of 6 mg dexamethasone given intramuscularly every 12 hours. A single course of antenatal corticosteroids should be administered to women with PROM before 32 weeks of gestation to reduce the risks of respiratory distress syndrome, prenatal mortality, and other morbidities. The efficacy of corticosteroid use at 32–33 completed weeks of gestation is unclear based on available evidence, but treatment may be beneficial, particularly if pulmonary immaturity is documented.

Data from trials involving the follow-up of children for as long as 12 years indicate that single-course antenatal corticosteroid therapy does not adversely affect physical growth or psychomotor development. Therefore, with few exceptions, antenatal corticosteroid therapy is indicated for women with anticipated preterm delivery at less than 34 weeks of gestation. The use of antenatal corticosteroid therapy after 34 weeks of gestation is not recommended unless there is evidence of fetal pulmonary immaturity. The use of antenatal corticosteroids for fetal maturation is an example of an intervention technology that yields substantial cost savings in addition to improving health.

Births at the Threshold of Viability

Early preterm birth or birth of an extremely low birth weight (LBW) infant (less than 1,000 g), especially those weighing less than 750 g or less than 26 weeks of gestation, poses a variety of complex medical, social, and ethical considerations. The effect of such births on the infants, their families, the health care system, and society is profound. Although the prevalence of such births is less than 1%, they account for nearly one half of all cases of perinatal mortality. Until recently, discussion of clinical management and ethical and economic considerations of extremely preterm births were hampered by conflicting and insufficiently detailed outcome data.

Information from large multicenter studies, such as those sponsored by the National Institute of Child Health and Human Development (NICHD), provides sufficiently detailed data to assist the perinatal team in developing an evidence-based approach to managing the extremely preterm infant. Survival rates are directly related to birth weight, as shown in Figure 6–1. However, the combination of birth weight, gestational age, and gender provides the best estimate of chance of survival (Fig. 6–2). Data stratified by week and day of gestation are particularly important for these infants because even a few days difference in age can be associated with a dramatic difference in expected outcome.

Neonatal Mortality

An effort should be made to provide families with information specific to the gestational age, estimated weight, and gender of their fetus. A multidisciplinary team approach to counseling may be helpful in ensuring that the information provided is consistent and represents a range of concerns and areas of clinical care. Counseling from a practitioner with additional experience and expertise in extremely preterm and LBW births is encouraged where available.

When gestational age, birth weight, and gender are combined (Fig. 6–2), it becomes evident that at each gestational age, a lower birth weight carries a higher mortality risk. This effect is most pronounced in the lower ranges of gestational age and birth weight. In addition, when infants of similar gestational age and weight are compared, mortality rates are higher for males than

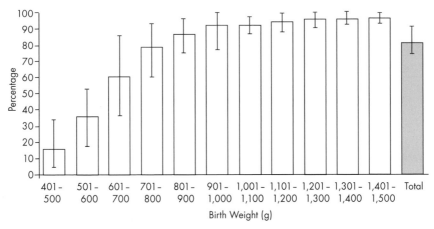

Fig. 6–1. Survival rates by birth rate, 1997–2002. Survival to discharge by birthweight in 100-g increments among infants born in National Institute of Child Health and Human Development Neonatal Research Network centers between January 1, 1997, and December 31, 2002, with center variability. (Fanaroff AA, Stoll BJ, Wright LL, Carlo WA, Ehrenkranz RA, Stark AR, et al. Trends in neonatal morbidity and mortality for very low birthweight infants. National Institutes for Child Health and Human Development Neonatal Research Network. Am J Obstet Gynecol 2007;196:147.e1–147.e8. Copyright © 2007, with permission from Elsevier.)

for females. For example, a male born at 24 weeks of gestation weighing 700 g has a predicted mortality rate of 51%, whereas a female of the same age and weight has a predicted mortality rate of 35%.

Neonatal Morbidity

A gestational-age-based population study of 3,785 extremely preterm newborns (gestational age 22–32 weeks) born between 1993 and 1998 within the NICHD Neonatal Research Network provided outcome data related to mental and psychomotor development, neuromotor function, and sensory and communication function at 18–22 months of corrected age. The infants were divided into early (22–26 weeks) or later (27–32 weeks) gestation, and into three epochs based on year of birth (1993–1994, 1995–1996, and 1997–1998). Overall survival and neurodevelopmental outcome improved over the three epochs. As expected, survival and neurodevelopmental outcome were better in the later-gestation infants. Male newborns had lower psychomotor scores and were significantly more likely to have cerebral palsy than female

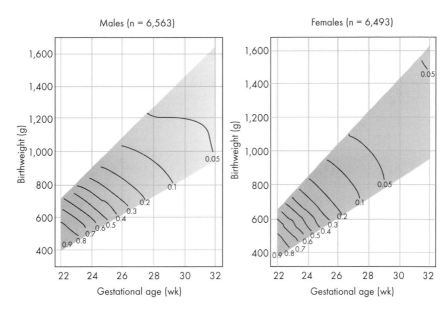

Fig. 6-2. Mortality by birth weight, gestational age, and gender. The limits of the shaded area indicate the upper 95th and lower 5th percentiles of birthweight for each gestational age. The curved lines indicate combinations of birthweight and gestational age with the same estimated probability of mortality (ie, 10-90%). The methods used underestimate mortality at 22 weeks and 23 weeks of gestation with a birthweight up to 600 g. (Fanaroff AA, Stoll BJ, Wright LL, Carlo WA, Ehrenkranz RA, Stark AR, et al. Trends in neonatal morbidity and mortality for very low birthweight infants. National Institutes for Child Health and Human Development Neonatal Research Network. Am J Obstet Gynecol 2007;196: 147.e1-147.e8. Copyright © 2007, with permission from Elsevier.)

newborns. A similar disadvantage for male newborns has been reported in other studies.

The major morbidities influencing later development in these children included chronic lung disease, severe brain injury (intraventricular hemorrhage and periventricular leukomalacia), necrotizing enterocolitis, nosocomial infection, and retinopathy of prematurity. Neurologic outcome at 18–22 months of corrected age by epoch and gestational age is shown in Table 6–1.

In the NICHD Neonatal Research Network multicenter prospective study, sample size was sufficient to overcome some of the limitations that hampered the clinical applicability of earlier longitudinal outcome studies. In the earlier gestational age group, approximately one third had a Bayley II Mental

Table 6–1. Neurodevelopmental Outcomes of Extremely Low Birth Weight Cohort Evaluated at 18 Months Corrected Age by Epoch and Gestational Age*

	1993–1994		1995–1996		1997–1998	
	22–26 weeks GA	27–32 weeks GA	22–26 weeks GA	27–32 weeks GA	22–26 weeks GA	27–32 weeks GA
Evaluated at 18 mo	665	444	716	538	910	512
CP	20.1	12.4	18.7	11.2	18.1	11.3
Moderate to severe CP	12.1	7.8	10.8	7.1	10.4	6.3
Bayley MDI less than 70	41.8	29.9	38.5	25.5	37.2	22.8
PDI less than 70	31.6	23.4	31.8	18.3	26	16.9
Blind unilateral[†]	4.2	2.1	2.5	1.1	1.6	0.8
Blind bilateral	2.3	1.4	1.5	0.4	1	0.4
Permanent hearing loss[‡]	3.4	1.7	2.3	0.8	1.8	1.8
Hydrocephalus with shunt	3	1.8	2.5	0.7	3.6	1
Seizures	5	5.2	4.5	6.2	3.4	3.9
NDI[§]	50.2	39.8	47.2	31.7	44.6	27.8

Abbreviations: CP, cerebral palsy; GA, gestational age; MDI, mental development index; NDI, neurodevelopmental impairment, PDI, psychomotor development index

*Data are expressed as percentages except where noted.

[†]Blindness is defined as blind with no functional vision.

[‡]Hearing loss requiring amplification in both ears.

[§]Includes the presence of any of the following factors: moderate to severe CP, MDI less than 70, PDI less than 70, blindness in both eyes, or hearing loss requiring amplification in both ears.

Modified from Vohr BR, Wright LL, Poole WK, McDonald SA. Neurodevelopmental outcomes of extremely low birth weight infants <32 weeks' gestation between 1993 and 1998. Pediatrics 2005;116:635–43.

Development Index score of less than 70 or a Psychomotor Developmental Index score of less than 70 (normal for both these indices is greater than 80), and 10% had moderate-to-severe cerebral palsy. The incidence of visual and hearing impairment decreased over the epochs, from approximately 10% in 1992–1993 to 5% in 1997–1998. Significant risk factors associated with cerebral palsy were grades III-IV intraventricular hemorrhage, periventricular leukomalacia and necrotizing enterocolitis. Risk factors for Mental Development Index or Psychomotor Developmental Index scores less than 70 included grades III-IV intraventricular hemorrhage, periventricular leukomalacia, chronic lung disease, use of postnatal prescription steroids (dexamethasone), necrotizing enterocolitis, a mother with less than a high school education, and male gender of the fetus.

In general, parents of anticipated extremely preterm infants can be counseled that the neonatal survival rate for newborns increases from 30% at 23 weeks of gestation to 75% at 25 weeks of gestation and from 11% at 401–500 g birth weight to 75% at 701–800 g birth weight. In addition, females generally have a better prognosis than males. Parents of anticipated extremely preterm infants can be counseled that infants delivered before 24 weeks of gestation are less likely to survive, and those who do survive are likely to have significant neurodevelopmental impairment. Disabilities in mental and psychomotor development, neuromotor function, or sensory and communication function are present in approximately one half of extremely preterm infants.

Maternal transport to a tertiary care center before delivery should be considered when possible. The effects of aggressive resuscitation at birth on the outcome of the extremely preterm fetus also are unclear. Therefore, management decisions regarding the extremely preterm fetus must be individualized. The effect of antenatal steroid use in the extremely preterm fetus is unclear; however, it is recommended that all women at risk of preterm birth at 34 weeks of gestation or less be considered candidates for a single course of corticosteroids. Recognizing regional differences, the decision to give steroids should be made in consultation between the patient, obstetrician, and neonatologist. Prospectively collected outcome data for extremely preterm fetuses are available. Whenever possible, data specific to the age, weight, and sex of the individual extremely preterm fetus should be used to aid management decisions made by obstetricians and parents of fetuses at risk for preterm birth before 26 completed weeks of gestation. This information may be developed by each institution and should indicate the population used in determining estimates of survivability.

Multifetal Pregnancy

In 2002, more than 130,000 infants were born of multifetal gestations in the United States. Since 1980, there has been a 65% increase in the frequency of twins and a 500% increase in triplet and high-order births. Most of this increase results from increased use of ovulation-induction agents and assisted reproductive technology (ART). Assisted reproductive technology has been associated with a 30-fold increase in multiple pregnancies compared with the rate of spontaneous twin pregnancies (1% in the general population). If the recommendations of the Society of Assisted Reproductive Technologies and the American Society for Reproductive Medicine regarding the number of embryos per transfer are adopted universally and followed, the number of high-order gestations should decline in the United States.

Although multifetal births account for only 3% of all live births, they are responsible for a disproportionate share of perinatal morbidity and mortality. They account for 17% of all preterm births (before 37 weeks of gestation), 23% of early preterm births (before 32 weeks of gestation), 24% of LBW infants (less than 2,500 g), and 26% of very LBW infants (less than 1,500 g). Although twins do have an increased risk of morbidity and mortality, a far greater proportion of triplet and high-order multiple gestations have poor outcomes. All survivors of preterm multifetal births have an increased risk of mental and physical handicap. Women should be counseled about the risk of high-order pregnancies before beginning ART (see "Multifetal Gestations" in Chapter 4). Methods to limit high-order multiple pregnancies include monitoring hormone levels and follicle number during superovulation and limiting transfer to fewer embryos in in vitro fertilization cycles.

Complications of Multifetal Pregnancy

Gestational Diabetes

The incidence of gestational diabetes in twin pregnancies is slightly higher than in singleton pregnancies, and the incidence in triplet pregnancies is higher than in twin pregnancies; 22–39% of triplet pregnancies are complicated by gestational diabetes, compared with 3–6% of twin pregnancies. Many aspects of the diagnosis and management of gestational diabetes in multiple gestations remain unexamined. The best time for testing, the ideal number of daily calories, the optimal weight gain, whether women treated with oral hypoglycemic agents for polycystic ovary syndrome should continue taking them, the best form of insulin to use, the best method of fetal surveillance, and the ideal time for delivery currently are unknown.

Hypertension and Preeclampsia

The incidence of preeclampsia is 2.6 times higher in twin gestations than in singleton gestations and is higher in triplet gestations than in twin gestations. When multiple gestation is complicated by preeclampsia, it is significantly more likely to occur earlier and to be severe. Gestational hypertension before 35 weeks of gestation, preeclampsia before 35 weeks of gestation, and hypertension with a diastolic blood pressure greater than 110 mm Hg occur 12.4 times more often, respectively, in twin gestations than in singleton gestations. Placental abruption is 8.2 times more likely. Multiple gestations resulting from ART seem to be at greater risk of developing hypertensive complications than spontaneous multiple gestations. If severe preeclampsia, HELLP syndrome, or another serious hypertensive complication develops before term, transfer to a tertiary care center may improve outcomes for both the woman and her fetuses.

Premature Delivery

Data from U.S. birth records indicate that 55–57% of all multiple gestations are delivered preterm, and 49–63% of these infants weigh less than 2,500 g. Births in 12% percent of twin pregnancies, 36% of triplet pregnancies, and 60% of quadruplet pregnancies occur before 32 weeks of gestation, during the period when perinatal morbidity and mortality are greatest. In addition to uterine overdistension, the same factors that may contribute to preterm birth in singleton pregnancies affect multiple gestations and may be more common: lower and upper genital tract infection; decidual hemorrhage (abruptio placenta); cervical incompetence; maternal medical complications; maternal stress; and fetal, placental, or uterine abnormalities. However, the identification of these risk factors has not led to the development of effective protocols or therapies to prevent preterm birth.

Growth Restriction

Fetuses of a multiple gestation generally do not grow at the same rate as singleton fetuses. One obvious etiology is placental pathology; multiple gestations are at increased risk to include at least one fetus with a suboptimal placental implantation site or abnormal umbilical cord morphology. Depending on the number of fetuses, a diminution in fetal growth may be discernible as early as 22 weeks of gestation. The long-held opinion that LBW infants from a multiple gestation do better than LBW singleton infants is not correct.

Discordant Growth

Discordant fetal growth is common in multiple gestations and usually is defined by a 20–25% reduction in the estimated fetal weight of the smallest fetus when compared with the largest. Most published studies examine discordance in twins; twin weight discordance is associated with structural malformations, stillbirth, intrauterine growth restriction, preterm birth, cesarean delivery for nonreassuring fetal heart pattern, umbilical arterial pH less than 7.1, admission to the neonatal intensive care unit, respiratory distress syndrome, and neonatal death within 7 days of delivery. The threshold at which discordant growth is most strongly associated with adverse outcomes is unclear, even in twin gestations.

Discordance can be caused by structural or genetic fetal anomalies, discordant infection, an unfavorable placental implantation or umbilical cord insertion site, placental damage (ie, partial abruption), or complications related to monochorionic placentation, such as twin–twin transfusion syndrome. All of these complications occur more frequently in high-order multiple gestations. The workup should include a review of all prenatal exposures, a specialized ultrasound examination, and, depending on the gestational age, tests of fetal well-being. The ultrasound examination should be performed by someone with skill and experience in evaluating multiple gestations. Likewise, a consultation with an obstetrician–gynecologist with expertise in the management of high-risk pregnancies, such as a maternal–fetal medicine specialist, may be helpful in determining further therapy for these cases when complications arise.

Death of One Fetus

No fetal monitoring protocol has been shown to predict most losses of a fetus in a multifetal pregnancy. In addition, authorities disagree about antepartum management once a demise has occurred. Some investigators have advocated immediate delivery of the remaining fetuses. However, if the death is the result of an abnormality of the fetus itself rather than maternal or uteroplacental pathology and the pregnancy is remote from term, expectant management may be appropriate. The most difficult cases are those in which fetal demise occurs in one fetus of a monochorionic twin pair. Because virtually 100% of monochorionic placentas contain vascular anastomoses that link the circulations of the two fetuses, the surviving fetus is at significant risk of sustaining permanent damage or death caused by the sudden hypotension that occurs at the time of the cotwin's demise. By the time the demise is discovered, the greatest harm has most likely already been done. Thus, there may be little or no benefit in immediate delivery, especially if the surviving fetuses are very preterm. In such cases, allowing the pregnancy to continue may provide the most benefit.

Twin–Twin Transfusion Syndrome

Twin–twin transfusion syndrome is believed to occur as the result of uncompensated arteriovenous anastomoses in a monochorionic placenta, which leads to greater net blood flow going to one twin at the expense of the other. The syndrome usually becomes apparent in the second trimester and can lead rapidly to PROM, preterm labor, or early mortality because of heart failure in either of the fetuses. A variety of therapies have been attempted, but serial therapeutic amniocenteses of the recipient twin's amniotic sac are used most frequently. This therapy is believed to work by favorably changing intraamniotic pressure and, thus, placental intravascular pressure, allowing redistribution of placental blood flow and normalization of amniotic fluid volumes in each sac. More aggressive therapies, which usually are considered only for very early, severe cases, include abolishing the placental anastomoses by endoscopic laser coagulation or selective feticide by umbilical cord occlusion. These cases should be managed in consultation with a maternal–fetal medicine specialist.

Timing of Delivery in Multiple Gestations

The nadir of perinatal mortality for twin pregnancies occurs at approximately 38 completed weeks of gestation and at 35 completed weeks of gestation for triplets; the nadir for quadruplet and other high-order multiple gestations is not known. Fetal and neonatal morbidity and mortality begin to increase in twin and triplet pregnancies extended beyond 37 and 35 completed weeks of gestation, respectively. If the fetuses are appropriate in size for gestational age with evidence of sustained growth and there is normal amniotic fluid volume and reassuring antepartum fetal testing in the absence of maternal complications, such as preeclampsia or gestational diabetes, the pregnancy can be continued. Alternatively, if the woman is experiencing morbidities that would improve with delivery but do not necessarily mandate delivery (eg, worsening dyspnea, inability to sleep, severe dependent edema, painful superficial varicosities), delivery may be considered at these gestational ages.

Fetal Loss

The rate of stillbirth, defined as fetal death at 20 weeks of gestation or greater, is 5–12 per 1,000 live births in the United States, depending on race and ethnicity. This is higher than the mortality caused by prematurity and sudden infant death syndrome combined. Studies of case series estimate that at least 50% of these stillbirths have an undetermined cause of death.

Fetal death usually is suspected by the woman when fetal movements cease. The physician is unable to hear fetal heart tones. Real-time ultrasonography is used to confirm the absence of cardiac activity. In experienced hands, real-time ultrasonography is 100% accurate in this regard.

Overall, 80–90% of patients enter spontaneous labor within 2 weeks of fetal death. This interval, called the latency period, can vary in individual cases. In general, the latency period is inversely proportional to the duration of the gestation when the demise occurred. The consumptive coagulopathy associated with prolonged retention of a dead fetus presumably results from the release of tissue factor (thromboplastin) from the fetus into the maternal circulation. A coagulopathy will be seen in approximately one fourth of women who retain a dead fetus for longer than 4 weeks. Because delivery almost always will be effected before 4 weeks, this is rarely encountered today.

After a stillbirth or neonatal death, proper management includes a careful perinatal and family history, a physical examination of the fetus or infant, and indicated laboratory studies. Both prostaglandins and oxytocin are effective for achieving delivery in this setting.

The general examination of the stillborn infant should be done promptly, noting any dysmorphic features and obtaining body measurements, including crown–rump, crown–heel, and foot lengths, as well as weight. Foot length is especially useful before 23 weeks of gestation. These measurements help estimate gestational age and evaluate intrauterine growth. Further documentation by frontal and profile photographs, with close-ups of specific abnormalities, is valuable for subsequent review and consultations. If reluctant to consent to a full autopsy, the family should be informed of the value of less-invasive methods of evaluation, including photographs, X-rays, and sampling of tissues, such as blood or skin. Even if parents have declined an autopsy, a description of any obvious abnormalities of the stillbirth should be included in the medical record.

When a full autopsy is performed, it should follow the guidelines for perinatal autopsy published by the College of American Pathologists (www.cap.org) or other standard references. The pathologist should be aware of the clinical history and suspected genetic diagnoses so that samples for cytogenetic, metabolic, and molecular studies may be taken.

Samples of amniotic fluid, umbilical cord blood, or amnion may be obtained for chromosomal and other relevant studies. Analysis of bile, vitreous humor, urine, and fetal tissue may be helpful if umbilical cord blood is unobtainable. Guidelines for the procurement of samples for chromosomal and genetic studies are outlined in Box 6–1.

Chromosomal analysis of amniotic fluid or chorionic villi ideally should be offered as soon as a fetal death is recognized. Although this information can be obtained at the time of delivery, the likelihood of obtaining a karyotype is

---

Box 6–1. Acceptable Cytologic Specimens

Obtain at least one of the following samples with sterile technique and instruments, then place in sterile tissue culture medium of lactated ringers solution and keep at room temperature:

- Amniotic fluid obtained by amniocentesis at time of prenatal diagnosis of demise, particularly valuable if delivery is not expected imminently

- Placental block 1 cm by 1 cm taken from below the cord insertion site on the unfixed placenta

- 1.5 cm umbilical cord segment

- Internal fetal tissue specimen, such as costochondral junction or patella; skin is not recommended.

---

decreased if there is a long interval between fetal death and delivery. This is especially true when dysmorphic features, inconsistent growth measurements, anomalies, or hydrops are present, or when a parent carries a balanced chromosomal rearrangement (eg, translocation or inversion) or has a mosaic karyotype.

The results of the autopsy, placental examination, laboratory tests, and cytogenetic studies should be communicated to the involved clinicians and to the family of the deceased infant in a timely manner. Further, the family should be counseled promptly after consensus is reached. Counseling before the evaluation is complete or before different opinions of the various caregivers have been resolved may increase feelings of guilt or anger in parents who have experienced a perinatal death. When there is an abnormal child or a genetic defect, these feelings often are magnified. Specific testing of the parents may be offered. The results of the tests are important even when no specific diagnosis is identified. A list of diagnoses excluded may be useful in counseling the parents. Whether or not there is a specific diagnosis, compassionate counseling of the parents and sensitivity to their needs are required. For more information on grief counseling, see "Death of a Neonate" in Chapter 8.

Obesity

The World Health Organization and the National Institutes of Health define overweight as a body mass index (BMI) of 25–29.9, obesity as a BMI of 30–34.9, and morbid obesity as a BMI greater than 35. The most recent National Health and Nutrition Examination Survey from 1999–2002 found that one third of adult women are obese. This problem is greatest among non-Hispanic black women (49%) compared with Mexican-American women (38%) and non-Hispanic white women (31%).

Obese women are at increased risk for several pregnancy complications. Obstetricians should evaluate all women for obesity by calculating a BMI and should provide education about the possible complications, nutrition, and exercise (see "Nutrition in Pregnancy" in Chapter 4 for more information).

Studies consistently report higher rates of preeclampsia, gestational diabetes, and cesarean delivery, particularly for failure to progress, in obese women compared with nonobese women. Operative and postoperative complications include increased rates of excessive blood loss, operative time greater than 2 hours, wound infection, endometritis, and thromboembolism.

Nutrition consultation should be offered to all obese women, and they should be encouraged to follow an exercise program. Screening for gestational diabetes mellitus should be performed during the first trimester or on presentation and repeated later in pregnancy if the initial screening result is negative. Because these women are at increased risk for emergent cesarean delivery and anesthetic complications, anesthesiology consultation before delivery is encouraged (please see "Cesarean Delivery" in Chapter 5).

It is important to discuss potential intrapartum complications, such as difficulty or impossibility of establishing fetal weight (even with ultrasound examination), inability to obtain interpretable external fetal heart rate and uterine contraction patterns, and the difficulty and dangers of performing an emergency cesarean delivery. If an anesthesiology consultation was not obtained antepartum, it should be conducted early in labor to allow adequate time for development of an anesthetic plan. If obese women require cesarean delivery, they should receive antibiotic prophylaxis even if surgery is scheduled and they have not labored.

It has been recommended that graduated compression stockings, hydration, and early mobilization be used during and after cesarean delivery in obese patients and that postpartum heparin therapy be used in patients thought to be at high risk for venous thromboembolism. There remains insufficient data to determine whether the benefits of heparin prophylaxis in this group of patients outweigh the risks.

Preeclampsia

Preeclampsia is a disorder characterized by hypertension, proteinuria, and edema occurring after 20 weeks of gestation. Preeclampsia complicates approximately 3–7% of pregnancies and is a major cause of maternal and perinatal morbidity and mortality. Efforts to prevent preeclampsia using low-dose aspirin or calcium supplementation have not been successful and are not recommended for routine use in pregnancy.

Treatment of preeclampsia should be directed toward ensuring the safety of the woman and delivery of a healthy, mature neonate. When preeclampsia is diagnosed during the intrapartum period, initial management should include assessing the condition of both the woman and the fetus and administering prophylaxis for maternal seizures. Although the most effective treatment is delivery, other considerations also affect management:

- Severity of preeclampsia
- Gestational age
- Maternal condition
- Fetal condition
- Presence of labor
- Availability of hospital staff and resources
- Capability of hospital staff

Mild preeclampsia before term often can be managed with in-hospital or careful home observation. The disease process is regarded as mild when the following conditions are present:

- Blood pressure levels equal to or greater than 140 mm Hg systolic or equal to or greater than 90 mm Hg diastolic that occur after 20 weeks of gestation in a woman with previously normal blood pressure levels
- Proteinuria, defined as urinary excretion of 0.3 g of protein or more in a 24-hour urine specimen

Preeclampsia is considered severe if one or more of the following criteria are present:

- Blood pressure levels of equal to or greater than 160 mm Hg systolic or equal to or greater than 110 mm Hg diastolic on two occasions at least 6 hours apart while the patient is on bed rest
- Proteinuria of 5 g or more in a 24-hour urine collection or 3+ or greater on two random urine samples collected at least 4 hours apart
- Oliguria of less than 500 mL in 24 hours
- Cerebral or visual disturbances

- Pulmonary edema or cyanosis
- Epigastric or right upper quadrant pain
- Impaired liver function
- Thrombocytopenia or evidence of hemolysis
- Fetal growth restriction in the setting of preeclampsia

The development of severe preeclampsia usually warrants delivery of the neonate, irrespective of gestational age or fetal maturity. The presence of hemolysis, elevated liver enzymes, and low platelet counts (HELLP) syndrome also is an indication for delivery to avoid jeopardizing the health of the woman. There is an increased risk of early-onset severe preeclampsia among women with the antiphospholipid antibody syndrome, and women with early development of severe preeclampsia should be evaluated for lupus anticoagulant and anticardiolipin antibodies. The value of screening for inherited thrombophilias such as factor V Leiden and prothrombin G20210A mutations, hyperhomocysteinemia, and deficiencies of antithrombin, protein S, and protein C in this setting is under investigation.

Fetuses of women with preeclampsia are at increased risk of a nonreassuring heart rate during labor. Once labor is established, the route of delivery is determined by obstetric factors. Augmentation or induction of labor can be used if needed.

Seizure Prophylaxis

Magnesium sulfate is the drug of choice for the prevention or treatment of eclamptic convulsions, and it is superior to phenytoin and diazepam for this purpose. Therapy with magnesium sulfate should be initiated intravenously with a loading dose followed by a continuous infusion. In most situations, clinical assessment of respirations, deep tendon reflexes, and urine output is adequate to monitor for maternal magnesium toxicity without the need to determine the actual maternal serum magnesium levels. If toxic serum levels or side effects are encountered, magnesium sulfate infusion must be discontinued, and calcium gluconate may be administered to reverse these effects.

Antihypertensive Therapy

Severe hypertension with a systolic blood pressure level of 180 mm Hg or greater and a diastolic blood pressure level of 110 mm Hg or greater increases the maternal risks of cerebrovascular accidents and congestive heart failure. Reducing the woman's diastolic blood pressure level to 90–100 mm Hg is recommended. Reducing the woman's severe systolic hypertension is just as important.

Hydralazine is the most widely used agent for the treatment of acute hypertension in pregnancy, has almost universal efficacy, and is extremely safe. Labetalol is equally effective, although it has a wide range of individual dosage requirements. The calcium antagonist nifedipine, when administered orally (not sublingually) to postpartum patients with severe preeclampsia, offers good blood pressure control and cardiorenal protection. Caution should be used to avoid maternal hypotension, regardless of which agent is selected to lower the blood pressure.

Fluid Balance

Patients with severe preeclampsia are at increased risk of fluid overload and pulmonary edema. Fluid intake and urine output should be assessed hourly before delivery. Total intravenous intake rarely should exceed 100–125 mL per hour. Because intrapartum oliguria is common (especially with oxytocin usage), its presence should not be treated with repetitive "bolus" crystalloid infusions. If oliguria of less than 30 cc per hour for 2 consecutive hours occurs, the woman should receive up to three 500 mL fluid boluses of crystalloid during labor. If oliguria persists after such infusions, her intravascular volume status may require accurate determination with invasive monitoring.

After delivery (especially cesarean delivery), oliguria most commonly is caused by hypovolemia. The initial management of postdelivery oliguria is directed at volume replacement with an infusion of 500 mL of crystalloid over 20 minutes. If oliguria persists after delivery and the woman is anemic, the need for a packed red blood cell transfusion should be considered. Repetitive bolus infusions of crystalloid solution in such patients without red blood cell replacement increase the risk of pulmonary edema and acute renal failure. In rare instances, oliguria that persists despite conservative measures is an indication for invasive hemodynamic monitoring to guide fluid, electrolyte, and blood replacement more accurately.

Deep Vein Thrombosis and Pulmonary Embolism

The risk of venous thromboembolic disease is increased during pregnancy and during the puerperium in association with increased venous stasis in the lower extremities and increased levels of circulating clotting factors and lower levels of free protein S. Risk factors for thromboembolism include cesarean delivery, operative vaginal delivery, maternal age, obesity, trauma, infection, and prolonged bed rest. Women with a personal or family history of venous thromboembolic disease should be evaluated for hereditary and acquired thrombophilic disorders, including:

- Antiphospholipid syndrome (lupus anticoagulant, anticardiolipin antibodies)

- Factor V Leiden gene mutation

- Prothrombin G20210A mutation

- Hyperhomocysteinemia, usually associated with methylenetetrahydrofolate reductase mutations

- Deficiencies of antithrombin, protein C, protein S

Women with a personal history of venous thromboembolism also should be tested for lupus anticoagulant and anticardiolipin antibodies.

The diagnosis of deep vein thrombosis is best made by compression ultrasound examination. There may be a role for D-dimer assessment as an initial "rule-out" screen in low-risk women. Most instances of pulmonary embolism are associated with symptoms such as dyspnea, tachypnea, pleuritic chest pain, and hemoptysis. The diagnosis is most likely in a patient who also has a reduced PAO_2 level (less than 80 mm Hg); however, a normal arterial blood gas analysis does not rule out a pulmonary embolus. In contemporary practice, the condition generally is diagnosed with a highly sensitive multidetector-row spiral computed tomography (CT) pulmonary angiography. Again, there may be a role for D-dimer assessment as an initial rule-out screen in women at low risk. Negative spiral CT results in women at high risk may be followed up with a lower extremity compression ultrasound examination or intravenous contrast pulmonary artery angiography.

Anticoagulation is the mainstay of therapy for deep vein thrombosis with or without pulmonary embolism. Acute thromboembolism associated with pregnancy requires an intravenous unfractionated heparin bolus of 5,000 international units (80 international units/kg) followed by continuous infusion of at least 30,000 international units for 24 hours, titrated to achieve full anticoagulation (ie, an activated partial thromboplastin test of 1.5–2.5 times control values).

Venous thrombosis or pulmonary embolism or both also may be treated effectively with low molecular weight heparin. Although laboratory testing appears not to be essential in the nonpregnant patient, the availability of low molecular weight heparin is affected by changes in maternal physiology. Therefore, it may be warranted to periodically reevaluate antifactor Xa levels during pregnancy in a woman on adjusted-dose full anticoagulation.

Intravenous unfractionated heparin is continued for at least 5–7 days or until the symptoms have resolved and there is no evidence of recurrence. Patients should continue therapeutic anticoagulation with either subcutaneous injections of unfractionated heparin or low molecular weight heparin for at least 3 months after the acute event. Warfarin should be used for anticoagulation postpartum and does not contraindicate breastfeeding. To avoid paradoxical thrombosis and skin necrosis from the early antiprotein C effect of warfarin, it is critical to maintain these women on therapeutic doses of unfractionated heparin or low molecular weight heparin for 5 days and until the international normalized ratio is in a therapeutic range (ie, 2–3).

Pregnant patients with a history of idiopathic thrombosis, thrombosis related to pregnancy or oral contraceptive use, or a history of thrombosis accompanied by an underlying thrombophilia other than homozygous for the factor V Leiden mutation, heterozygous for both the factor V Leiden and the prothrombin G20210A mutation, or AT-III deficiency should be offered antepartum and postpartum low-dose heparin prophylaxis.

In patients receiving once-daily prophylactic low-dose low molecular weight heparin, regional anesthesia should not be offered until at least 10–12 hours after the last injection of low molecular weight heparin. In addition, low molecular weight heparin should be withheld for at least 2 hours after the removal of an epidural catheter. The safety of regional analgesia in patients receiving twice-daily therapeutic low molecular weight heparin has not been studied sufficiently, and it is not known whether delaying regional analgesia for 24 hours after the last injection is adequate. Because the onset of labor often is difficult to predict, it may be reasonable to convert patients receiving low molecular weight heparin to unfractionated heparin as they approach term (eg, 36–38 weeks of gestation).

Trauma During Pregnancy

Trauma and other forms of violence are the leading causes of death in women of reproductive age and among the leading causes of nonobstetric maternal death. Physical trauma is estimated to complicate 1 of every 12 pregnancies. Obstetricians are uniquely qualified to play a vital role in the management of trauma during pregnancy. They understand the effects of altered maternal physiology and anatomy on the management of trauma and its effects on the fetus. The obstetrician's role in ensuring both maternal and fetal well-being is paramount in the management of pregnant trauma victims. Whether acting as a consultant or as a primary physician when seeing a pregnant trauma victim, the obstetrician should provide maternal–fetal care that is timely and systematic to ensure maternal medical stabilization and fetal evaluation.

Evaluation

Pregnancy should not restrict the use of any of the usual diagnostic, pharmacologic, or resuscitative procedures or maneuvers provided to trauma victims. The possibility of domestic violence or intimate-partner violence should be considered (see "Domestic Violence" in Chapter 4). The more seriously injured the woman, the more important it is to follow a methodical evaluation that ensures her complete assessment and stabilization. Serious or life-threatening maternal injuries can be overlooked if maternal evaluation is not thorough during stabilization. The finding of nonreassuring fetal status by heart rate monitoring or ultrasonography may alert the clinician to more severe maternal injuries than were initially appreciated. To prevent supine hypotension syndrome, deflection of the uterus off the inferior vena cava and abdominal aorta can be obtained by placing the patient in the lateral decubitus position. This position should be maintained throughout evaluation.

After stabilization, a more detailed secondary survey of the patient, including a thorough ultrasound evaluation of the pregnancy, should be performed. Ultrasonography in this setting can be useful to determine estimated gestational age, placental location, fetal cardiac status, amniotic fluid volume, and the presence of maternal intraabdominal fluid.

Once the woman's condition has been stabilized, continuous fetal monitoring is recommended when the fetus's gestational age approaches viability. Monitoring and further evaluation are warranted if uterine contractions, a nonreassuring fetal heart rate pattern, vaginal bleeding, significant uterine tenderness or irritability, serious maternal injury, or rupture of the amniotic membranes is present. Monitoring periods of 2–6 hours usually are adequate if there are no uterine contractions, uterine tenderness, or bleeding. Abruptio placentae usually becomes apparent shortly after injury.

Use of open peritoneal lavage to diagnose intraperitoneal hemorrhage has been shown to be safe, sensitive, and specific during pregnancy, particularly in association with abdominal signs and symptoms of intraperitoneal bleeding, altered sensorium, major thoracic injury, unexplained shock, and multiple major orthopedic injuries. This procedure is unnecessary if clinically obvious intraperitoneal bleeding is present or if ultrasound findings are highly suggestive of free blood in the peritoneal cavity.

Treatment

In general, aggressive exploratory laparotomy is advocated for gunshot wounds and other penetrating trauma to the abdomen during pregnancy. Laparotomy alone is not an indication to perform cesarean delivery. The fetus usually tolerates surgery and anesthesia well if adequate oxygenation and uterine perfusion are maintained. The uterus should be carefully inspected for injury at the time of laparotomy.

Administration of 300 µg of anti-D immune globulin within 72 hours of injury should protect nearly all (90%) D-negative trauma victims with substantial abdominal trauma and possible D isoimmunization. The Kleihauer–Betke test or a similar quantitative assay of fetal–maternal hemorrhage may be used to detect a fetomaternal transfusion of greater than 30 mL that requires additional anti-D immune globulin.

After evaluation and hospital discharge, the patient should be instructed to seek care if she develops vaginal bleeding, leakage of fluid, decreased fetal movement, or severe abdominal pain. Measures to prevent the recurrence of trauma also should be discussed.

After 5 minutes of unsuccessful maternal cardiac resuscitation, perimortem cesarean delivery is recommended, as it may facilitate maternal resuscitative efforts and reduce the risks of fetal compromise and death. Postmortem cesarean delivery more than 10–15 minutes after maternal death is unlikely to result in neonatal survival. If a fetus does survive, there is a high risk of adverse neurodevelopmental sequelae.

Maternal Hemorrhage

Hemorrhage remains one of the leading causes of maternal mortality and a cause of substantial morbidity. Facilities that provide labor and delivery services should be prepared to manage maternal hemorrhage. Proper preparation and resources to manage maternal hemorrhage in a timely manner can be lifesaving. Policies to ensure the rapid availability of blood products for transfusion in the event of hemorrhage must be in place.

Hemorrhagic Shock

Obstetric hemorrhage can be of a volume large enough to precipitate a state of generalized circulatory failure, resulting in decreased tissue perfusion that progresses to hypoxia, acidosis, and irreversible tissue damage. The goal of therapy should be timely intervention to identify and remedy the cause of hemorrhage in conjunction with reversing the effects leading to shock.

Postpartum Hemorrhage

Factors associated with obstetric hemorrhage include uterine atony (the most common cause of postpartum hemorrhage), uterine inversion, obstetric lacerations, retained placental fragments, placentation abnormalities (such as placenta accreta and succenturiate placental lobe), and maternal coagulopathy. An attempt should be made to identify patients with known risk factors for postpartum hemorrhage. Most postpartum hemorrhage occurs immediately or soon after delivery. Maternal postpartum observation should be tailored to the need for timely identification of signs of excessive blood loss, including hypotension and tachycardia. Maternal vital signs and the amount of vaginal bleeding should be evaluated continuously. The uterine fundus should be identified and massaged and its size and degree of contraction noted. A dilute solution of oxytocin (20 units/L), routinely administered intravenously after delivery, reduces the incidence of postpartum hemorrhage resulting from uterine atony. Labor and delivery areas should have 15-methyl prostaglandin F_2, misoprostol and ergot alkaloids readily available for further treatment of uterine atony. Any bleeding lacerations of the genital tract should be sutured. If perineal or pelvic pain is present, the patient should be evaluated for a genital tract hematoma.

Appropriate maneuvers, including medical therapy, may fail to control postpartum hemorrhage. Uterine packing (eg, No. 24 Foley catheter with a 30 mL balloon inflated with 60–80 mL of saline) and radiographic embolization of the appropriate pelvic vessels may be appropriate. Exploratory laparotomy and ligation of the uterine arteries, the utero-ovarian arteries, or the infundibulopelvic vessels is highly effective as a treatment of atony. Good results also have been achieved with plication stitches of the uterus itself, such as the B-Lynch suture. The responsible physician and obstetric support staff must be prepared to initiate surgical management when it is deemed necessary. Because of the rich collateral circulation in the pelvis, surgical ligation of the internal iliac (hypogastric) arteries often fails to control hemorrhage and may result in delay of definitive therapy or prevent subsequent radiologic embolization procedures. Puerperal hysterectomy may be indicated to control hemorrhage in cases of intractable bleeding from uterine atony, uterine rupture, placenta accreta, or leiomyomas. The incidence of placenta accreta has increased steadily, and patients with placenta previa and previous uterine incisions are at increased risk of severe hemorrhage at the time of placental separation. The antenatal use of ultrasonography and magnetic resonance imaging may help to make the diagnosis of placenta accreta before delivery and facilitate planning and surgical management.

Transfusion

Transfusion therapy is used to prevent or treat hemorrhagic shock and its consequences. Blood loss estimated to be 1,500 mL or greater on average represents approximately 25% of a pregnant woman's total estimated blood volume (6,000 mL). This assumes that normal pregnancy volume expansion has occurred, which may not occur with preeclampsia. In many clinical circumstances, a pregnant patient might benefit from transfusion of red blood cells before the blood loss has reached such levels. The circulating blood volume must be maintained in the pregnant patient, and therapy should be directed at the prevention of inadequate cardiac output and resultant decreased tissue perfusion. Component therapy, including fresh-frozen plasma, cryoprecipitate, and platelets, should be available if needed for correction of clotting factor deficiencies.

Some women have a religious objection to the receipt of any blood product. Written policies to guide the management of these patients during treatment are advisable, and the woman's autonomy should be respected.

Before Delivery

The goal of red blood cell transfusion therapy is to avoid irreversible tissue damage caused by hypoperfusion from inadequate circulating blood volume. In the obstetric patient, the need for adequate blood volume is made more pressing by the presence of the fetus.

The end point of red blood cell transfusion therapy before delivery varies with the clinical situation. A hematocrit level of 30% or greater generally has been recommended as a goal of therapy in a pregnant woman who is actively bleeding or who is at continued risk for considerable obstetric hemorrhage, such as in the presence of placenta previa. In a clinically stable patient who has responded appropriately to therapy, however, the decision to transfuse should be based on individual circumstances. Recombinant human erythropoietin is extremely expensive but may be useful to treat severe but nonacute anemia, particularly in patients who refuse transfusion.

After Delivery

If active bleeding has ceased after delivery, transfusion can be withheld unless there is evidence of symptomatic anemia, hypovolemia, decreased tissue perfusion, or decreased urinary output (less than 30 mL/h). The patient's compensatory mechanisms of increased erythropoiesis and plasma volume expansion, along with iron supplementation, often will suffice to correct the red blood cell deficit.

When obstetric hemorrhage is diagnosed, packed red blood cells should be typed and cross-matched (prior typed and screened red blood cells are equally safe), and the hospital's blood bank personnel should be notified of the potential for massive transfusion. Until the blood loss is controlled by medical or surgical therapy, it is advisable to ensure the ready availability of packed red blood cell units for use if rapid transfusion is required. Obstetric blood loss of greater than 1,500 mL, or of lesser amounts because of placental causes, may result in inadequate coagulation in otherwise healthy patients.

Endometritis

Postpartum endometritis occurs in 1–3% of vaginal deliveries and in 10–50% of cesarean deliveries. Risk factors for endometritis include cesarean delivery, prolonged rupture of membranes, prolonged labor with multiple vaginal examinations, intrapartum fever, and lower socioeconomic status.

Prophylaxis Against Postcesarean Infection

A short course of prophylactic antibiotics significantly lowers the risk of endometritis and abdominal wound infection after both elective and nonelective (ie, after rupture of membranes or labor of any duration) cesarean deliveries. Intravenous administration of an antibiotic before the procedure has been demonstrated to be more effective than administration immediately after umbilical cord clamping. For procedures lasting less than 2 hours, a single dose is as effective as a longer course of therapy. If excessive intraoperative blood loss occurs, a second dose may be indicated. A first-generation cephalosporin, such as cefazolin, is as effective as other broad-spectrum agents and is less expensive. Broad-spectrum antibiotics should be reserved for therapy rather than for prophylaxis.

Management

Endometritis usually is diagnosed within a few days after delivery. Infection often is caused by several organisms, including aerobic streptococci (group B β-hemolytic streptococci and the enterococci), gram-negative aerobes (especially *Escherichia coli*), gram-negative anaerobic rods (especially *Bacteroides bivius*), and anaerobic cocci (*Peptococcus* species and *Peptostreptococcus* species). Clinically, endometritis is characterized by fever, uterine tenderness, malaise, tachycardia, abdominal pain, or foul-smelling lochia. Of these, fever is the most characteristic and may be the only sign early in the course of infection.

A woman with postpartum fever should be evaluated by pertinent history, physical examination, blood count, and urine culture. Blood cultures rarely influence therapeutic decisions but could be indicated if septicemia is suspected. Cervical, vaginal, or endometrial cultures need not be routinely performed because the results might not indicate the infecting organism.

Principles for managing postpartum endometritis are as follows:

- Parenteral, broad-spectrum antibiotic treatment should be initiated according to a proven regimen and continued until the patient is afebrile. A combination of clindamycin and gentamicin, with the addition of ampicillin in refractory cases, is recommended for cost-effective therapy.

- Response usually is prompt. If fever persists, a search for alternative etiologies, including pelvic abscess, wound infection, septic pelvic thrombophlebitis, inadequate antibiotic coverage, and retained placental tissue, should be performed.

- Because postpartum endometritis may have neonatal implications, information about the mother's condition should be provided to the neonate's health care provider.

Resources

American College of Obstetricians and Gynecologists. Prevention of deep vein thrombosis and pulmonary embolism. ACOG Practice Bulletin 21. Washington, DC: ACOG; 2000.

American College of Obstetricians and Gynecologists. Thromboembolism in pregnancy. ACOG Practice Bulletin 19. Washington, DC: ACOG; 2000.

Antenatal corticosteroid therapy for fetal maturation. ACOG Committee Opinion No. 273. American College of Obstetricians and Gynecologists. Obstet Gynecol 2002;99:871–3.

Antenatal corticosteroids revisited: repeat courses. NIH Consens Statement 2000;17(2): 1–18.

Antiphospholipid syndrome. ACOG Practice Bulletin No. 68. American College of Obstetricians and Gynecologists. Obstet Gynecol 2005;106:1113–21.

Assessment of risk factors for preterm birth. ACOG Practice Bulletin No. 31. American College of Obstetricians and Gynecologists. Obstet Gynecol 2001;98:709–16.

Chronic hypertension in pregnancy. ACOG Practice Bulletin No. 29. American College of Obstetricians and Gynecologists. Obstet Gynecol 2001;98:177–85.

Diagnosis and management of preeclampsia and eclampsia. ACOG Practice Bulletin No. 33. American College of Obstetricians and Gynecologists. Obstet Gynecol 2002;99: 159–67.

Effect of corticosteroids for fetal maturation on perinatal outcomes. NIH Consens Statement 1994;12(2):1–24.

Management of preterm labor. ACOG Practice Bulletin No. 43. American College of Obstetricians and Gynecologists. Obstet Gynecol 2003;101:1039–47.

Multiple gestation: complicated twin, triplet, and high-order multifetal pregnancy. ACOG Practice Bulletin No. 56. American College of Obstetricians and Gynecologists. Obstet Gynecol 2004;104:869–83.

Obesity in pregnancy. ACOG Committee Opinion No. 315. American College of Obstetricians and Gynecologists. Obstet Gynecol 2005;106:671–5.

Perinatal care at the threshold of viability. ACOG Practice Bulletin No. 38. American College of Obstetricians and Gynecologists. Obstet Gynecol 2002;100:617–24.

Perinatal risks associated with assisted reproductive technology. ACOG Committee Opinion No. 324. American College of Obstetricians and Gynecologists. Obstet Gynecol 2005;106:1143–6.

Placenta accreta. ACOG Committee Opinion No. 266. American College of Obstetricians and Gynecologists. Obstet Gynecol 2002;99:169–70.

Postpartum hemorrhage. ACOG Practice Bulletin No. 76. American College of Obstetricians and Gynecologists. Obstet Gynecol 2006;108:1039–47.

Premature rupture of membranes. ACOG Practice Bulletin No. 80. American College of Obstetricians and Gynecologists. Obstet Gynecol 2007;109:1007–19.

Safety of Lovenox in Pregnancy. ACOG Committee Opinion No. 276. American College of Obstetricians and Gynecologists. Obstet Gynecol 2002;100:845–6.

Shinwell ES, Karplus M, Reich D, Weintraub Z, Blazer S, Bader D, et al. Early postnatal dexamethasone treatment and increased incidence of cerebral palsy. Arch Dis Child Fetal Neonatal Ed 2000;83:F177–81.

Spong CY, Erickson K, Willinger M, Hankins GD, Schulkin J. Stillbirth in obstetric practice: report of survey findings. J Matern Fetal Neonatal Med 2003;14:39–44.

chapter 7

Care of the Neonate

Delivery Room Care

Neonatal Resuscitation

Both routine assessment and resuscitation of the newborn at delivery should be provided in accordance with the principles of the American Heart Association and the American Academy of Pediatrics (AAP) Neonatal Resuscitation Program. Although the guidelines for neonatal resuscitation focus on delivery room resuscitation, most of the principles are applicable throughout the neonatal period and early infancy. Each hospital should have policies and procedures addressing the care and resuscitation of the newborn, including the qualifications of physicians and staff who provide this care. A program should be in place that ensures the competency of these individuals as well as their periodic credentialing. At every delivery, there should be at least one person whose primary responsibility is the newborn and who is capable of initiating resuscitation, including positive-pressure ventilation and chest compressions. Either that person or someone else who is immediately available should have the skills required to perform a complete resuscitation, including endotracheal intubation and the use of medications. Approximately 10% of infants require some assistance at birth, and approximately 1% require extensive assistance. Recognition and immediate resuscitation of a distressed neonate requires an organized plan of action and the immediate availability of qualified personnel and equipment. Responsibility for identification and resuscitation of a distressed neonate should be assigned to a qualified individual, who may be a physician, certified nurse midwife, advanced practice neonatal nurse, labor and delivery nurse, nurse anesthetist, nursery nurse, physician assistant, or respiratory therapist. The provision of services and equipment for resuscitation should be planned jointly by the medical and nursing directors of the departments involved in resuscitation of the newborn, usually the departments of obstetrics, anesthesia, and pediatrics. A physician, usually a pediatrician, should be designated to assume primary responsibility for initiating, supervising, and reviewing the plan for management of newborns requiring resuscitation in the delivery room. The following issues should be considered in this plan:

- A list should be developed of maternal and fetal complications that require the presence in the delivery room of someone qualified in all aspects of newborn resuscitation.

- Individuals qualified to perform neonatal resuscitation should demonstrate the following capabilities:

  — Ability to rapidly and accurately evaluate the newborn condition

  — Knowledge of the pathogenesis of risk factors predisposing for the need for resuscitation (eg, hypoxia, drugs, hypovolemia, trauma, anomalies, infections, and preterm birth), as well as specific indications for resuscitation

  — Skills in airway management, including bag and mask ventilation, laryngoscopy, endotracheal intubation and suctioning of the airway, chest compressions, emergency administration of drugs and fluids, and maintenance of thermal stability. Recognition and decompression of a tension pneumothorax by needle aspiration also is a desirable skill.

  — Skill in placing an umbilical venous catheter. This is especially important because most medications needed for resuscitation should be given by this route.

- Procedures should be developed to ensure the readiness of equipment and personnel and to provide for periodic review and evaluation of the effectiveness of the system.

- Contingency plans should be created for multiple births and other unusual circumstances.

- Guidelines should be developed for documentation of the resuscitation, including interventions, medications, and the time of each intervention.

- Procedures should be developed for transfer of responsibility for care.

Apgar Score

The Apgar score is useful for describing the status of the newborn at birth and his or her subsequent adaptation to the extrauterine environment, but it should not be used to determine the need for resuscitation or the steps to be taken. Resuscitation, when it is indicated, should be initiated before the 1-minute Apgar score is obtained. Apgar scores (Fig. 7–1) should be assigned at 1 minute and 5 minutes after birth, and if the 5-minute Apgar score is less than 7, additional scores should be assigned every 5 minutes for up to 20 minutes. The AAP Committee on Fetus and Newborn has recommended the use of an assisted Apgar Scoring System that documents the assistance the infant is receiving at the time of assignment of the score.

Steps in Delivery Room Management

Newly born infants who do not require resuscitation should be identified by rapid assessment of four characteristics:

1. Is the baby full term?
2. Is the amniotic fluid clear of meconium and evidence of infection?
3. Is the baby breathing or crying?
4. Does the baby have good muscle tone?

If the answers to these questions are "yes," the baby does not need resuscitation and should not be separated from the mother. If the answer to any of these questions is "no," the infant should receive one or more of the following categories of action (see Fig. 7–2 for a detailed treatment algorithm):

- Initial steps in stabilization (warmth, positioning, clearing the airway, drying, stimulating, and repositioning)
- Oxygen administration
- Positive pressure ventilation
- Chest compressions
- Administration of epinephrine or volume expansion or both

Maintenance of Body Temperature

Immediately after delivery, the vigorous term infant can be dried and placed skin-to-skin with the mother, both covered with a blanket. The premature infant or any infant who requires resuscitation should be dried completely with prewarmed towels to reduce evaporative heat loss and should be placed on a preheated radiant warmer. The radiant warmer will reduce heat loss and allow easy access to the newborn during resuscitation procedures. The premature infant is at particular risk for cold stress. In addition to increasing the temper-

Apgar Score

Gestational age: _____ weeks

Sign	0	1	2	1 min	5 min	10 min	15 min	20 min
Color	Blue or Pale	Acrocyanotic	Completely Pink					
Heart rate	Absent	Less than 100 min	Greater than 100 min					
Reflex irritability	No response	Grimace	Cry or active withdrawal					
Muscle tone	Limp	Some flexion	Active motion					
Respiration	Absent	Weak cry, hypoventilation	Good, crying					
			Total					

Comments:

Resuscitation

Min	1	5	10	15	20
Oxygen					
PPV/NCPAP					
ETT					
Chest compressions					
Epinephrine					

Fig. 7-1. The expanded Apgar score form. Record the score in the appropriate place at specific time intervals. The additional resuscitative measures (if appropriate) are recorded at the same time that the score is reported using a check mark in the appropriate box. Use the comment box to list other factors including maternal medications and/or the response to resuscitation between the recorded times of scoring. Abbreviations: ETT, endotracheal tube; PPV/NCPAP, positive-pressure ventilation/nasal continuous positive airway pressure. (The Apgar Score. ACOG Committee Opinion No. 333. American College of Obstetricians and Gynecologists. Obstet Gynecol 2005;106:1141–2.)

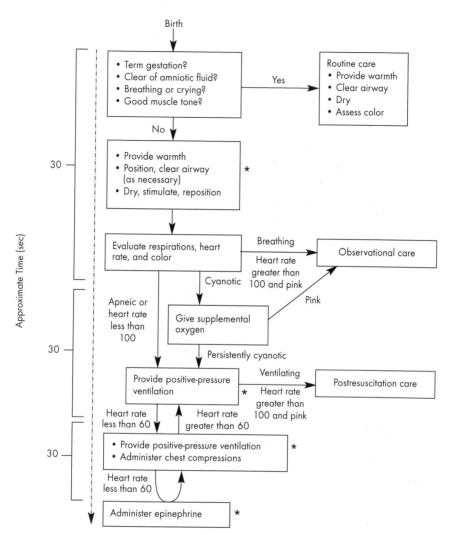

Fig. 7–2. Neonatal resuscitation algorithm. *Endotracheal intubation may be considered at several steps. American Academy of Pediatrics, American Heart Association. Neonatal resuscitation textbook. 5th ed. Elk Grove Village (IL): AAP; Dallas (TX): AHA; 2006.

ature of the delivery room, the use of a preheated radiant warmer and warmed towels to dry the infant off, other special measures should be considered, including the use of portable warming pads under the towels. For the very premature infant (less than 28 weeks of gestation), consider placing her, below the neck, in a food-grade reclosable one-gallon polyethylene bag that has been cut on the end to allow the head to pass through. The infant is placed in this bag before drying and should remain in the bag from the neck down until arrival in the nursery. Temperature must be monitored to avoid the risk of hyperthermia with this technique.

Management of Meconium-Stained Amniotic Fluid

Previously, the management of a newborn with meconium-stained amniotic fluid included intrapartum suctioning of the oropharynx and nasopharynx at the perineum after delivery of the head. Current evidence does not support this practice, as routine intrapartum oropharyngeal and nasopharyngeal suctioning does not prevent or alter the course of meconium aspiration syndrome. If meconium is present and the newborn is depressed, the clinician should intubate the trachea and suction to remove meconium or other aspirated material from beneath the glottis. When using mechanical suction apparatus, the suction pressure should be set such that negative pressure does not exceed 100 mm Hg. If the newborn is vigorous, defined as having strong respiratory efforts, good muscle tone, and a heart rate greater than 100, there is no evidence that tracheal suctioning is necessary. Furthermore, injury to the vocal cords is more likely to occur in attempting to intubate a vigorous newborn.

Positioning

The newborn can be positioned on either the back or the side, with the neck slightly extended. This "sniffing" position readily aligns the posterior pharynx, larynx, and trachea for optimal air entry, both with spontaneous breaths and bag or mask ventilation. The newborn's mouth and nose may be wiped with a towel or suctioned gently to remove excess mucus or blood. Although clear mucus routinely is suctioned from the mouth in most centers, there is no evidence to support the value of this practice. Vigorous suctioning of the posterior pharynx should be avoided because this may produce significant reflex bradycardia and may damage the oral mucosa, leading to interference with suckling because of pain.

Stimulation

Drying and suctioning the newborn infant provide stimulation and, for most newborns, this is all that is needed. However, if the infant does not have adequate respirations, some additional tactile stimulation may be needed. Acceptable methods of stimulation include slapping or flicking the soles of the feet and gently rubbing the newborn's back, trunk, or extremities. If the baby does not respond to one or two slaps, flicks to the feet, or rubbings of the back, positive-pressure ventilation should be initiated.

Ventilation

The normal newborn breathes within seconds of delivery and usually has established regular respirations within 1 minute after delivery. A newborn who is apneic or gasping or whose heart rate is less than 100 beats per minute requires positive-pressure ventilation. For most newborns, bag and mask ventilation is effective, can serve to initiate spontaneous respirations, and is the only resuscitation maneuver required.

Endotracheal intubation may be performed at various points during resuscitation, and the timing of intubation is determined by many factors, one of which is the skill of the resuscitator. Individuals not adept at intubation should obtain assistance and focus on providing effective ventilation with bag and mask rather than using valuable time trying to intubate. Indications for intubation include the following list:

- The presence of meconium in a depressed infant
- Poor response to bag or mask ventilation
- Enhancing coordination of ventilations and chest compressions when chest compressions are necessary

Other indications for intubation include extreme prematurity, need for surfactant administration, and a suspected or known diaphragmatic hernia.

Chest Compressions

If the heart rate does not increase promptly after effective ventilation with oxygen, chest compressions should be instituted while ventilation is continued. If there is no response in the heart rate after 30 seconds of effective chest compressions, appropriate drug therapy (and volume expansion, if indicated) should be instituted.

Medications

The use of medications for resuscitation of the newborn rarely is necessary in the delivery room and should be considered only after ventilation and chest compressions have been initiated and the heart rate remains low. A list of drugs for resuscitation, with their doses, should be readily available, preferably in a prominent place in the resuscitation area. National Resuscitation Program reference charts that provide this information as well as a flow diagram of the resuscitation procedure are available from the AAP for use in the delivery room and on code carts.

Epinephrine. Epinephrine is indicated when the heart rate remains less than 60 beats per minute, despite adequate ventilation and chest compressions. The recommended dose is 0.1–0.3 mL/kg of a 1:10,000 solution given intravenously, preferably through an umbilical venous catheter placed emergently in the delivery room. Previously, it was recommended that initial doses of epinephrine be given through the endotracheal tube because this can be done rapidly, but the efficacy of this route is unproven and use of this route results in lower and unpredictable blood levels that may not be effective. Some clinicians may choose to give an endotracheal tube dose while the umbilical venous catheter is being placed; if this route is being used, the dose should be 0.3–1 mL/kg of a 1:10,000 preparation.

Volume expanders. Volume expanders should be considered when a baby is not responding to resuscitation and there is evidence of blood loss. The recommended volume expander is normal saline, with a dose of 10 mL/kg given intravenously. It is given by the most accessible route, which in the delivery room is usually the umbilical vein. The infusion should not be given rapidly because this may increase the risk of intracranial hemorrhage, especially in the premature infant.

Narcotic agonists. Respiratory depression may result from narcotics administered to the mother before delivery, but this is infrequent. When suspected, the initial response, as in any case of apnea, should be positive-pressure ventilation. A narcotic antagonist should be considered only if severe respiratory depression persists after positive-pressure ventilation has improved the heart rate and color, and the mother received narcotics within 4 hours of delivery. If indicated, the recommended dose and concentration of naloxone is 0.1 mg/kg of a 1 mg/mL preparation, preferably given either intravenously or intramuscularly. Naloxone is contraindicated in an infant born to a narcotic-addicted mother. An infant who receives naloxone should be monitored because the effect of the narcotic may last longer than the length of time that the naloxone is effective, and repeated doses may be required.

Assessment of the Newborn in the Delivery Room

After delivery, the newborn must be assessed for individual needs to determine the best location for care. A healthy-appearing newborn may be admitted to the observation–admission–transition area of the well-baby nursery in preparation for rooming-in with the mother. An infant with known or anticipated medical needs may be admitted to the level II intermediate-care nursery or level III intensive-care area in the same hospital if it is a specialty or subspecialty hospital or may be transferred to a hospital that provides the appropriate specialty or subspecialty care (see "Specialty Care Facility" and "Subspecialty Care Facility" in Chapter 2 and "Transport Procedure" in Chapter 3).

If the newborn's condition is stable and does not require further intervention, immediate and sustained skin-to-skin contact between the mother and her infant can be provided. If the mother has chosen to breastfeed, the newborn should be placed at the breast in the delivery room within the first hour after delivery, as initial skin-to-skin contact has been associated with a longer duration of breastfeeding. Such contact maintains the infant's body temperature and facilitates the opportunity for breastfeeding soon after delivery. Generally, healthy newborns should remain with their mothers. The nursing staff in the delivery room, recovery room, or labor–delivery–recovery–postpartum area should be trained in assessing and recognizing problems in the newborn.

Newborns who have depressed breathing, depressed activity, or cyanosis at birth and require some intervention in the delivery room but make a prompt response, or those with symptoms including mild respiratory distress, are at risk for developing problems and should be frequently evaluated during the immediate neonatal period. This may take place in an observation–admission–transition nursery, where frequent vital signs can be obtained and the nursing staff is familiar with the signs and symptoms of an infant who is in distress. If the vital signs stabilize and the infant has no other risk factors, these newborns can then room-in with their mothers.

Infants who require more extensive resuscitation are at risk for developing subsequent complications and may require ongoing support. These infants should be managed in an area where ongoing evaluation and monitoring are available. This may take place in the birth hospital, if there is an appropriate facility, or may require transport to another hospital for a higher level of care.

Immediate plans for the newborn should be discussed with the parents (or other support person), preferably before leaving the delivery room. Whenever possible, the parents should have the opportunity to see and touch the newborn before transfer to a nursery or before transfer to another facility. The physician or other responsible person delivering the newborn also should be advised of the status and plans for the newborn, including potential transfer or admission to a level II specialty-care nursery or level III neonatal intensive care unit.

Infant Identification

The possibility of newborns being switched in the hospital requires strict guidelines to prevent these events. Human error continues to be the major cause of infant-switch events, and establishing procedures with multiple checks or electronic matching systems will minimize this risk. Infant identification procedures should begin in the delivery room with matching bands for the infant and the mother. The nurse in the delivery room should be responsible for preparing and securely fastening these identification bands on the newborn and the mother while the newborn is still in the delivery room. These identical bands should indicate the mother's admission number, the infant's sex, the date and time of birth, and other information specified in hospital policy. Footprinting and fingerprinting alone are not adequate methods of patient identification. The birth records and identification bands should be checked and verified for accuracy before the newborn leaves the delivery room. When the newborn is taken to the nursery, both the nurse accompanying the newborn and the admitting nurse should check and again verify the identification bands and birth records. Policies and procedures requiring personnel to match identification bands each time the infant is taken to the mother while in the hospital and at discharge will minimize the risk of errors. If the condition of the newborn does not allow placement of identification bands (eg, extreme preterm birth), the identification bands should accompany the infant and should be placed on the incubator or warmer to be attached as soon as is practical.

With multiple births, each of the newborns should be identified as to birth order (eg, A, B, C or 1, 2, 3) and the corresponding umbilical cords should be identified according to hospital policy (eg, use of different number of clamps). This will ensure that umbilical cord blood specimens will be labeled correctly and can be correlated with the correct newborn. All umbilical cord blood samples must be labeled with an indication that these are samples of the newborn's umbilical cord blood and not that of the mother. The birth order may or may not correlate with the number assigned to the fetus in utero.

Communication of Information

Care of the newborn is aided by effective communication of information about the mother and her fetus to the pediatrician or other health care provider. With an uncomplicated pregnancy, labor, and delivery, the information on the medical record accompanying the newborn, if complete, may be sufficient. The obstetric staff should record the following information, which also should be available on a medical record that accompanies the newborn during any transfer of responsibility for care:

- The mother's name, medical record number, blood type, serology result, rubella status, hepatitis B test result, and human immunodeficiency virus (HIV) status

- Any history of substance use or any other known socially high-risk circumstances, such as unstable housing, adolescent mother, maternal psychiatric disease, domestic violence, or history of previous child abuse or neglect

- Other maternal test results, if obtained, that are relevant to neonatal care, such as colonization with group B streptococci or intrapartum maternal antibiotic therapy (including type and doses of antibiotics)

- Maternal illness potentially affecting the pregnancy, evidence of chorioamnionitis, and maternal medications (including tocolytics and corticosteroids)

- Complications of pregnancy associated with abnormal fetal growth, fetal anomalies, or abnormal results from tests of fetal well-being and the corresponding interpretation

- Information regarding the delivery (eg, method and duration of labor), complications of labor (eg, nonreassuring fetal heart rate), duration of rupture of amniotic membranes, presence or absence of meconium in amniotic fluid, or need for resuscitation

- Situations in which lactation may be compromised, such as history of breast surgery, trauma, or previous lactation failure

The obstetric staff should communicate problems before and after delivery in a timely manner to the physician or other health care provider who will be caring for the newborn. For some high-risk pregnancies, a neonatal consultation during the antepartum period may be helpful in obstetric management and may assist the parents in understanding what to expect for their newborn. This is of particular importance when fetal abnormalities are significant or a very preterm newborn is expected.

Assessment of the Infant in the Nursery

Intrauterine Growth Status

The newborn's gestational age can be estimated from the mother's menstrual history or the results of an ultrasound examination before 20 weeks of gestation (see "Estimated Date of Delivery" in Chapter 4) and from the nursery assessment of gestational age (Fig. 7–3). The gestational age should be assigned by

Neuromuscular maturity

	-1	0	1	2	3	4	5
Posture							
Square window (wrist)	>90°	90°	60°	45°	30°	0°	
Arm recoil		180°	140–180°	110–140°	90–110°	<90°	
Popliteal angle	180°	160°	140°	120°	100°	90°	<90°
Scarf sign							
Heel to ear							

Physical maturity

Skin	Sticky, friable, transparent	Gelatinous, red, translucent	Smooth, pink, visible veins	Superficial peeling or rash or both, few veins	Cracking, pale areas, rare veins	Parchment, deep cracking, no vessels	Leathery, cracked, wrinkled
Lanugo	None	Sparse	Abundant	Thinning	Bald areas	Mostly bald	
Plantar surface	Heel–toe 40–50 mm:-1 <40 mm:-2	<50 mm, no crease	Faint red marks	Anterior transverse crease only	Creases on anterior 2/3	Creases over entire sole	
Breast	Imperceptible	Barely perceptible	Flat areola– no bud	Stripped areola, 1–2 mm bud	Raised areola, 3–4 mm bud	Full areola, 5–10 mm bud	
Eye/ear	Lids fused loosely (-1), tightly (-2)	Lids open, pinna flat, stays folded	Slightly curved pinna; soft; slow recoil	Well-curved pinna, soft but ready recoil	Formed and firm, instant recoil	Thick cartilage, ear stiff	
Genitals male	Scrotum flat, smooth	Scrotum empty, faint rugae	Testes in upper canal rare rugae	Testes descending, few rugae	Testes down, good rugae	Testes pendulous, deep rugae	
Genitals female	Clitoris prominent, labia flat	Prominent clitoris, small labia minora	Prominent clitoris, enlarging minora	Majora & minora equally prominent	Majora large, minora small	Majora cover clitoris & minora	

Maturity rating

Score	Weeks
-10	20
-5	22
0	24
5	26
10	28
15	30
20	32
25	34
30	36
35	38
40	40
45	42
50	44

Fig. 7–3. The expanded new Ballard Score includes extremely preterm infants and has been refined to improve accuracy in more mature infants. (Ballard JL, Khoury JC, Wedig K, Wang L, Eilers-Walsman BL, Lipp R. New Ballard Score, expanded to include extremely premature infants. J Pediatr 1991;119:417–23.)

the physician after all data, both pediatric and obstetric, have been assessed. Any marked discrepancy between the presumed duration of pregnancy by obstetric assessment and the physical and neurologic findings in the newborn should be documented on the medical record.

Growth parameters should be plotted on a birth weight–gestational age record. Determination of gestational age and its relationship to weight can be used to identify newborns at risk for postnatal complications. For example, newborns who are either large or small for their gestational ages are at relatively increased risk for hypoglycemia and polycythemia, and appropriate tests (eg, serum glucose screen or hematocrit determination) are indicated.

Risk Assessment

No later than 2 hours after birth, nursery personnel should evaluate the newborn's status and assess risks. Risks can be assessed through the history as documented on the antepartum and intrapartum records, as well as from the gestational age assessment and growth parameter determination. If the newborn's physician (or other health care provider) is not present at the delivery, he or she should be notified of the admission and of the status of the newborn within a time frame established by institutional policy.

Nursery policies should delineate those conditions (eg, low birth weight or small for gestational age) that require specific actions by nurses or immediate notification of a physician. Clinical conditions such as maternal substance use, maternal fever or infection, or low Apgar scores at 5 minutes or more are associated with increased risk for neonatal illness and should prompt immediate notification of the physician. The obstetrician should be notified of the newborn's status in a timely manner, particularly if problems or complications arise.

If immediate attention is not indicated, the newborn's physician or other health care provider, as defined by institutional policy, should examine the apparently normal newborn no later than 24 hours after delivery and within

24 hours before discharge from the hospital. This may be accomplished with one physical examination. The results of the examination should be recorded on the newborn's medical record and discussed with the parents.

Transitional Care

After an initial evaluation of the newborn's condition, a care plan should be established, and the newborn should be carefully observed during the subsequent stabilization–transition period (the first 6–12 hours after birth). If the infant is healthy and stable, the care plan should allow ongoing contact of the mother and the infant during this period. Temperature, heart and respiratory rates, skin color, adequacy of peripheral circulation, type of respiration, level of consciousness, tone, and activity should be monitored and recorded at least once every 30 minutes until the newborn's condition has remained stable for 2 hours. Rooming-in for the mother and her infant is optimal because it allows unrestricted contact and feeding. Hospital staff easily can assess the infant's status in the mother's room until discharge.

The newborn should be observed for any of the following signs of illness:

- Temperature instability
- Change in activity, including refusal of feedings
- Unusual skin color
- Abnormal cardiac or respiratory rate and rhythm
- Abdominal distension or bilious vomiting
- Excessive lethargy and sleeping
- Delayed or abnormal stools—The normal, term newborn passes meconium within the first 24 hours after birth. If a term newborn has not passed meconium by 48 hours after birth, the lower gastrointestinal tract may be obstructed.
- Delayed voiding—Urine is normally passed within the first 12 hours after birth. Failure to void within the first 24 hours may indicate genitourinary obstruction or abnormality.

Eye Care

Prophylaxis against gonococcal ophthalmia neonatorum is mandatory for all newborns, including those born by cesarean delivery. A variety of topical agents appear to be equally efficacious. Acceptable prophylactic regimens are an application of a 1 cm ribbon of sterile ophthalmic ointment containing erythromycin (0.5%) or tetracycline (1%) in each lower conjunctival sac. Care should be taken to ensure that the agent reaches all parts of the conjunctival sac. The eyes should not be irrigated with saline or distilled water after application of any of these agents; however, after 1 minute, excess solution or ointment can be wiped away with sterile cotton. Application should be given shortly after birth, but may be delayed up to 1 hour until after the initial breastfeeding.

Vitamin K

Every newborn should receive a single parenteral dose of natural vitamin K1 oxide (phytonadione) (0.5–1 mg) to prevent vitamin K-dependent hemorrhagic disease of the newborn. The administration of this dose traditionally has been given within 1 hour of birth but may be delayed until after the first breastfeeding in the delivery room. Although oral administration of vitamin K might be efficacious in prevention of early hemorrhagic disease of the newborn, it has not been shown to be as efficacious as parenteral administration for the prevention of late hemorrhagic disease. In addition, there is no commercial oral vitamin K preparation approved for use in the United States.

Weighing

Each newborn should be weighed shortly after birth, or after the first breastfeeding, and daily thereafter. The newborn must be kept warm during weighing. The scale pan should be covered with clean paper before each newborn is weighed.

Clothing

Most newborns require only a cotton shirt or gown without buttons in addition to a soft diaper once thermal stability has been established. A supply of soft, clean, cotton clothing, bed pads, sheets, and blankets should be kept at the bedside. Nontoxic dyes should be used to mark clothing, blankets, or other items used in the care of newborns. A cap prevents excess heat loss from the head.

Skin Care

Skin care, including bathing, may be important for the health and appearance of the individual newborn and for infection control within the nursery. Removal of blood and secretions from the skin after delivery may minimize the risk of infection with potentially contaminating microorganisms, such as hepatitis B virus, herpes simplex virus, and HIV. Because bathing can be associated with significant heat loss, the first bath should be postponed until the newborn's thermal stability is ensured unless indicated by maternal infection risk factors, particularly HIV. The medical and nursing services of each hospital should develop guidelines regarding the time of the first bath, measures to protect against excessive heat loss, circumstances and methods of skin cleansing, and the roles of personnel and parents.

The effects on the newborn's skin should be considered in selecting skin care techniques. Some agents are absorbed and may be toxic; others change skin flora and may increase the risk of infection. Whole-body bathing of the newborn may not be necessary. Localized skin care or techniques that minimize exposure to water may reduce the newborn's heat loss. Sterile cotton sponges (not gauze) soaked with warm water may be used to remove blood and meconium from the newborn's face, head, and body. Alternatively, the newborn can be cleansed with a mild, non-medicated soap and then rinsed with water. After washing by either method, the infant should be dried carefully, with particular attention to the head.

For the remainder of the newborn's stay in the hospital nursery, local skin care of the buttocks and perianal regions with warm water and cotton, a mild soap and water, or baby wipes at diaper changes should be adequate. Ideally, agents used on the newborn's skin should be dispensed in single-use containers, or each newborn should have a personal dispenser.

Various antiseptic compounds for skin care have been studied to determine their safety and effectiveness in preventing colonization and infection in newborns. Hexachlorophene, although relatively effective against gram-positive bacteria, particularly *Staphylococcus aureus*, should not be used routinely for bathing newborns because of its potential for neurotoxic effects in newborns. Although iodophors are good antiseptics, they have not been proved to be both safe and effective for routine skin care. Chlorhexidine gluconate, a compound that is poorly absorbed through intact skin, is useful for bathing or for localized skin care.

Umbilical Cord Care

No single method of umbilical cord care has been proved to be superior in preventing colonization and disease. Current methods include the local application of antimicrobial agents, such as triple-dye, iodophor ointment, or hexachlorophene powder. The skin absorption and toxicity of triple-dye in newborns have not been studied carefully. Alcohol used alone is not effective in preventing umbilical cord colonization and omphalitis.

Circumcision

Existing scientific evidence demonstrates potential medical benefits of newborn male circumcision; however, these data are not sufficient to recommend routine neonatal circumcision. The exact incidence of complications after circumcision is not known, but data indicate that the rate is low and that the most common complications are local infection and bleeding. Given this understanding, parents should make the determination in the interest of the newborn. To make an informed choice, the parents of all male newborns should be given accurate and unbiased information on circumcision and be given an opportunity to discuss this decision. Information sheets for parents about circumcision are available through the AAP.

Analgesia must be provided if circumcision is performed. Swaddling, sucrose by mouth, and acetaminophen administration may reduce the stress response but are not sufficient for the operative pain and cannot be recommended as the sole method of analgesia. Although local anesthesia and combination preparations of lidocaine and prilocaine provide some anesthesia benefit, both ring blocks and dorsal penile blocks have been proved to be more effective.

Written instructions for care of the circumcision site are suggested. Postprocedure care of the circumcised infant should include cleaning and protecting the site from infection and irritation. With each diaper change, the penis should be cleaned with warm water, and petroleum jelly can be placed over the surgical site. The jelly can be placed on a bandage or clean gauze pad and applied directly on the penis or placed on the diaper in the area with which the penis comes into contact. The petroleum jelly is not necessary for healing, but it keeps the site from sticking to the diaper and causing irritation and bleeding when the diaper is removed. This will be necessary for approximately 4–7 days after circumcision.

If the family decides against circumcision, the uncircumcised penis is easy to keep clean. Because of physiologic adhesions, the foreskin usually does not retract fully for several years and should not be forced. Gentle washing of the genital area while bathing is sufficient for normal hygiene.

Preventive Care

Hepatitis Immunization

Each hospital should establish procedures to assess the newborn's status regarding hepatitis exposure and timely, appropriate intervention and immunization (see "Hepatitis B Virus" in Chapter 9). Early hepatitis B immunization is recommended for all medically stable infants with birth weights greater than 2 kg, irrespective of maternal hepatitis B status. In infants born to mothers with negative hepatitis B serology, it is preferable that the initial dose is administered before discharge from the nursery.

Universal Newborn Screening

Newborn screening is a preventive public health procedure that should be available to all newborns. Advances in technology have expanded newborn screening capabilities. The panel of diseases or abnormalities that are subjected to universal screening is determined and implemented by the local and state health authority or agency and, although all states have newborn screening programs, there is wide variation between states for diseases screened. Currently, there is an effort to develop national guidelines for newborn screening that would be uniform for every state.

An adequate neonatal screening program includes education, laboratory tests, administration, follow-up, management, and evaluation components. A comprehensive screening program includes the following components:

- Education of parents and practitioners about newborn screening and their participation in the activity
- Reliable acquisition and transportation of adequate specimens
- Reliable and prompt performance of screening tests
- Prompt retrieval and follow-up of individuals with abnormal test results
- Appropriate further testing of individuals with abnormal test results to establish an accurate diagnosis
- Appropriate intervention and treatment of affected individuals
- Education, genetic counseling, and psychosocial support for families with affected newborns

Every hospital should establish routines to ensure that all newborns are screened in accordance with state law. Some newborns with disorders included in the newborn screening battery will not be identified even with a properly conducted screening test because of individual or biologic variations, very early discharge, or administrative or laboratory error.

If the initial specimen is obtained from the infant before 12–24 hours after delivery, then a second specimen should be obtained at 1–2 weeks of age to decrease the probability that phenylketonuria and other disorders with metabolite accumulation will be missed as a consequence of early testing. Repeat testing also should be performed if clinically indicated, regardless of the initial screening results. An adequate specimen must be provided to the laboratory for accurate testing. Umbilical cord blood is never an appropriate specimen because it will be inaccurate for detection of disorders in which metabolite accumulation occurs after birth and after the initiation of feeding.

Premature infants, neonates receiving parenteral feeding, or neonates being treated for illness should have a newborn screening test performed at or near 7 days of age, regardless of feeding status. A repeat specimen should be obtained in these infants when enteral feedings are adequate. Nurseries should develop protocols for these infants that comply with state regulations.

The responsibility for transmitting the screening test results to the physician or other health care providers should rest with the authority or agency that performed the test. Screening test status should be entered into the patient's medical record. The pediatrician and other health care providers should recognize the need for careful documentation of newborn screening test results for each infant entering the practice.

Hearing Screening

The prevalence of newborn hearing loss is approximately 1–2 per 1,000 live births, with an incidence of 1 per 1,000 in the normal newborn nursery population and 20–40 per 1,000 in the newborn intensive care unit population. In accordance with the recommendations of the AAP Task Force on Newborn and Infant Hearing and the Joint Committee on Infant Hearing, every hospital with an obstetric service should develop and implement a universal newborn hearing screening program to ensure appropriate screening, tracking and follow-up, identification, intervention, and evaluation. A protocol for screening should be developed at each hospital, defining how each step in the program will be carried out. Screening should be performed with a physiologic measure, using either an automated auditory brainstem response, an otoacoustic emission, or a combination of the two. Every effort should be made to complete screening before discharge from the hospital. Many programs use a two-step screening protocol, in which all infants have an initial screening test with either automated auditory brainstem response or otoacoustic emission. If they pass the screening test, no further testing is done; if they fail the first screening test, a repeat screening test is performed before discharge, usually with automated auditory brainstem response. The failure rate for newborn hearing screening (ie, the referral rate for diagnostic hearing testing after completion of screening) should be less than 4%.

In hospitals where universal newborn hearing screening is not fully implemented, infants should be evaluated if they have the following risk factors:

- Family history of hereditary childhood sensorineural hearing loss
- In utero infection, such as cytomegalovirus (CMV), rubella, syphilis, herpes, or toxoplasmosis
- Craniofacial anomalies, including infants with morphologic abnormalities of the pinnae and ear canals
- Birth weight less than 1,500 g
- Hyperbilirubinemia at a serum level requiring exchange transfusion
- Ototoxic medications, including, but not limited to, aminoglycosides used in multiple courses or in combination with loop diuretics
- Bacterial meningitis
- Apgar score of 0–4 at 1 minute or 0–6 at 5 minutes after birth
- Mechanical ventilation lasting 5 days or longer
- Stigmata or other findings associated with a syndrome known to include a sensorineural or conductive hearing loss

Screening infants with these indications will identify only 50% of all newborns with significant hearing loss.

All infants who pass the newborn hearing screening test, and particularly those with any risk factor, should be reevaluated periodically throughout childhood with objective measures of hearing (see the AAP periodicity table). A significant number of children may develop progressive or late-onset hearing loss, and continued surveillance is essential to identify these children in a timely manner.

All infants who fail the newborn screening test should receive complete diagnostic testing by qualified pediatric specialists by 3 months of age, with intervention provided by 6 months of age. Tracking and close follow-up are essential to ensure that children receive the appropriate and necessary evaluation and intervention. Ongoing evaluation of the screening program also is essential for quality assessment.

Screening for Hyperbilirubinemia

In most infants, jaundice is a benign condition, but in some infants who develop severe hyperbilirubinemia, it may result in death or encephalopathy. To minimize the risk in term or late preterm infants (those 35 weeks of gestation or more), it is recommended that a systematic assessment be made before discharge for the risk of severe hyperbilirubinemia, a plan for treatment be developed (when indicated), and early follow-up after discharge be arranged based on the risk assessment (see Chapter 8). Each nursery should develop policies and procedures for hyperbilirubinemia screening. These policies should consider the following elements:

- Promotion and support of successful breastfeeding
- Protocols for identification and evaluation of hyperbilirubinemia
- Provision for measurement of the total serum bilirubin or transcutaneous bilirubin concentration in infants jaundiced in the first 24 hours
- Recognition that visual estimation of the degree of jaundice can lead to errors, especially in darkly pigmented infants
- Interpretation of all bilirubin levels according to the infant's age in hours (see Chapter 8)
- Recognition that infants born at less than 38 weeks of gestation, especially those who are breastfed, are at higher risk of developing hyperbilirubinemia and require closer surveillance and monitoring
- Performance of a systematic assessment on all infants before discharge for the risk of severe hyperbilirubinemia
- Provision of both written and verbal information to parents about newborn jaundice
- Provision of appropriate follow-up based on the time of discharge and the risk assessment
- Treatment of newborns, when indicated, with phototherapy or exchange transfusion (For more information, see "Hyperbilirubinemia" in Chapter 8.)

Visiting Policies

The father or other support person should be encouraged to remain with the mother throughout the intrapartum and postpartum periods. Flexible and liberal visiting policies for families are encouraged.

Some institutions offer sibling classes to prepare other children in a family for the event of childbirth. Contact with the mother and newborn in the hospital helps prepare siblings for the new family member and is reassuring for younger children. The presence of siblings may be appropriate in labor, at delivery, or in the postpartum period, as local policy permits. The children must be accompanied by an adult to help them understand what is occurring and to remove them if circumstances demand.

Physical contact of siblings with infants is a topic of ongoing concern because of the possible transmission of viral infectious diseases. If siblings are allowed to have direct contact with the newborn, the visit may take place in the mother's private room or, if the mother is not in a private room, in a special sibling visitation area. Thorough hand hygiene as practiced at the institution should be required before physical contact with the infant. Parents should share the responsibility of preventing the exposure of their newborn to a sibling with a contagious illness by providing accurate information about illness or exposures. Contact of the newborn with children other than siblings should be avoided.

An institution that allows sibling visitation should have clearly defined, written policies and procedures that are based on currently available information. Basic guidelines for sibling visits that may serve as the basis for policy formulation are listed as follows:

- Sibling visits should be encouraged for both healthy and ill newborns.
- Before the visit, a member of the hospital staff should interview the parents to assess the current health of each sibling visitor. No child with fever or symptoms of an acute illness, such as upper respiratory infection or gastroenteritis, should be allowed to visit. Siblings who recently have been exposed to a known communicable disease (eg, chickenpox) should not be allowed to visit.
- Children should be prepared in advance for their visit.
- Children should only visit their sibling.
- Children should practice hand hygiene according to the unit guidelines before patient contact.
- Throughout the visit, sibling activity should be supervised by parents or a responsible adult.

Because available data on the risks and benefits of sibling visitation are limited, continued evaluation and reporting are needed. Evaluation should include both psychologic and infectious-disease factors. Institutions offering controlled sibling visitation in neonatal intensive care units have noted no adverse effects, although chickenpox exposures have occurred, but more study is needed before a general recommendation can be made.

Security

The threat of infant abduction requires that hospitals have active programs to prevent these events. Prevention of infant abduction is minimized by policies that include educating staff about the risk factors for abduction, educating parents about safe procedures for release of their infant, and controlling access to the postpartum area. Each institution should develop a newborn security system, which may include the use of electronic sensor devices. When the newborn is rooming-in, the parents should be instructed to release their infant only to an individual with a picture ID badge, and they should question why and where their infant is being taken. Access to the labor and delivery area as well as the postpartum area should be controlled.

Discharge

The hospital stay of the mother and the newborn should be long enough to allow identification of problems and to ensure that the mother is sufficiently recovered and prepared to care for herself and her newborn at home. Many neonatal cardiopulmonary problems related to the transition from the intrauterine to the extrauterine environment usually become apparent during the first 12 hours after birth. Other neonatal problems, such as jaundice, ductal-dependent cardiac lesions, and gastrointestinal obstruction, may require a longer period of observation by skilled and experienced personnel. Likewise, significant maternal complications, such as endometritis, may not become apparent during the first day after delivery. The length of stay, therefore, should be based on the unique characteristics of each mother–infant dyad, including the health of the mother, the health and stability of the newborn, the ability and confidence of the mother to care for herself and her newborn, the adequacy of support systems at home, and access to appropriate follow-up care. All efforts should be made to keep mothers and newborns together and to ensure simultaneous discharge.

The timing of discharge from the hospital should be the decision of the physicians caring for the mother and her newborn. This should be made in consultation with the family and should not be based on arbitrary policies established by third-party payers.

A shortened hospital stay (less than 48 hours after delivery) for healthy, term newborns can be accomplished but is not appropriate for every mother and newborn. Institutions should develop guidelines through their professional staff in collaboration with appropriate community agencies, including third-party payers, to establish hospital-stay programs for mothers and their healthy, term newborns. State and local public health agencies also should be involved in the oversight of existing hospital-stay programs for quality assurance and monitoring.

The following minimum criteria should be met before a newborn is discharged from the hospital after an uncomplicated pregnancy, labor, and delivery. It is unlikely that the fulfillment of these criteria and conditions can be met in less than 48 hours after birth. If discharge is considered before 48 hours, it should be limited to infants born with uncomplicated antepartum, intrapartum, and postpartum courses for both mother and newborn; singleton vaginal births between 38 weeks and 42 weeks of gestation; infants with birth weights appropriate for gestational age; and meeting other discharge criteria as follows:

- The infant's vital signs are documented to be normal and stable for the 12 hours before discharge, including a respiratory rate of fewer than 60 breaths per minute, a heart rate of 100–160 beats per minute, and an axillary temperature of 36.5–37.4°C (97.7–99.3°F) in an open crib with appropriate clothing.

- The infant has urinated and has passed at least one stool spontaneously.

- The infant has completed at least two successful feedings
  — If bottle feeding, documentation has been made that the infant is able to coordinate sucking, swallowing, and breathing while feeding.
  — If breastfeeding, an actual feeding should be observed by a caregiver knowledgeable in breastfeeding, and latch-on, swallowing, and infant satiety should be documented in the medical record.

- Physical examination reveals no abnormalities that require continued hospitalization.

- There is no evidence of excessive bleeding at the circumcision site for at least 2 hours.

- The clinical significance of jaundice, if present before discharge, has been determined, and appropriate management or follow-up plans have been put in place.

- The mother's (or, preferably, both parents') knowledge, ability, and confidence to provide adequate care for the infant are documented by the fact that the following training and information has been received:
  — Appropriate urination and stooling frequency for the infant
  — Umbilical cord, skin, and newborn genital care, as well as temperature assessment and measurement with a thermometer
  — Signs of illness and common newborn problems, particularly jaundice

- A car safety seat appropriate for the infant's maturity and medical condition that meets Federal Motor Vehicle Safety Standard 213 has been obtained and is available at hospital discharge.

- Family members or other support persons, including health care providers, such as the family pediatrician or his or her designees, who are familiar with newborn care and are knowledgeable about lactation and the recognition of jaundice and dehydration, are available to the mother and the infant after discharge.

- Instructions to follow in the event of a complication or emergency have been provided.

- Maternal and infant laboratory tests are available and have been reviewed, including:

  — Maternal syphilis, hepatitis B virus surface antigen (HBsAg), and HIV status

  — Umbilical cord or newborn blood type and direct Coombs' test result, if clinically indicated

  — Screening tests, in accordance with state requirements. If a test was performed before 24 hours of milk feeding, a system for repeating the test during the follow-up visit must be in place in accordance with local or state policy.

- Initial hepatitis B vaccine has been administered or an appointment scheduled for its administration as indicated by the infant's risk status and according to the current immunization schedule.

- Hearing screening has been completed per hospital protocol.

- Family, environmental, and social risk factors have been assessed. When these or other risk factors are present, the discharge should be delayed until they are resolved or a plan to safeguard the newborn is in place. Such factors may include, but are not limited to:

  — Untreated parental substance use or positive urine toxicology test results in the mother or the newborn

  — History of child abuse or neglect

  — Mental illness in a parent who is in the home

  — Lack of social support, particularly for single, first-time mothers

  — No fixed home

  — History of domestic violence, particularly during this pregnancy

— Adolescent mother, particularly if other risk factors are present

— Barriers to adequate follow-up, such as lack of transportation, lack of access to telephone communication, and non-English speaking parents

- A physician-directed source of continuing medical care for both the mother and the infant has been identified. For newborns discharged before 48 hours after delivery, an appointment has been made for the infant to be examined within 48 hours of discharge. If this cannot be ensured, discharge should be deferred until a mechanism for follow up is identified. The follow-up visit can take place in a home or clinic setting, as long as the personnel examining the infant are competent in newborn assessment and the results of the follow-up visit are reported to the infant's physician or designees on the day of the visit.

The follow-up visit is designed to fulfill the following functions:

- Weigh the infant, assess the infant's general health, hydration, and degree of jaundice, and identify any new problems

- Review feeding patterns and technique, including observation of breast-feeding for adequacy of position, latch-on, and swallowing, and obtain historical evidence of adequate stool and urine patterns

- Assess quality of mother–infant interaction and details of newborn behavior

- Reinforce maternal or family education in infant care, particularly regarding feeding and sleep position

- Review results of laboratory tests performed at discharge

- Perform screening tests in accordance with state regulations and other tests that are clinically indicated, such as serum bilirubin

- Verify the plan for health care maintenance, including a method for obtaining emergency services, preventive care and immunizations, periodic evaluations and physical examinations, and necessary screening

This follow-up visit should be considered an independent service to be reimbursed as a separate package and not part of a global fee for labor, delivery, and routine nursery services.

Education and Psychosocial Factors

The reduction in the average length of a newborn's hospital stay has compromised the opportunity for parent education. Traditional methods of individual teaching of parents by nurses cannot be accomplished within the shortened hospital stay.

This requires that other methods of education be developed, including prenatal classes, audiovisual materials, printed materials, and online education programs. Audiovisual materials that have been reviewed and approved by the obstetric and pediatric staff, printed materials, and education by a variety of hospital personnel (eg, postpartum and nursery nurses, registered dietitians and nutritionists, lactation specialists, and physical therapists) can be helpful to parents. Many educational resources can be made available via the Internet. There is a parent-education site on the AAP web site (www.aap.org), and many individual hospitals have their own web sites with appropriate information. Other beneficial activities are group or individual educational sessions held regularly during the postpartum period to teach and discuss patient self-care, including exercises and self-examination of the breasts; parent–infant relationships; care of the newborn, including bathing and feeding; and child growth and development. Family-planning techniques appropriate to the patient's needs and desires also should be explained in detail (see "Postpartum Considerations" in Chapter 5).

The educational activities should include information explaining the rapid changes in physiology that occur in the newborn. Parents should be familiar with normal and abnormal changes in wake–sleep patterns, temperature, respiration, voiding, stooling, and the appearance of the skin, including jaundice. They also should observe and become familiar with the behavior, temperament, and neurologic capabilities of the newborn. Awareness of newborn cardiopulmonary resuscitation techniques also may be helpful.

During the postpartum hospital stay, health care personnel can provide the mother with professional assistance when she is most likely to be uncomfortable and can help her to anticipate how she may feel once she is home. The mother may be unsure of the normal physical changes that occur after delivery and of her ability to care for the newborn. The mother should be evaluated when she is with her newborn to identify any problems she is having so that appropriate instructions can be provided before and after discharge. Prenatal instructions given to prepare the family for the newborn's care at home also should be reinforced.

Both in-hospital and community agencies often are available to assist the family. Information on public and private groups that provide services to families with newborns, and the circumstances under which these organizations may be asked for such assistance, should be available in the hospital. Information may be obtained from the following sources:

- The in-hospital social service department, as an integral part of the interdisciplinary effort to coordinate hospital and discharge activities, to obtain public or private assistance, and to render psychosocial support

- Members of the home care service, for home visits to assess the parents' child-rearing skills, the home environment, the mother's emotional stability, and the infant's status and development (under the physician's direction, home care nurses may administer drugs or provide other types of therapy)
- Groups that lend support and provide education on special activities (eg, breastfeeding)

Sleep Position and Sudden Infant Death Syndrome

Sudden infant death syndrome (SIDS) is a leading cause of newborn mortality after 1 month and before 1 year of age in the United States. There are several modifiable risk factors that have been identified, including prone sleeping, soft sleep surfaces, loose bedding, overheating, and bed sharing. Investigations on the hazards of prone sleeping and reviews of the epidemiology of SIDS with attention to sleep position have resulted in the recommendation that healthy infants not be placed in the prone position for sleeping. Supine positioning (lying wholly on the back) carries the lowest risk of SIDS and is preferred; although the side position is safer than the prone position, there remains a significantly higher risk of SIDS in the side position and it should not be used. Infants should be placed supine when resting, sleeping or when left alone, and all caregivers, baby sitters, and child-care centers should have this emphasized to them by the parent. Hence, mothers must be educated about this during their hospital stay. "Tummy time" should be encouraged for awake playtime and when under direct observation by the parent. Additionally, parents should be instructed to avoid excessively loose or soft bedding materials by which the infant's airway may become occluded. Overheating may be an independent risk factor or may be associated with the use of additional clothing or blankets. Bed sharing or cosleeping is of concern because of the risk of suffocation through overlaying, as well as the risk of entrapment, wedging, falling, or strangulation on an adult bed. Proponents of bed sharing propose that breastfeeding, especially nocturnal breastfeeding, is enhanced, and some mothers will choose to cosleep. Cosleeping is associated with an increased risk for SIDS, although the risk is greater when the infant cosleeps with children or other adults rather than with the mother. The Task Force on Sudden Infant Death Syndrome recommends a separate but proximate sleeping environment because SIDS has been shown to be decreased when the infant sleeps in the same room as the mother.

For infants with gastroesophageal reflux disease, obstructive sleep apnea, or certain congenital malformations, the physician should recommend specific sleep positioning. Preterm infants in the newborn intensive care unit should be placed supine as determined by physician judgment as far in advance of discharge as possible.

Decreases in deaths caused by SIDS have been documented in countries where parents have changed from placing infants in prone positions to back positions for sleeping. Cardiorespiratory monitoring has not been demonstrated to decrease the incidence of SIDS, and home cardiorespiratory monitoring should not be prescribed to prevent SIDS. No serious adverse effects to the newborn because of supine positioning have been reported. There has been an increase in the diagnosis of cranial asymmetry or positional plagiocephaly temporally related to the "Back to Sleep" positioning recommendation. This can be minimized by encouraging tummy time when awake as well as alternating the supine head position during sleep.

Follow-up Care

The physical and psychosocial status of the mother and her infant should be subject to ongoing assessment after discharge. The mother needs personalized care during the postpartum period to hasten the development of a healthy mother–infant relationship and a sense of maternal confidence. Support and reassurance should be provided as the mother masters and adapts to her maternal role. Involving the other parent or other close support person and encouraging participation in the infant's care not only can provide additional support to the mother but also can enhance the relationship between the newborn and the family.

The postpartum period is a time of developmental adjustment for the whole family. Family members have new roles and relationships, and an effort should be made to assess the progress of the family's adaptation. If a family member finds it difficult to assume the new role, the health care team should arrange for sensitive, supportive assistance. This is particularly important for adolescent mothers, for whom it may be necessary to mobilize multiple resources within the community.

The frequency of follow-up visits for normal infants varies with patient, locale, and community practices. The intervals should be consistent with the AAP's guidelines on preventive health care. Regular follow-up visits and good records of development should be maintained.

Physicians and other professionals who provide follow-up care to women and infants should be aware of and look for the following physical, social, and psychologic factors associated with child abuse:

- Preterm birth
- Neonatal illness with long periods of hospitalization, especially in neonatal intensive care units
- Single parenthood
- Adolescent motherhood
- Closely spaced pregnancies
- Infrequent family visits to hospitalized infants
- Substance use

Infants and parents with such a history or with other factors associated with child abuse require closer follow-up than does the average family. The interaction of the parents, especially the mother with the infant, should be evaluated periodically. The infant or child who fails to thrive may be a victim of neglect, if not outright abuse, and a causal relationship between neglect and failure to thrive always should be suspected. In every state, providers of health care to children are legally obligated to report suspected child abuse.

Adoption

Health care for infants who are to be adopted should focus on the needs of the child, the adoptive family, and the birth parents. These infants may have acute and long-term medical, psychologic, and developmental problems because of their genetic, emotional, cultural, psychosocial, or medical backgrounds. The pediatrician should perform a careful medical assessment of the infant and should counsel the adopting family appropriately. Just as a birth family cannot be certain that its biologic child will be healthy, an adoptive family cannot be guaranteed that a child will not have future health problems. Most adopted children, even those from high-risk backgrounds, are healthy. Those with certain disorders and special problems, however, also can be adopted successfully. The risks should be defined and explained carefully to the family so that problems can be anticipated and addressed expediently.

The pediatrician's role is not to judge the advisability of a proposed adoption but to apprise the prospective parents and any involved agency clearly and honestly of any special health needs detected at examination or anticipated in the future. Physicians evaluating a newborn for adoption should obtain an extensive history from the birth parents and enter these data into the formal medical record. There may never again be a comparable opportunity to obtain this information. If the pediatrician is unable to interview the parents personally, an adoption agency social worker who is trained to do a skilled genetic and medical interview should obtain a complete prenatal and postpartum history. The prenatal history should include information on the birth parents' lifestyle that may affect the fetus at birth or later in development. Physicians and adoption agency social workers should be trained to obtain lifestyle information in a manner that is sensitive to psychologic and cultural issues. Such information includes parental use of alcohol or other drugs and history of sexual practices that increase the risk of sexually transmitted diseases in both birth parents. The increased risk of genetically inherited disorders by infants of incestuous mating may require special consultations. After reviewing whatever history is available, the pediatrician should examine the adopted child carefully and perform metabolic, genetic, and other assessments as indicated.

Physicians must be careful with semantics when dealing with the adoptive family. This is an "adoptive family," not only an "adopted child." The term "parents" applies to the parents in the adoptive family; the birth parents are those who conceived the child. Real or natural parent(s) are confusing terms that should be eliminated because they may reflect negatively on adoptive families and imply a temporary or less-than-genuine relationship between adoptive families and their children.

The physician should be aware of state laws regarding adoption procedures. Hospital nurseries should have policies regarding the handling of adoptions in accordance with these laws. Policies should reflect sensitivity toward both the adoptive family as well as the birth parents. Although adoption is generally an elective decision initiated by the birth parents, the birth parents often need support adjusting to the separation from their infant.

Neonatal Nutrition

Breastfeeding

There are diverse and important advantages to infants, mothers, families, and society for breastfeeding and the use of human milk for infant feeding. These include health, nutritional, immunologic, developmental, psychologic, social, economic, and environmental benefits. Human milk supports optimal growth and development of the infant while decreasing the risk of a variety of acute and chronic diseases.

Prenatal counseling and education regarding methods of newborn feeding may allow correction of misperceptions about feeding methods. Virtually all mothers who are hesitant to breastfeed can do so successfully with appropriate counseling, education, and knowledgeable support. If, after these interventions, the mother chooses not to breastfeed, she should be supported in her decision.

Initiation of Breastfeeding

The successful management of breastfeeding begins during pregnancy. Prenatal care should include discussion of prior breastfeeding experience, feeding plans, and breast care. Ascertainment of history of breast surgery, trauma, or prior lactation failure is important because these situations may present special challenges to successful breastfeeding. The integration of breastfeeding into the total care of the newborn in the first months of life should be discussed.

The mother should be offered the opportunity and be encouraged to breastfeed her newborn as soon as possible after delivery. A healthy newborn is capable of latching on to a breast without specific assistance within the first hour after birth, and breastfeeding should be initiated in the first hour of life unless medically contraindicated. Infants should be placed in direct skin-to-skin contact with their mother immediately after delivery and should remain there until the first feeding is completed.

Rooming-in with the mother should be expected and supported because this facilitates breastfeeding. From the time of delivery to discharge from the hospital, the mother and her infant should be together continuously. The mother should be encouraged to offer the breast whenever the infant shows early signs of hunger, such as increased alertness, increased physical activity, mouthing, or rooting, and not to wait until the infant cries because crying is a late indicator of hunger.

When awake, the newborn should be encouraged to feed frequently (8–12 times per day) until satiety (usually 10–15 minutes on each breast) to help stimulate milk production. In the early weeks after birth, nondemanding infants may need to be aroused to feed if 4 hours have elapsed since the last nursing. Usually, it is wise to alternate the breast used to initiate the feeding and to equalize the time spent at each breast over the day. When satisfied, the newborn will fall asleep or unlatch.

Supplements including water, glucose water, formula, and other fluids should not be given to the breastfeeding infant unless ordered by the physician for a medical indication. Supplementation of the breastfed infant is best accomplished with formula or expressed breast milk. Intermittent bottle-feeding of a breastfed newborn may lessen the success of breastfeeding and, if the newborn's appetite is partially satisfied by water or formula supplements, the newborn will take less from the breast, and milk production will be diminished.

Monitoring the Breastfed Newborn

During the newborn hospitalization, formal evaluation of breastfeeding, including observation of position, latch, and milk transfer, should be done by trained caregivers and documented at least twice a day. The mother should be encouraged to record the time and duration of each feeding, as well as urine and stool output, during the early days of breastfeeding to help facilitate the evaluation process both in the hospital and at home after discharge.

The breastfeeding newborn infant should be seen by a pediatrician or other knowledgeable and experienced health care professional at 3–5 days of age or within 48 hours of discharge, with a second ambulatory visit at 2–3 weeks of age, unless indicated earlier, to monitor progress. The initial visit should include infant weight, physical examination (especially for jaundice and hydration), maternal history of breast problems, including pain or engorgement, elimination patterns (expect 3–5 urine eliminations and 3–4 stool eliminations per day by 3–5 days of age and 4–6 urine eliminations and 3–6 stool eliminations per day by 5–7 days of age), and a formal observed evaluation of breastfeeding, including position, latch, and milk transfer.

Weight loss beyond 3 days of age, weight loss of more than 7% of birth weight, or failure to regain birth weight by 2 weeks of age in the term infant requires a careful evaluation of the feeding techniques being used and the adequacy of breastfeeding. Some mothers may experience a delay in milk "coming in," such as that associated with retained placental fragments. If unrecognized, this failure of lactation may lead to significant neonatal dehydration, hypernatremia, and hyperbilirubinemia. First-time breastfeeding mothers are most likely to have difficulty in recognizing failure of lactation and its associated signs and consequences. Examining both the mother and baby regularly while in the hospital and after discharge to document effective milk production and milk transfer is essential. Exclusive breastfeeding is ideal nutrition and sufficient to support optimal growth and development for the healthy term infant for approximately 6 months after delivery. In families with a strong history of allergy, breastfeeding is likely to be especially beneficial. Newborns weaned before the age of 12 months should not receive cow's milk feedings; instead, they should receive iron-fortified newborn formula.

Contraindications to Breastfeeding

Contraindications to breastfeeding include certain maternal infectious diseases and maternal medications. Endometritis or mastitis that is being treated with antibiotics is not a contraindication to breastfeeding. A mother with active herpes simplex virus infection may breastfeed her infant if she has no vesicular lesions in the breast area, as long as the mother observes careful hand hygiene (see "Handwashing" in Chapter 10). A mother who has herpes simplex lesions on a breast should not breastfeed her infant on that breast until the lesion is cleared.

Despite the demonstrated benefits of breastfeeding, there are some situations in which breastfeeding is not in the best interest of the newborn. These include the newborn with galactosemia, who must be fed non-lactose based formula, the newborn whose mother uses illegal drugs, or the newborn whose mother is positive for human T-cell lymphotrophic virus type I or II. The newborn whose mother has untreated active tuberculosis initially should not have direct contact with the mother, either breast or bottle feeding, but may breastfeed after the mother has received adequate therapy and is considered noninfectious. Even though the mother should not nurse the infant, her milk can be expressed and given to the infant, except in the rare case of tuberculous mastitis. The infant should be examined for infection and provided with appropriate treatment. In the United States and other developed countries where formula is safe and readily available, women infected with HIV should not breastfeed their infants. Mothers who have received radioactive materials should not breastfeed as long as there is radioactivity in the milk, and mothers who are receiving antimetabolites or chemotherapy should not breastfeed until the medication has cleared from the milk.

Conditions That Are Not Contraindications to Breastfeeding

Certain conditions have been shown to be compatible with breast feeding, including maternal test results that are positive for HBsAg, if the infant receives both hepatitis B vaccine and hepatitis B immune globulin, although breastfeeding need not be delayed while waiting for the administration of hepatitis B vaccine and hepatitis B immune globulin; positive maternal test results for hepatitis C (either hepatitis C virus antibody or hepatitis C virus-RNA-positive blood) because there have been no reported cases of transmission via breast milk; maternal fever, unless because of a previously listed contraindicated condition; and maternal seropositivity (not recent convertors) for CMV, if the infant is term. Newborns born to women who are CMV seronegative but who seroconvert during lactation can develop symptomatic disease with sequelae caused by acquisition of CMV through breastfeeding. Pasteurization of milk inactivates CMV, and freezing milk at -20°C (-4°F) will decrease viral titers but does not eliminate CMV reliably.

The effects on the newborn of medications taken by a nursing mother have been closely studied. The AAP Committee on Drugs reviewed the current data on the transfer of drugs and other chemicals into human milk (Tables 7–1 to 7–6). There are only a few drugs taken by the mother that are absolute contraindications to breastfeeding. Physicians are encouraged to review available data and recommendations from reputable sources before advising against breastfeeding when mothers are taking medications. The mother should discuss the use of these medications with her obstetrician and child's physician if she wishes to continue breastfeeding. The physicians must determine whether the drug therapy really is necessary, whether safer drugs are available, and whether the infant's drug exposure may be minimized by having the woman take the medication after feedings. If the drug presents a risk to the infant, the infant should be carefully monitored to detect any adverse effects, and consideration should be given to measuring blood concentrations. Oral contraceptives may be used by breastfeeding mothers once lactation has been established.

Table 7–1. Cytotoxic Drugs That May Interfere With Cellular Metabolism of the Nursing Infant

Drug	Reason for Concern, Reported Sign or Symptom in Infant, or Effect on Lactation
Cyclophosphamide	Possible immune suppression, unknown effect on growth or association with carcinogenesis, neutropenia
Cyclosporine	Possible immune suppression, unknown effect on growth or association with carcinogenesis
Doxorubicin*	Possible immune suppression, unknown effect on growth or association with carcinogenesis
Methotrexate	Possible immune suppression, unknown effect on growth or association with carcinogenesis, neutropenia

*Drug is concentrated in human milk.

American Academy of Pediatrics. Transfer of drugs and other chemicals into human milk. Pediatrics 2001;108:776–89.

Table 7–2. Drugs of Abuse for Which Adverse Effects on the Infant During Breastfeeding Have Been Reported*

Drug	Reported Effect or Reasons for Concern
Amphetamine[†]	Irritability, poor sleeping pattern
Cocaine	Cocaine intoxication—irritability, vomiting, diarrhea, tremulousness, seizures
Heroin	Tremors, restlessness, vomiting, poor feeding
Marijuana	Only one report in literature, no effect mentioned, very long half-life for some components
Phencyclidine	Potent hallucinogen

*The Committee on Drugs strongly believes that nursing mothers should not ingest drugs of abuse because they are hazardous to the nursing infant and to the health of the mother.

[†]Drug is concentrated in human milk.

American Academy of Pediatrics. Transfer of drugs and other chemicals into human milk. Pediatrics 2001;108:776–89.

Table 7–3. Radioactive Compounds That Require Temporary Cessation of Breastfeeding*

Compound	Recommended Time for Cessation of Breastfeeding
Copper 64 (^{64}Cu)	Radioactivity in milk present at 50 h
Gallium 67 (^{67}Ga)	Radioactivity in milk present for 2 wk
Indium 111 (^{111}In)	Very small amount present at 20 h
Iodine 123 (^{123}I)	Radioactivity in milk present up to 36 h
Iodine 125 (^{125}I)	Radioactivity in milk present for 12 d
Iodine 131 (^{131}I)	Radioactivity in milk present 2–14 d, depending on study
Iodine[131]	If used for treatment of thyroid cancer, high radioactivity may prolong exposure to infant
Radioactive sodium	Radioactivity in milk present 96 h
Technetium 99m (^{99m}Tc), ^{99m}Tc macro-aggregates, ^{99m}Tc O$_4$	Radioactivity in milk present 15 h to 3 d

*Consult nuclear medicine physician before performing diagnostic study so that radionuclide that has the shortest excretion time in breast milk can be used. Before the study, the mother should pump her breast and store enough milk in the freezer for feeding the infant; after the study, the mother should pump her breast to maintain milk production but discard all milk pumped for the required time that radioactivity is present in milk. Milk samples can be screened by radiology departments for radioactivity before resumption of nursing.

American Academy of Pediatrics. Transfer of drugs and other chemicals into human milk. Pediatrics 2001;108:776–89.

Table 7–4. Drugs for Which the Effect on Nursing Infants Is Unknown but May Be of Concern*

Drug	Reported or Possible Effect
Antianxiety	
Alprazolam	None
Diazepam	None
Lorazepam	None
Midazolam	—
Perphenazine	None
Prazepam†	None
Quazepam	None
Temazepam	—
Antidepressants	
Amitriptyline	None
Amoxapine	None
Bupropion	None
Clomipramine	None
Desipramine	None
Dothiepin	None
Doxepin	None
Fluoxetine	Colic, irritability, feeding and sleep disorders, slow weight gain
Fluvoxamine	—
Imipramine	None
Nortriptyline	None
Paroxetine	None
Sertraline†	None
Trazodone	None
Antipsychotic	
Chlorpromazine	Galactorrhea in mother, drowsiness and lethargy in infant, decline in developmental scores
Chlorprothixene	None
Clozapine†	None
Haloperidol	Decline in developmental scores
Mesoridazine	None
Trifluoperazine	None

(continued)

Table 7–4. Drugs for Which the Effect on Nursing Infants Is Unknown but May Be of Concern* (continued)

Drug	Reported or Possible Effect
Others	
Amiodarone	Possible hypothyroidism
Chloramphenicol	Possible idiosyncratic bone marrow suppression
Clofazimine	Potential for transfer of high percentage of maternal dose, possible increase in skin pigmentation
Lamotrigine	Potential therapeutic serum concentrations in infant
Metoclopramide†	None described, dopaminergic blocking agent
Metronidazole	In vitro mutagen, may discontinue breastfeeding for 12–24 h to allow excretion of dose when single-dose therapy given to mother
Tinidazole	See metronidazole

*Psychotropic drugs, the compounds listed under anti-anxiety, antidepressant, and antipsychotic categories, are of special concern when given to nursing mothers for long periods. Although there are very few case reports of adverse effects in breastfeeding infants, these drugs do appear in human milk and, thus, could conceivably alter short-term and long-term central nervous system function. See discussion in text of psychotropic drugs.

†Drug is concentrated in human milk relative to simultaneous maternal plasma concentrations.

American Academy of Pediatrics. Transfer of drugs and other chemicals into human milk. Pediatrics 2001;108:776–89.

Table 7–5. Drugs That Have Been Associated With Significant Effects on Some Nursing Infants and Should Be Given to Nursing Mothers With Caution*

Drug	Reported Effect
Acebutolol	Hypotension, bradycardia, tachypnea
5-Aminosalicylic acid	Diarrhea (one case)
Atenolol	Cyanosis, bradycardia
Bromocriptine	Suppresses lactation, may be hazardous to the mother
Aspirin (salicylates)	Metabolic acidosis (one case)
Clemastine	Drowsiness, irritability, refusal to feed, high-pitched cry, neck stiffness (one case)
Ergotamine	Vomiting, diarrhea, convulsions (doses used in migraine medications)
Lithium	One third to one half therapeutic blood concentration in infants
Phenindione	Anticoagulant—increased prothrombin and partial thromboplastin time in one infant; not used in United States

(continued)

Table 7–5. Drugs That Have Been Associated With Significant Effects on Some Nursing Infants and Should Be Given to Nursing Mothers With Caution* *(continued)*

Drug	Reported Effect
Phenobarbital	Sedation; infantile spasms after weaning from milk containing phenobarbital, methemoglobinemia (one case)
Primidone	Sedation, feeding problems
Sulfasalazine (salicylazosulfapyridine)	Bloody diarrhea (one case)

*Blood concentration in the infant may be of clinical importance.

American Academy of Pediatrics. Transfer of drugs and other chemicals into human milk. Pediatrics 2001;108:776–89.

Table 7–6. Food and Environmental Agents: Effects on Breastfeeding

Agent	Reported Sign or Symptom in Infant or Effect on Lactation
Aflatoxin	None
Aspartame	Caution if mother or infant has phenylketonuria
Bromide (photographic laboratory)	Potential absorption and bromide transfer into milk
Cadmium	None reported
Chlordane	None reported
Chocolate (theobromine)	Irritability or increased bowel activity if excess amounts (greater than or equal to 16 oz/d) consumed by mother
Chlorophenothane, benzene hexachlorides, dieldrin, aldrin, hepatachlorepoxide	None
Fava beans	Hemolysis in patient with G-6-PD deficiency
Fluorides	None
Hexachlorobenzene	Skin rash, diarrhea, vomiting, dark urine, neurotoxicity, death
Hexachlorophene	None; possible contamination of milk from nipple washing
Lead	Possible neurotoxicity
Mercury, methylmercury	May affect neurodevelopment

(continued)

Table 7–6. Food and Environmental Agents: Effects on Breastfeeding (*continued*)

Agent	Reported Sign or Symptom in Infant or Effect on Lactation
Methylmethacrylate	None
Monosodium glutamate	None
Polychlorinated biphenyls and polybrominated biphenyls	Lack of endurance, hypotonia, sullen, expressionless facies
Silicone	Esophageal dysmotility
Tetrachloroethylene cleaning fluid (perchloroethylene)	Obstructive jaundice, dark urine
Vegetarian diet	Signs of B_{12} deficiency

American Academy of Pediatrics. Transfer of drugs and other chemicals into human milk. Pediatrics 2001; 108:776–89.

Human Milk Collection and Storage

There are many situations in which a mother might be separated from her infant, necessitating her to express and store her breast milk. A mother who is in school or employed outside of the home can maintain exclusive breast-milk feeding by providing expressed milk to be given in her absence. Therefore, it is important to encourage and support mothers in providing their infants with expressed milk. All mothers who provide breast milk for their newborns should be instructed in the proper techniques of milk collection to minimize bacterial contamination. Careful hand hygiene is critical before handling the breast, the equipment, or the milk. Previous practices of washing the breast and discarding the first expressed milk did not result in a decrease in colonization of the milk. Although manual expression, when performed correctly, yields relatively clean milk, many women prefer to use a breast pump. All parts of the pump that are in contact with the milk should be washed carefully with hot, soapy water, rinsed thoroughly, and allowed to dry after each use.

Mothers who have tested positive for HBsAg should not provide stored breast milk for their infants while in the nursery because of the risk to other newborns. Although mothers who are HBsAg positive may breastfeed their infants after the infants have received hepatitis B immune globulin and vaccine, it is preferable not to store breast milk that is potentially contaminated with hepatitis B virus in the nursery.

Fresh expressed breast milk can be refrigerated in sterile glass or plastic containers or plastic bags made specifically for breast milk storage and optimally should be used within 24 hours. Expressed breast milk should be discarded if not frozen or used within 24 hours. If it must be stored for longer periods, it can be frozen in the freezing compartment of a refrigerator for 2–3 weeks or in a deep freeze at -20°C plus or minus 2°C (-4°F plus or minus 3.6°F) for several months.

Frozen expressed breast milk should be thawed quickly under running water, using precautions to avoid contamination from the water, or thawed gradually in the refrigerator at 4°C (39.2°F). It should not be left at room temperatures for long periods, nor should it be subjected to extremely hot water or to microwave ovens. The very high temperatures that may be reached with the latter methods can destroy valuable components of the breast milk and result in thermal injury to the infant. Once the breast milk has been thawed, it may be refrigerated for up to 24 hours.

When using expressed breast milk in the nursery, it is essential to have policies and procedures for storing breast milk, appropriately identifying the breast milk, and checking the milk before giving it to an infant.

Banked Donor Milk

Banked human milk may be a suitable alternative for infants whose mothers are unable or unwilling to provide their own milk. Human milk banks in North America follow national guidelines for quality control of screening and testing of donors and pasteurize all milk before distribution. Fresh human milk from unscreened donors is not recommended because of concerns about infectious disease transmission. Women who donate breast milk for other newborns should be interviewed carefully regarding past and current infectious diseases, use of drugs and medicines, and other factors that may impair the quality or safety of the breast milk that they provide. Before they are accepted as milk donors, they should be tested for HIV, HBsAg, hepatitis C, and tuberculosis. Women with positive test results should not be accepted as donors. These tests should be repeated periodically for donors who continue to provide milk or who seek reinstatement as a donor. The potential risks should be explained to mothers whose newborns are to receive donated milk. Decisions regarding the use of fresh, unpasteurized CMV-seropositive donor milk for preterm newborns should consider both the potential benefits of human milk and the risk of CMV transmission.

Formula Preparation

If a mother chooses not to breastfeed or is medically unable to breastfeed her infant, the infant should receive a standard infant formula. Cow's milk should not be given for the first 12 months. Formula selection should be directed by the physician, and new formulas should be reviewed by the appropriate hospital committees and the director of the nursery before use. For mothers who intend to breastfeed their newborns, distribution of formula packages on discharge should be discouraged. For mothers who intend to feed their newborns with formula, the distribution of formula packages on discharge should be consistent with the physician's written orders.

Most hospitals now use prepared formula units with separate nipples that are readily attached to the bottles just before use. These units need not be refrigerated and may be stored in a convenient, clean, cool area. The sterile cap should be kept on the nipple until the infant is ready to be fed.

If there is a special area where nipples are uncapped and placed on the bottle, it should be kept very clean and should be used only for formula preparation. Alternatively, nipples may be uncapped and attached to bottles at the mother's bedside just before feeding. The formula and nipple unit should be used as soon as possible, certainly within 4 hours after the bottle is uncapped, and then discarded.

Vitamin and Mineral Supplementation

The vitamin D content of human milk is low, and rickets can occur in deeply pigmented breastfed infants or in those with inadequate exposure to sunlight. As adequate exposure to sunlight is difficult to guarantee, and because supplementation at the recommended dose is safe, vitamin D supplementation at 200 international units per day should begin during the first 2 months of life. Fluoride supplementation for both breastfed and bottle-fed newborns can begin at age 6 months.

Although the iron content of human milk is low, the bioavailability is high—50% of the iron is absorbed by newborns who are breastfed exclusively. Breastfed newborns should be given supplemental elemental iron (2–3 mg/kg/d) or iron-containing complementary foods when they reach 6 months of age. Iron-containing formulas with up to 12 mg of elemental iron per liter of formula should be used for all formula-fed newborns. Further iron supplementation is not necessary. Newborns consuming commercial newborn formulas do not need vitamin and mineral supplementation for the first 6 months of life.

Resources

Adoption. ACOG Committee Opinion No. 368. American College of Obstetricians and Gynecologists. Obstet Gynecol 2007;109:1507–10.

American Academy of Pediatrics. Pediatric nutrition handbook. 5th ed. Elk Grove (IL): AAP; 2004.

American Academy of Pediatrics. Redbook: 2006 report of the Committee on Infectious Diseases. 27th ed. Elk Grove Village (IL): AAP; 2006.

American Academy of Pediatrics, American College of Obstetricians and Gynecologists. Breastfeeding handbook for physicians. Elk Grove Village (IL): AAP; Washington DC: ACOG; 2006.

American Academy of Pediatrics, American Heart Association. Neonatal resuscitation textbook 5th ed. Elk Grove Village (IL): AAP; Dallas (TX): AHA; 2006.

The Apgar score. ACOG Committee Opinion No. 333. American College of Obstetricians and Gynecologists, American Academy of Pediatrics. Obstet Gynecol 2006;107: 1209–12.

Apnea, sudden infant death syndrome, and home monitoring. Committee on Fetus and Newborn. American Academy of Pediatrics. Pediatrics 2003;111:914–7.

Ballard JL, Khoury JC, Wedig K, Wang L, Eilers-Walsman BL, Lipp R. New Ballard Score, expanded to include extremely premature infants. J Pediatr 1991;119:407–23.

Borchers D. Families and adoption: the pediatrician's role in supporting communication. American Academy of Pediatrics Committee on Early Childhood, Adoption & Dependent Care. Pediatrics 2003;112:1437–1441.

Breastfeeding: maternal and infant aspects. ACOG Committee Opinion No. 361. American College of Obstetricians and Gynecologists. Obstet Gynecol 2007;109: 279–80.

Bull M, Agran P, Laraque D, Pollack SH, Smith GA, Spivak HR, et al. American Academy of Pediatrics. Committee on Injury and Poison Prevention. Safe transportation of newborns at hospital discharge. Pediatrics 1999;104:986–7. Reaffirmed 2003.

The changing concept of sudden infant death syndrome: diagnostic coding shifts, controversies regarding the sleeping environment, and new variables to consider in reducing risk. American Academy of Pediatrics Task Force on Sudden Infant Death Syndrome. Pediatrics 2005;116:1245–55.

Circumcision. ACOG Committee Opinion No. 260. American College of Obstetricians and Gynecologists. Obstet Gynecol 2001;98:707–8.

Circumcision policy statement. American Academy of Pediatrics. Task Force on Circumcision. Pediatrics 1999;103:686–93. Re-affirmed Pediatrics 116:796, 2005.

Controversies concerning vitamin K and the newborn. American Academy of Pediatrics Committee on Fetus and Newborn. Pediatrics 2003;112:191–2. Reaffirmed 2006.

Cunniff C. Prenatal screening and diagnosis for pediatricians. American Academy of Pediatrics Committee on Genetics. Pediatrics 2004;114:889–94.

Edwards ES, Howell RR, Lloyd-Puryear MA, editors. A look at newborn screening: today and tomorrow [entire issue]. Pediatrics 2006;117(suppl).

Erenberg A, Lemons J, Sia C, Trunkel D, Ziring P. Newborn and infant hearing loss: detection and prevention. American Academy of Pediatrics Task Force on Newborn and Infant Hearing, 1998–1999. Pediatrics 1999;103:527–30.

Gartner LM, Greer FR. Prevention of rickets and vitamin D deficiency: new guidelines for vitamin D intake. Section on Breastfeeding and Committee on Nutrition. American Academy of Pediatrics. Pediatrics 2003;111:908–10.

Gartner LM, Morton J, Lawrence RA, Naylor AJ, O'Hare D, Schanler RJ, et al. Breastfeeding and the use of human milk. American Academy of Pediatrics Section on Breastfeeding. Pediatrics 2005;115:496–506.

Hospital discharge of the high-risk neonate–proposed guidelines. American Academy of Pediatrics. Committee on Fetus and Newborn. Pediatrics 1998;102:411–7. Reaffirmed 2001.

Hospital stay for healthy term newborns. American Academy of Pediatrics Committee on Fetus and Newborn. Pediatrics 2004;113:1434–6.

Human Milk Banking Association of North America. Best practice for expressing, storing and handling human milk in hospitals, homes and child care settings. Raleigh (NC): HMBANA; 2005.

Iron fortification of infant formulas. American Academy of Pediatrics. Committee on Nutrition. Pediatrics 1999;104:119–23.

Kaye CI. Newborn screening fact sheets. American Academy of Pediatrics. Committee on Genetics. Pediatrics 2006;118:e934–63.

Management of hyperbilirubinemia in the newborn infant 35 or more weeks of gestation. American Academy of Pediatrics Subcommittee on Hyperbilirubinemia [published erratum appears in Pediatrics 2004;114:1138]. Pediatrics 2004;114:297–316.

Maternal and Child Health Bureau. Newborn screening: toward a uniform screening panel and system report for public comment. Rockville (MD): MCHB; 2005. Available at: http://mchb.hrsa.gov/screening. Retrieved December 18, 2006.

National Institute of Child Health and Human Development. Report of the workshop on acute perinatal asphyxia in term infants. NIH publication 96-3823. Washington, DC: NICHD; 1996.

Newborn screening. ACOG Committee Opinion No. 287. American College of Obstetricians and Gynecologists. Obstet Gynecol 2003;887–9.

Persing J, James H, Swanson J, Kattwinkel J. Prevention and management of positional skull deformities in infants. American Academy of Pediatrics Committee on Practice and Ambulatory Medicine, Section on Plastic Surgery and Section on Neurological Surgery. Pediatrics 2003;112:199–202.

Read JS. Human milk, breastfeeding, and transmission of human immunodeficiency virus type I in the United States. American Academy of Pediatrics Committee on Pediatric AIDS. Pediatrics 2003;112:1196–1205.

Recommended childhood and adolescent immunization schedule: United States, 2005. American Academy of Pediatrics Committee on Infectious Diseases. Pediatrics 2005; 115:182.

The role of the primary care pediatrician in the management of high-risk new born infants. American Academy of Pediatrics. Committee on Practice and Ambulatory Medicine and Committee on Fetus and Newborn. Pediatrics 1996;98:786–8.

Safe transportation of premature and low birth weight infants. American Academy of Pediatrics. Committee on Injury and Poison Prevention and Committee on Fetus and Newborn. Pediatrics 1996;97:758–60.

Stark AR. Levels of neonatal care. American Academy of Pediatrics Committee on Fetus and Newborn [published erratum appears in Pediatrics 2005;115:1118]. Pediatrics 2004; 114:1341–7.

The transfer of drugs and other chemicals into human milk. American Academy of Pediatrics Committee on Drugs. Pediatrics 2001;108:776–9.

Wiswell, T, Gannon CM, Jacob J, Goldsmith L, Szyld E, Weiss K, et al. Delivery room management of the apparently vigorous meconium–stained neonate: results of the multicenter, international collaborative trial. Pediatrics 2000:105;1–7.

Vain NE, Szyld EG, Prudent LM, Wiswell TE, Aguilar AM, Vivas NI. Oropharyngeal and nasopharyngeal suctioning of meconium-stained neonates before delivery of their shoulders: multicentre, randomised controlled trial. Lancet 2004;364:597–602.

Year 2000 position statement: principles and guidelines for early hearing detection and intervention programs. Joint Committee on Infant Hearing. Pediatrics 2000;106: 789–817.

chapter 8

Neonatal Complications

Because of advances in knowledge and controversies surrounding certain issues, some neonatal conditions and treatments require particular attention. Whenever possible, therapies should be based on the best evidence available, preferably from well-designed, randomized, controlled trials.

Hyperbilirubinemia

Although bilirubin may be toxic to the central nervous system and may cause neurologic impairment, the factors that determine the toxicity of bilirubin to the brain cells of neonates are many, complex, and incompletely understood. Factors include those that affect serum albumin concentration and the binding of bilirubin to albumin, the penetration of bilirubin into the brain, the presence of comorbidities, gestational age, postnatal age, and the vulnerability of brain cells to the toxic effects of bilirubin. In addition, the interrelationships between serum bilirubin concentrations and kernicterus (a condition characterized by a definitive neurologic syndrome, with bilirubin staining and neuronal injury within specific brainstem nuclei) and residual bilirubin encephalopathy (brain damage caused by bilirubin) are not clear. Whether hyperbilirubinemia causes mild neurologic impairment less severe than frank bilirubin encephalopathy is not known nor is it known at what bilirubin concentration or under what circumstances the risk of brain damage exceeds that of treatment. In addition to uncertainty about the cause and effect of the disorder, differences in patient populations, geographic locations, and practice settings contribute to variations in the management of hyperbilirubinemia.

Bilirubin Toxicity

A direct association between severe and increasing unconjugated hyperbilirubinemia, kernicterus, and bilirubin encephalopathy has been demonstrated in neonates with erythroblastosis fetalis. In the past, survivors often manifested serious sequelae, particularly the athetoid form of cerebral palsy, hearing loss, paralysis of upward gaze, and dentoalveolar dysplasia. In most studies of otherwise healthy term neonates without hemolysis, total serum bilirubin concentrations of less than 25 mg/dL (428 micromoles per liter) have not been associated with either cognitive or serious neurologic abnormalities. The historical data and subsequent studies demonstrate that a total serum bilirubin greater than 30 mg/dL (513 micromoles per liter) carries a decidedly higher risk of kernicterus. No specific total serum bilirubin threshold for neurotoxicity has been established.

Studies of preterm neonates have failed to identify a specific serum bilirubin concentration as a risk factor for kernicterus. Autopsy findings of yellow-stained cerebral tissues in very low birth weight (VLBW) neonates whose bilirubin concentrations never exceeded 10 mg/dL (171 micromoles per liter) have been reported. More recently, studies in VLBW infants suggested that the incidence of kernicterus in this group is uncommon even if bilirubin is allowed to increase above a level previously considered to be harmful. Thus, the relationship of serum bilirubin and neurodevelopmental outcome in the VLBW infant is unclear. Some published guidelines for the management of jaundice in such neonates have suggested early phototherapy and exchange transfusion for bilirubin concentrations of as low as 10 mg/dL (171 micromoles per liter). Several studies of preterm neonates, however, have failed to confirm a relationship between serum bilirubin concentrations and later neurodevelopmental handicap, particularly if serum bilirubin concentrations did not exceed 20 mg/dL (342 micromoles per liter). In the studies reporting kernicterus in preterm neonates at low bilirubin concentrations, noteworthy clinical findings were a lack of the classic encephalopathic syndrome and the concurrent presence of other disorders that had the potential to result in a central nervous system insult—respiratory failure with hypoxia and hypercarbia, sepsis, and intraventricular hemorrhage. Therefore, the management decision for exchange transfusion for prevention of kernicterus in the preterm neonate should include consideration of other coexisting pathophysiologic processes.

Detection and Management of Jaundice

A key recommendation in the American Academy of Pediatrics' (AAP) clinical practice guideline on hyperbilirubinemia is to assess every newborn for risk of severe hyperbilirubinemia before discharge. All nurseries should have protocols for assessing the risk. The guideline recommends two methods of assessment:

1) predischarge measurement of total serum bilirubin or transcutaneous bilirubin and 2) application of clinical risk factors for predicting severe hyperbilirubinemia. Jaundice that persists beyond 2 weeks requires further investigation, including measurement of both total and direct serum bilirubin concentrations. Elevation of the direct serum bilirubin concentration always requires further investigation and possible intervention.

Ten principles for preventing and managing hyperbilirubinemia include:

- Promote and support successful breastfeeding

- Establish nursery protocols for the jaundiced newborn and permit nurses to obtain total serum bilirubin levels without a physician's order

- Measure the total serum bilirubin or transcutaneous bilirubin in an infant who is jaundiced in the first 24 hours

- Recognize that visual diagnosis of jaundice is unreliable, particularly in a darkly pigmented infant

- Interpret all total serum bilirubin levels according to the infant's age in hours, not days

- Recognize that a late preterm (35–37 weeks of gestation) infant is at much higher risk of hyperbilirubinemia than a term infant

- Perform a predischarge, systematic assessment on all infants for the risk of severe hyperbilirubinemia

- Provide parents with information about newborn jaundice

- Provide follow-up based on time of discharge and risk assessment

- When indicated, treat the newborn with phototherapy or exchange transfusion (see Fig. 8–1).

Term and Late Preterm Neonates With Hemolytic Disease

Clinical observation of term neonates with hemolytic disease has confirmed that the occurrence of clinical kernicterus is highly unlikely if serum unconjugated bilirubin concentrations are less than 20 mg/dL (342 micromoles per liter). The AAP guideline addresses therapy for infants with hemolysis (Fig. 8–2).

Term and Late Preterm Neonates Without Hemolytic Disease

There are no properly designed studies, or even observational data, on preterm or term neonates without hemolytic disease on which to base clinical guidelines for the treatment of neonates with serum bilirubin concentrations of less than

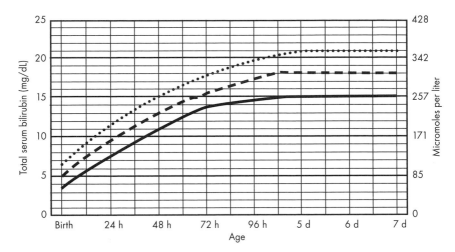

••••• Infants at lower risk (equal to or greater than 38 wk of gestation and well)
— — Infants at medium risk (equal to or greater than 38 wk of gestation with risk factors or
        35–37% wk gestation and well)
——— Infants at higher risk (35–37% wk of gestation with risk factors)

Fig. 8–1. Guidelines for phototherapy in hospitalized infants at 35 weeks of gestation or older. These guidelines are based on limited evidence, and the levels shown are approximations. The guidelines refer to the use of intensive phototherapy, which should be used when the total serum bilirubin level exceeds the line indicated for each category. Infants are designated as "higher risk" because of the potential negative effects of the conditions listed on albumin binding of bilirubin, the blood-brain barrier, and the susceptibility of the brain cells to damage by bilirubin. Use total bilirubin. Do not subtract direct reacting or conjugated bilirubin. Risk factors are isoimmune hemolytic disease, G6PD deficiency, asphyxia, significant lethargy, temperature instability, sepsis, acidosis, or albumin less than 3 g/dL (if measured). For well infants 35–37% wk of gestation total serum bilirubin levels can be adjusted for intervention around the medium risk line. It is an option to intervene at lower total serum bilirubin levels for infants closer to 35 wk of gestation and at higher total serum bilirubin levels for those closer to 37% wk of gestation. It is an option to provide conventional phototherapy in the hospital or at home with total serum bilirubin levels 2–3 mg/dL (35–50 micromoles per liter) below those shown, but home phototherapy should not be used in any infant with risk factors. (Management of hyperbilirubinemia in the newborn infant 35 or more weeks of gestation. American Academy of Pediatrics. Subcommittee on Hyperbilirubinemia [published erratum appears in Pediatrics 2004;114:1138]. Pediatrics 2004;114:297–316.)

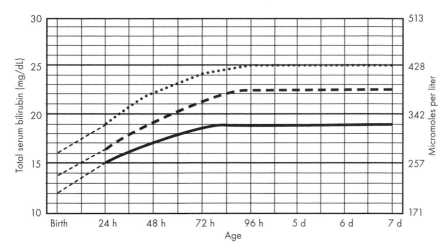

Fig. 8-2. Guidelines for exchange transfusion in infants at 35 weeks of gestation or older. These suggested levels represent a consensus of most of the committee but are based on limited evidence, and the levels shown are approximations. During birth hospitalization, exchange transfusion is recommended if the total serum bilirubin level increaes to these levels despite intensive phototherapy. For readmitted infants, if the total serum bilirubin level is above the exchange level, repeat total serum bilirubin measurement every 2-3 hours and consider exchange if the total serum bilirubin level remains above the levels indicated after intensive phototherapy for 6 hours. The dashed lines for the first 24 hours indicate uncertainty because of a wide range of clinical circumstances and a range of responses to phototherapy. Immediate exchange transfusion is recommended if the infant shows signs of acute bilirubin encephalopathy (hypertonia, arching, retrocollis, opisthotonos, fever, or high pitched cry) or if the total serum bilirubin level is equal to or greater than 5 mg/dL (85 micromoles per liter) above these lines. Risk factors are isoimmune hemolytic disease, G6PD deficiency, asphyxia, significant lethargy, temperature instability, sepsis, and acidosis. Measure serum albumin level and calculate bilirubin/albumin ratio. Use total bilirubin. Do not subtract direct reacting or conjugated bilirubin. If the infant is well and at 35-37% wk of gestation (medium risk), total serum bilirubin levels for exchange can be individualized based on actual gestational age. (Management of hyperbilirubinemia in the newborn infant 35 or more weeks of gestation. American Academy of Pediatrics. Subcommittee on Hyperbilirubinemia [published erratum appears in Pediatrics 2004;114:1138]. Pediatrics 2004;114:297-316.)

20 mg/dL (342 micromoles per liter). Follow-up data for apparently healthy term neonates whose serum bilirubin concentrations were as high as 25 mg/dL (428 micromoles per liter) showed no apparent ill effects from these concentrations. On the basis of these observations, the AAP guideline is based on limited evidence for phototherapy and exchange transfusion in infants born at 35 weeks of gestation or more (Fig. 8–1 and Fig. 8–2).

Preterm Neonates

In the past, some physicians recommended, as a result of the aforementioned autopsy studies, initiating phototherapy early and performing exchange transfusions in selected preterm neonates who have serum bilirubin concentrations as low as 10 mg/dL (171 micromoles per liter). However, this approach cannot guarantee the prevention of kernicterus. A threshold for an adverse serum bilirubin that affects neurodevelopmental outcome of preterm infants is not known at this time. Because extremely preterm infants often are critically ill, having variable but low albumin concentrations and immature blood–brain barriers, bilirubin-induced brain injury may be more likely at lower bilirubin concentrations than in term infants. Therefore, it is not possible to give specific recommendations for a specific lower bilirubin threshold at which to initiate treatment in preterm infants, other than it would appear prudent to commence treatment earlier than in term infants.

Relationship Between Breastfeeding and Jaundice

Breastfeeding has a significant effect on the level as well as the duration of unconjugated hyperbilirubinemia compared with formula feeding. This relationship is seen in two ways. The first is known as breast milk jaundice, characterized as an extension of physiologic jaundice beyond the first week of age. Although formula-fed infants generally have serum bilirubin levels less than 1.5 mg/dL (25.6 micromoles per liter) by 10–14 days of age, breastfed infants commonly have levels greater than 5 mg/dL (85.5 micromoles per liter) for several weeks after delivery. This increased unconjugated hyperbilirubinemia is caused by an as yet unidentified factor in human milk that promotes an increase in intestinal absorption of bilirubin. Jaundice persisting beyond the first week of life should be monitored to ensure that it is unconjugated hyperbilirubinemia, that the concentration of bilirubin is not increasing, and that other pathologic causes for the jaundice are not present.

A second way in which breastfeeding is related to hyperbilirubinemia is a pathologic one, which is a result of an inadequate intake of human milk in breastfed infants. This breastfeeding failure, or "breast-non-feeding jaundice," most often occurs in association with a primiparous or first-time breast-feeding mother with a late preterm infant. Early hospital discharge is an additional risk factor. Because of inadequate milk production, which is unrecognized by the woman and health care providers, the infant may lose up to 30% of its birth weight over the initial 7–14 days of life and develop marked hyperbilirubinemia following hospital discharge. It is unlikely that dehydration itself is an important cause of hyperbilirubinemia. It is more likely that caloric deprivation and its effect on the enterohepatic circulation of bilirubin is primarily responsible. There have been reports of mortality and kernicterus associated with this type of lactation failure. Proper education and support of the mother and the infant, along with early and continued follow-up after hospital discharge to evaluate the feeding process and the health of the neonate, are essential in preventing such problems. If failure of milk production is confirmed, infants promptly should be provided necessary medical evaluation and support (including appropriate rehydration) and changed to newborn formula because establishing lactogenesis at that point is unlikely to be successful.

Some evidence indicates that frequent breastfeeding (8–12 times per 24 hours) may reduce the incidence of hyperbilirubinemia. Supplementing nursing with water or dextrose-water will not decrease serum bilirubin concentrations in jaundiced, healthy, breastfeeding neonates. When an indirect serum bilirubin concentration is elevated by some pathologic cause, there is no reason to discontinue breastfeeding. However, if the serum unconjugated bilirubin level in a breastfed, term, healthy infant is increasing and is higher than 20 mg/dL (171 micromoles per liter), the physician has several options to reduce the level. Breastfeeding may be continued and the infant may be treated with phototherapy while infant and mother undergo thorough evaluation and assistance with the feeding process. Alternatively, breastfeeding may continue and the infant may be supplemented with newborn formula. Finally, complete substitution of breast milk with infant formula for 24–48 hours almost always will result in a rapid decrease in serum bilirubin concentrations. This can be combined with phototherapy. Women who must cease nursing temporarily should be given positive and enthusiastic support. They should be encouraged to maintain lactation by using a breast pump or manual expression during the period of interrupted nursing. They also should be reassured that the nutritional value of their milk is not compromised by the use of these methods.

Hydration

There is no evidence that excess fluid administered to the neonate decreases the serum bilirubin concentration. Some neonates who are admitted to the hospital with high bilirubin concentrations also may be mildly dehydrated and may need supplemental fluid intake to correct dehydration. In the absence of dehydration, routine supplementation (with dextrose-water) of neonates receiving phototherapy is not indicated. However, in sick, VLBW neonates receiving phototherapy, excess evaporative water loss is known to occur and frequently necessitates increased fluid intake, environmental humidity, or both for replacement or prevention of ongoing losses.

Phototherapy

Phototherapy is effective in reducing serum bilirubin concentrations in neonates with nonhemolytic jaundice. Phototherapy is less effective in neonates with ABO and CDE (Rh) group hemolytic disease, reducing, but not eliminating, the need for exchange transfusions in these neonates. Exchange transfusion is the treatment of choice when the bilirubin concentration appears to pose an imminent threat to the health of the neonate.

There is no standardized method for delivering phototherapy. However, detailed recommendations on phototherapy can be found in the hyperbilirubinemia practice parameters from the AAP. Commonly used phototherapy units contain daylight, cool white, blue, or "special blue" fluorescent tubes. Other units use tungsten-halogen lamps in different configurations, either free-standing or as part of a radiant-warming device. Fiber optic systems have been developed that deliver high-intensity light via a fiber optic blanket.

The efficacy of phototherapy is influenced by the energy output (irradiance) in the blue spectrum (measured in microwatt per centimeter squared), the spectrum of light source, and the surface area of the neonate exposed to the light source. The irradiance of a unit should be monitored and bulbs changed as needed to maintain maximum energy output. It is acceptable to interrupt phototherapy during feeding or brief parental visits. Intensive phototherapy can be achieved by use of blue lights, decreasing the distance of the source from the neonate and increasing the surface area exposed to the lights. The neonate's temperature should be monitored frequently while phototherapy is being applied.

Although phototherapy has many biologic effects, it has no known lasting toxic effects in the human neonate. Because experiments in animals have documented retinal damage from phototherapy, the neonate's eyes should be covered with opaque patches during exposure to phototherapy light. Known potential complications from improper monitoring of eye-patch placement include exposure to high-energy light, malposition and obstruction of the nares, inadequate securing of the patch that allows lid opening and resultant corneal abrasion, and conjunctivitis from use without intermittent removal to assess the condition of the covered tissues.

The determination of a neonate's suitability for early discharge requires heightened awareness of the normal course of physiologic hyperbilirubinemia. Recent data suggest that there is some predictability to the progressive increase in serum bilirubin concentrations from nonpathologic sources. It is suggested that for neonates who are otherwise candidates for early discharge, a predischarge serum bilirubin determination can be helpful in predicting risk for a subsequent increase to more concerning concentrations. A neonate with early onset jaundice (within the first 24 hours) should have hemolysis excluded as a cause before being considered for early discharge. After the newborn is discharged from the birthing hospital, the mother and child should receive a seamless continuation of care as outlined in the AAP guideline.

Some neonates with uncomplicated nonhemolytic jaundice may be treated with phototherapy at home. Guidelines should be developed by each institution to define criteria for neonates who are eligible for home phototherapy. Home care requires appropriate follow-up and supervision by a health care professional with access to serum bilirubin determinations as clinically indicated. With proper instruction of the parents or guardians, phototherapy can be provided by using a freestanding device or a fiber optic blanket. If serum bilirubin concentrations do not decrease in response to conventional phototherapy, admission to the hospital may be indicated for more intensive phototherapy or exchange transfusion and for evaluation of the underlying cause (Fig. 8–1 and Fig. 8–2).

Clinical Considerations in the Use of Oxygen

The hazards associated with nonindicated administration of supplemental oxygen to preterm neonates have been recognized for many years. Studies conducted in the 1950s indicated that prolonged oxygen therapy without clinical indication was associated with increased rates of retinopathy of prematurity, formerly called retrolental fibroplasia. The ensuing blanket restriction of ambient oxygen therapy resulted in a marked decrease in retinopathy of prematurity at the cost of an increase in morbidity and mortality. Current practice includes the prudent use of supplemental oxygen as needed, based on an objective determination of oxygen requirements.

When supplemental oxygen therapy is considered, the potential risks, in terms of both hypoxia and hyperoxia, should be weighed. Clinical judgment of physical signs alone as a guide to the amount of supplemental oxygen needed is acceptable for short periods, emergencies, or abrupt clinical changes. However, ongoing use of supplemental oxygen should be guided by an objective assessment of patient oxygenation.

Administration and Monitoring

In an emergency, high concentrations of supplemental oxygen may be administered by a face mask, nasal prongs, or endotracheal tube. When a neonate requires oxygen therapy beyond the emergency period, the oxygen should be warmed and humidified and the concentration or flow should be monitored and regulated. Supplemental oxygen can be delivered via endotracheal tube, oxygen hood, nasal prongs, or incubator. Oxygen analyzers should be calibrated in accordance with manufacturers' recommendations. Orders for oxygen therapy should include desired ambient concentration, flow, or both. The concentration or flow rate of oxygen should be checked routinely. Alternatively, orders should be written to adjust fraction of inspired oxygen (FIO_2) or flow within a stated range to maintain oxygen saturation within specific limits. There should be an institutional guideline for ordering, delivering, and documenting oxygen therapy and monitoring.

An important development in the care of neonates who require oxygen therapy is the ability to monitor oxygenation continuously with noninvasive techniques. The pulse oximeter measures oxyhemoglobin saturation and the transcutaneous oxygen analyzer provides an indirect measurement of PaO_2. Because neither technique measures PaO_2 directly, they should be used as adjuncts to, rather than substitutes for, arterial blood gas sampling, especially in neonates with moderate to severe respiratory distress.

Periodic or continuous measurement of PaO_2 in samples from an umbilical or peripheral artery catheter is the most reliable method of assessing the effectiveness of oxygen therapy. If an indwelling arterial catheter is not in place, peripheral artery puncture can be used, but this is painful and repeated sampling from these sites is not always possible. Oxygenation is not accurately estimated in arterialized capillary samples. However, arterialized capillary sampling provides fairly reliable estimates of arterial pH and $PaCO_2$. The combined use of continuous, transcutaneous oxygen saturation monitoring and intermittent percutaneous arterial or arterialized blood gases to guide oxygen therapy is an attractive pragmatic strategy when invasive arterial catheters are not in place.

In neonates whose condition is unstable, noninvasive measurements should be correlated with PaO_2 as often as every 8–24 hours. More frequent analyses of arterial blood gas may be indicated for the assessment of pH and $PaCO_2$. In neonates whose condition is stable, correlation with arterial blood gas samples may be performed when clinically indicated.

The use of either pulse oximetry or transcutaneous oxygen measurement may shorten the time required to determine optimum inspired oxygen concentration and ventilator settings in the acute care setting. Both measurements are particularly useful in monitoring oxygen therapy in neonates who are recovering from respiratory distress or who require long-term supplemental oxygen. Pulse oximetry is particularly advantageous for long-term monitoring of oxygen therapy because transcutaneous oxygen measurements underestimate oxygenation in older neonates with bronchopulmonary dysplasia (BPD) and may cause burns. Pulse oximetry also is widely available.

In consideration of the current, but incomplete, understanding of the effects of oxygen administration, the following recommendations are offered:

- Supplemental oxygen should be used for specific indications, such as cyanosis, low PaO_2, or low oxygen saturation.

- The continuous use of supplemental oxygen, other than for resuscitation, should be monitored by assessments of PaO_2, oxygen saturation, or both.

- Oxygenation monitoring should be available whenever oxygen is continuously administered to newborns.

- For neonates who require oxygen therapy for acute care, measurements of blood pH and $PaCO_2$ should accompany measurements of PaO_2. In addition, a record of blood gas measurements, noninvasive measurements of oxygenation, details of the oxygen delivery system (eg, ventilator, continuous positive airway pressure, nasal cannula, hood, mask, settings), and ambient oxygen concentrations (FIO_2, liter of flow per minute, or both) should be maintained.

- The optimal range for oxygen saturation and PaO_2 that balances tissue metabolism, growth and development, and toxicity has not been elucidated fully for preterm infants receiving supplemental oxygen. Oxygen saturation values between 85–95% and PaO_2 values between 50 mm Hg and 80 mm Hg are examples of ranges pragmatically determined by some clinicians to guide oxygen therapy in preterm infants. Additional research to determine the "optimal" oxygenation ranges for oxygen saturation and PaO_2 is needed. Of note, even with careful monitoring, oxygen saturation and PaO_2 may fluctuate outside specified ranges, particularly in neonates with cardiopulmonary disease.

- Regular and periodic (every 1–4 hours) measurement and recording of the concentration of oxygen delivered to the neonate receiving supplemental oxygen is recommended.

- Except for an emergency situation, air–oxygen mixtures should be warmed and humidified before being administered to newborns.

Retinopathy of Prematurity

A myriad of factors, including but not limited to hyperoxia, may contribute to the pathogenesis of retinopathy of prematurity. Prematurity, low birth weight, twin gestation, severity of illness, prolonged ventilatory support (especially when accompanied by episodes of hypoxia and hypercapnia) and clinical conditions, including acidosis, shock, sepsis, apnea, anemia, chronic lung disease, intraventricular hemorrhage, patent ductus arteriosus, and vitamin E deficiency, also have been associated with retinopathy of prematurity.

To date, a safe level of PaO_2 in relation to retinopathy of prematurity has not been established. Retinopathy of prematurity has occurred in preterm neonates who have never received supplemental oxygen therapy and in neonates with cyanotic, congenital heart disease in whom PaO_2 levels never exceeded 50 mm Hg. Conversely, retinopathy of prematurity has not developed in some preterm neonates after prolonged periods of hyperoxemia. Data have demonstrated no additional progression of active prethreshold retinopathy of prematurity when supplemental oxygen was administered at pulse oximetry saturations between 96% and 99%. Further, continuous, close monitoring of transcutaneous oxygen tension has not resulted in a decrease in the incidence of retinopathy of prematurity when compared with intermittent transcutaneous monitoring. However, recent data in extremely low birth weight infants between 23 weeks and 29 weeks of gestation suggest that oxygen saturation in the lowest range (70–90%) compared with highest range (88–98%) was associated with significantly less threshold retinopathy of prematurity. A one-year follow-up showed similar neurodevelopmental outcome. Randomized, controlled-trial studies will need to be done before this lower range of oxygenation can be recommended.

On the basis of published data, the following statements regarding retinopathy of prematurity and oxygen use are warranted:

- Retinopathy of prematurity is not preventable in some neonates, especially extremely premature neonates.

- Many factors other than hyperoxia contribute to the pathogenesis of retinopathy of prematurity.

- Transient hyperoxemia alone cannot be considered sufficient to cause retinopathy of prematurity.

- Strict adherence to existing guidelines for supplemental oxygen therapy will not completely prevent complications or side effects.

- An ophthalmologist with experience in retinopathy of prematurity and indirect ophthalmoscopy should examine the retinas of all preterm neonates born at 30 weeks of gestation or less or weighing less than 1,500 g at birth, as well as selected infants between 1,500–2,000 g birth weight with an unstable clinical course who are thought to be at risk by their attending pediatrician or neonatologist. The examination should be performed at 4–6 weeks of chronologic age or at 31–33 weeks postmenstrual age (gestational age at birth plus chronologic age), as determined by the neonate's attending pediatrician or neonatologist. The use of a digital, wide-field camera system to photograph retinas of neonates at high risk is being evaluated and may prove valuable to facilitate analysis by experienced off-site ophthalmologists.

- Table 8–1 represents a suggested schedule for timing of initial eye examinations based on postmenstrual age and chronologic (postnatal) age to detect retinopathy of prematurity before it becomes severe enough to result in retinal detachment and to allow for earlier intervention, while minimizing the number of examinations, which potentially are traumatic to the baby.

- The timing of follow-up examinations is best determined from the findings of the first examination, using the International Classification of Retinopathy of Prematurity. Treatment generally should be accomplished, when possible, within 72 hours of diagnosed treatable disease so as to minimize the risk of retinal detachment. The retinal findings requiring strong consideration of ablative treatment recently have been revised as follows:

  —Zone I retinopathy of prematurity: any stage with plus disease

  —Zone I retinopathy of prematurity: stage 3, no plus disease

  —Zone II: stage 2 or 3 with plus disease

Table 8–1. Timing of First Eye Examination Based on Gestational Age at Birth*

Gestational Age at Birth (wk)	Age at Initial Examination (wk)	
	Postmenstrual	Chronologic
22[†]	31	9
23[†]	31	8
24	31	7
25	31	6
26	31	5
27	31	4
28	32	4
29	33	4
30	34	4
31[‡]	35	4
32[‡]	36	4

*Shown is a schedule for detecting prethreshold retinopathy of prematurity with 99% confidence, usually well before any required treatment.

[†]This guideline should be considered tentative rather than evidence-based for infants with a gestational age of 22–23 weeks because of the small number of survivors in these gestational-age categories.

[‡]If necessary

Screening examination of premature infants for retinopathy of prematurity. Section on Ophthalmology, American Academy of Pediatrics; American Academy of Ophthalmology; American Association for Pediatric Ophthalmology and Strabismus. Pediatrics 2006;117:572–6.

- If a neonate at risk for retinopathy of prematurity is transferred to another hospital or discharged home during the period of susceptibility for development or progression of the disease, monitoring examinations by an experienced ophthalmologist must be continued.
- A systematic program for tracking and scheduling ophthalmologic examinations of preterm neonates at risk for retinopathy of prematurity is useful and strongly encouraged to reduce vision loss from retinopathy of prematurity that usually responds to timely treatment.

Substance Abuse

The use of illicit substances by women of childbearing age has led to an increased number of neonates having had in utero exposure and subsequent risk of adverse effects from a variety of drugs. Both licit substances, such as alcohol and tobacco, and illicit "street drugs" have the potential to adversely affect fetal growth and development and postnatal adaptation. Fetal drug exposure often is unrecognized because of the lack of overt symptomatology or structural abnormality following birth. In such circumstances, neonates may be discharged to homes where they are at increased risk for a variety of medical and social problems, including abuse and neglect. Women who use illicit substance(s) are at risk for human immunodeficiency virus (HIV), acquired immunodeficiency syndrome (AIDS), herpes, hepatitis, and syphilis, each of which can have significant adverse effects on the fetus and newborn. In addition, these women may have received little or no prenatal care, further increasing risks for the fetus.

Illicit drugs may reach the fetus via placental transfer or may reach the newborn through breast milk. The specific effect on the fetus and newborn varies with the respective substances. An opiate-exposed fetus may experience withdrawal in utero when the woman undergoes withdrawal, either voluntary or under supervision, or after birth when the delivery of the drug by way of the placenta ceases. Although the incidence of breastfeeding by substance-using women is low in general, nursing women should be counseled about the adverse effects of substance use.

Universal screening of women and newborns for substance abuse using biologic specimens is not recommended. However, every pregnant woman should be assessed for use of alcohol, tobacco, and illicit drugs. Such information should be used to develop a clinical care plan for the pregnant mother, either counseling to stop or referral to a drug-treatment program, if necessary, and careful follow-up postpartum. Identification of substance-exposed newborns is determined primarily by clinical indicators in the prenatal period, including maternal and newborn presentation, history of substance use or abuse, medical history, or toxicology results. Screening of meconium provides a more comprehensive and accurate indication of exposure over a longer gestational period than does screening of neonatal urine. Physicians and nursery staff should be competent in the recognition of signs of neonatal withdrawal. There are a number of useful systematic scoring schemata for assessing severity, and each nursery unit should have a written policy for implementation of a scoring system for neonatal withdrawal and appropriate treatment.

Documentation of in utero illicit substance exposure and alcohol use by the mother should preclude early discharge following birth. Appropriate planning for discharge and subsequent follow-up care requires social work assessment and may include referral for child protective services if there is a concern about the future well-being of the neonate.

Long-term effects on learning and school performance, behavioral problems, and emotional instability of children exposed to illicit drugs, alcohol, and tobacco in utero remain major concerns. There is evidence that all drugs of abuse have an effect on the endogenous neurotransmitter systems of the brain. Exposure during development may alter the development and functions of these systems, and this may have a long-lasting effect on behavioral and cognitive outcomes. Environmental factors also place drug-exposed children at high risk for physical, sexual, and emotional abuse, neglect, and developmental delay. Long-term follow-up is indicated from medical, developmental, and social aspects. Pediatricians, therefore, should work with state social service agencies and state legislatures to extend the assistance now available through child protective services. Until this is accomplished, pediatricians should consider recruiting the assistance of the local child protective services agency to provide multidisciplinary treatment and support for the affected woman, child, and family. In general, a coordinated multidisciplinary approach in the development of a plan without criminal sanctions has the best chance of helping children and families.

Respiratory Distress Syndrome

Respiratory distress syndrome (RDS) is associated with preterm birth-related surfactant deficiency. Multiple randomized, controlled clinical trials have demonstrated the benefits of surfactant replacement therapy, including reduction in the severity of RDS, improvement in survival without BPD, and limitation of pulmonary complications. However, surfactant therapy has no effect on coexistent morbidities, such as necrotizing enterocolitis, nosocomial infections, patent ductus arteriosus, intraventricular hemorrhage, and BPD. Long-term outcome of treated neonates has shown neither beneficial nor adverse effects on growth and neurodevelopment.

Antenatal corticosteroid administration stimulates structural maturation of the fetal lung and, like postnatal surfactant replacement, improves survival and reduces the incidence of RDS. Antenatal corticosteroids coupled with postnatal surfactant replacement have additive effects. Therefore, both antenatal steroid administration to women at risk for preterm delivery and postnatal surfactant administration to infants at high risk for RDS are important treatment considerations to optimize outcomes for preterm infants.

Surfactant replacement has proved efficacious for infants with respiratory distress associated with primary surfactant deficiency (eg, RDS) and secondary surfactant deficiency (eg, meconium aspiration, persistent pulmonary hypertension, sepsis, and pneumonia). Preterm infants at high risk for primary surfactant deficiency have reduced mortality and morbidity when surfactant is administered soon after birth. Preterm and term infants with moderate to severe respiratory failure caused by surfactant deficiency and who require mechanical ventilation also may benefit from surfactant treatment.

Surfactant replacement with both animal-derived (natural) and synthetic surfactant preparations have shown efficacy for respiratory distress because of surfactant deficiency. Animal-derived surfactant products are derived from bovine and porcine sources and are similar in efficacy. None have been associated with long-term immunologic or infectious complications. First-generation synthetic surfactant preparations are less effective than animal-derived surfactants, in part because of their inability to mimic the spreading and recycling functions of surfactant-associated proteins. Second-generation synthetic surfactant preparations contain recombinant surfactant proteins or peptides that mimic the function of surfactant-associated proteins. Clinical studies comparing animal-derived and second-generation synthetic surfactants are progressing.

Surfactant replacement therapy given to newborn infants with respiratory failure often is associated with multisystem organ dysfunction that requires specialized care. Caring for these neonates in nurseries that do not have the full range of required capabilities may affect overall outcome adversely. Therefore, infants with respiratory failure requiring surfactant therapy should be managed in neonatal intensive care nurseries that have the expertise to provide comprehensive care for sick newborn infants.

Surfactant replacement is an effective therapy for neonates at high risk for or with respiratory failure associated with surfactant deficiency. Systems of neonatal health care must adapt to advances in the science and application of surfactant therapy. The following recommendations should be incorporated into neonatal care systems:

- Surfactants should be administered by clinicians with the technical and clinical expertise to respond to rapid changes in lung volume and compliance and complications of surfactant instillation into the airway.

- Surfactant therapy should be provided by experienced personnel, within facilities or during transport, who are capable of managing multisystem disorders in sick neonates.

- An institutionally approved guideline for administering surfactant therapy should be a component of a quality-assessment program.

- Surfactant replacement therapy should be directed by physicians who are trained in the respiratory management of sick neonates and have knowledge and experience in mechanical ventilation.

- Nursing and respiratory therapy personnel who are experienced in the management of sick neonates, including the use of mechanical ventilation, should be available when surfactant therapy is administered.

- The equipment necessary for managing and monitoring the condition of sick neonates, including that needed for mechanical ventilation, should be available when surfactant therapy is administered.

- Radiology and laboratory support to manage a broad range of needs of sick neonates should be immediately available in facilities where surfactant therapy is prescribed.

- At institutions that do not meet these requirements to offer surfactant therapy, and when timely transfer of a high-risk newborn to an appropriate institution cannot be achieved, surfactant therapy may be given but only under supervision of a physician by clinicians who are skilled in endotracheal intubation and surfactant administration. Neonates should be transferred, if appropriate, from such institutions as soon as feasible to a center with appropriate facilities and trained staff to care for multisystem morbidity in sick neonates.

Hemorrhagic and Periventricular White Matter Brain Injury

Clinical Considerations

Neonates born at 32 weeks of gestation or less or at birth weights of 1,500 g or less are those at highest risk for hemorrhagic and other injury to the brain. Both the incidence and severity increase with decreasing gestational age. The vulnerability of the preterm infant arises from the vascular and cellular immaturity of the developing brain and may be compounded by inadequate protective cerebral autoregulation of blood flow during the frequent periods of physiologic instability characteristic of this group of newborns. Periventricular–intraventricular hemorrhage, which is the most frequent hemorrhagic lesion, ranges from a small, germinal matrix bleed to varying amounts of intraventricular blood to massive intraparenchymal hemorrhage or hemorrhagic infarction. Most periventricular–intraventricular hemorrhage occurs in the first 72 hours after birth. Posthemorrhagic hydrocephalus secondary to intraventricular hemorrhage is apparent within 2–4 weeks after delivery in most cases but occasionally can develop later. Periventricular leukomalacia is the most frequent white matter lesion identified. Residual lesions following brain injury include minimal to extensive cystic lesions in the periventricular white matter and ventriculomegaly secondary to diffuse cerebral atrophy. Porencephaly may develop following severe, localized ischemic or hemorrhagic infarction. These lesions evolve over the course of several weeks after the precipitating insult. Both hemorrhagic and other brain injury can occur in the same neonate, although the pathophysiologic processes are different.

Screening and Follow-up

Portable bedside cranial ultrasonography is the most frequent imaging modality used to diagnose and follow the evolution of brain injury. There can be great variability in interpretation. The quality of the images is affected by the choice of equipment and the expertise of the ultrasonographer in obtaining consistent positioning of the sensor.

It is recommended that each center establish a protocol for screening cranial ultrasound examinations in neonates who are at risk. In the absence of the need to diagnose for clinical reasons, the initial study can be performed between 3 postnatal days and 14 postnatal days. Follow-up studies to monitor for the evolution of severity or emergence of a complication may be timed based on the clinical course and the known progression of such. Current experience suggests that the best correlation with subsequent risk for neurodevelopmental sequelae is found from results of studies performed at approximately 36–40 weeks postmenstrual age or before discharge. However, to date there has been no recommendation for routine cranial magnetic resonance imaging for all preterm infants who are at risk.

Prevention

As yet, no single intervention has been found to consistently prevent either periventricular–intraventricular hemorrhage or other lesions, although many approaches have been tried. A coordinated perinatal approach to reduce the severity and effect of episodes of hemodynamic instability, including avoiding hypocapnia, is important. Prenatal betamethasone for acceleration of fetal lung maturation also decreases the incidence and severity of periventricular–intraventricular hemorrhage in susceptible fetuses. For this reason, the use of betamethasone is preferred over the use of dexamethasone for antenatal corticosteroid administration.

Hypoxic Cardiorespiratory Failure

Hypoxic cardiorespiratory failure in neonates born at term or late preterm may complicate heterogenous conditions such as primary persistent pulmonary hypertension, RDS, aspiration of meconium, pneumonia, sepsis, and congenital diaphragmatic hernia. Hypoxemia, hypercarbia, and acidosis generally are reversible with administration of oxygen, mechanical ventilation, inotropic agents, intravascular volume expansion, supportive care, and antibiotics. Term and late preterm neonates who fail to respond to these interventions may benefit from rescue therapies targeting specific physiologic abnormalities that may accompany hypoxic respiratory failure, such as surfactant deficiency (surfactant replacement) and pulmonary hypertension (inhaled nitric oxide). In small, randomized trials involving infants with meconium aspiration syndrome, persistent pulmonary hypertension, and sepsis, surfactant replacement reduced mortality and the need for extracorporeal membrane oxygenation (ECMO) without an increase in morbidity. Inhaled nitric oxide is a selective pulmonary vasodilator. Prospective, randomized clinical trials have shown that inhaled nitric oxide improves oxygenation and reduces the need for ECMO in term infants. Response to inhaled nitric oxide is optimized when the lungs are adequately recruited; high frequency ventilation often is successful for this purpose, especially in infants with homogenous lung disease.

The use of inhaled nitric oxide in preterm infants is the subject of ongoing investigation. Preterm infants with hypoxic respiratory failure may have improved oxygenation with inhaled nitric oxide. However, the acute improvement in oxygenation has not been accompanied by consistent improvement in survival and lower risk of BPD. Preterm neonates also may experience more toxicity than term and late preterm neonates. Until additional information becomes available, preterm infants should receive inhaled nitric oxide within the context of research protocols.

Extracorporeal membrane oxygenation is the use of prolonged (days to weeks) cardiopulmonary bypass for infants with hypoxic respiratory or cardiac failure who are failing to respond to maximal and less-invasive therapies. Criteria for initiating transfer and ECMO are complex because gestational age, size, diagnosis, severity of cardiorespiratory failure, clinical course, presence of complications, postnatal age, proximity of ECMO centers, risk of transport, and parental preferences all must be considered. In general, however, a neonate with respiratory failure who is deteriorating and has an oxygenation index greater than 25 (oxygenation index = [mean airway pressure/PaO_2] $\times$ FIO_2 $\times$ 100) has a moderately high risk of requiring ECMO. Consultation and possible transfer to an ECMO center is advised when the oxygenation index reaches 25. Neonates with oxygenation index calculations greater than 35–45 are at high risk for dying without ECMO. Extracorporeal membrane oxygenation should be considered unless contraindications exist; such contraindications may include gestational age less than 34–35 weeks, birth weight less than 2,000 g, profound hypoxic–ischemic encephalopathy, large intracranial hemorrhage, congenital anomalies associated with grave prognosis, or nonreversible pulmonary or cardiac disorder.

Lung rest during ECMO allows pulmonary and cardiac recovery with reduced risk of secondary injury from exposure to high oxygen and ventilator support. Extracorporeal membrane oxygenation is highly invasive and accompanied by risks associated with systemic anticoagulation, mechanical complications, and the cannulation procedures. Risks of hemorrhage and death are very high in preterm infants treated with ECMO. Therefore, the decision to transfer or begin ECMO must balance the risks and benefits of less invasive treatments to that of ECMO. Extracorporeal membrane oxygenation generally is reserved for late preterm and term infants who are failing to respond to less-invasive and lower-risk interventions.

Improved survival without an increase in morbidity for neonates receiving ECMO has been demonstrated in clinical trials. Medical complications may include BPD, feeding problems, gastroesophageal reflux, and slow growth. Significant neurologic abnormality, developmental delay, or neurocognitive disability occurs in approximately 15% of ECMO survivors evaluated at 5 years of age. Seizures; hearing loss; visual disturbances; learning disability; and social, attention, and behavioral problems are complications seen among many neonatal patients with complex medical courses, including those treated with inhaled nitric oxide and ECMO. Because of the risk for these adverse outcomes and the emergence of subtle disabilities during the school-age and adolescent years, it is recommended that infants who have been critically ill, especially those who survive with the use of rescue therapies such as ECMO, be followed by developmental specialists throughout childhood.

It is critical that neonates with hypoxic cardiorespiratory failure receive care in institutions that have appropriately skilled personnel—including physicians, nurses, and respiratory therapists who are qualified to use multiple modes of ventilation—and readily accessible radiologic and laboratory support. Neonates who are not benefiting from conventional therapies should be transferred in a timely manner to the appropriate level III neonatal intensive care unit (NICU) capable of providing alternative treatments.

Management of Anemia in Preterm Neonates

Anemia of prematurity results from multiple factors and varies with the degree of immaturity, postnatal age, nutritional status and intake, and the nature and severity of neonatal illness. Appropriate management requires accurate assessment of the roles of the various etiologies, with therapeutic interventions determined by that assessment. At times, the need for adequate oxygen-carrying capacity necessitates packed red blood cell transfusion on an acute basis while awaiting response to other interventions to correct the anemia-producing process. However, transfusion poses risk of the transmission of pathogens, particularly with exposure to multiple donors.

Current evidence indicates that most anemias occurring in the first 2–3 weeks after delivery mainly result from the volume of blood sampling obtained for clinical management. The balance of oxidative substrate (polyunsaturated free fatty acids), antioxidants (eg, vitamin E), and prooxidants (eg, iron) in the diet during growth also may play a role in red blood cell survival. As growth accelerates with advancing postnatal age, depletion of iron stores begins to affect erythropoiesis. Underlying these factors is the VLBW neonate's limited capacity to increase erythropoietin production in response to anemia. This further decreases red blood cell production and increases the likelihood of dilutional anemia from an expanding blood volume.

Controlled clinical trials have shown that adherence to protocols with strict indications for transfusion reduced both the volume of blood transfused and donor exposure without adverse clinical consequences. Prophylactic use of recombinant human erythropoietin in clinical trials, both administered early in the neonatal course and initiated after several weeks, has demonstrated a limited reduction in the number of transfusions and the volume of transfused blood; the effect of reduced donor exposure has not been studied in most trials. In none of these studies was the need for transfusion eliminated altogether.

It would seem prudent from the available evidence to recommend that a multipronged approach to limiting transfusion be used, particularly in VLBW neonates. Both the causation as well as the correction of anemia of prematurity must be addressed. This includes judicial use of blood sampling (using noninvasive oxygen monitoring extensively), maintenance of optimal nutritional intake, adherence to a protocol with strict indications for transfusion of packed red blood cells, and establishment of a system of blood banking that limits donor exposure to the maximum possible extent. Routine use of human recombinant erythropoietin for all preterm neonates is not recommended at this time.

However, there may be specific groups of VLBW neonates (eg, Jehovah's Witnesses) in whom its use would be beneficial.

Bronchopulmonary Dysplasia

Bronchopulmonary dysplasia, or chronic lung disease, complicates the recovery of some preterm infants with RDS and neonates of any gestational age with severe pulmonary insufficiency or hypoplasia who require prolonged respiratory support. In extremely preterm infants, many of whom have mild lung disease caused by the maturational effects of antenatal steroids, postnatal surfactant replacement, and gentle ventilation strategies, BPD evolves because of complex interactions between normal developmental processes and factors that adversely affect lung morphogenesis and alveolarization (such as hyperoxia, hypoxia, poor nutrition, corticosteroid use, and inflammatory mediators). Disruption in lung development in these extremely preterm infants is characterized pathologically by alveolar and capillary hypoplasia and reduction in gas exchange surface area and is referred to as the "new" BPD. Newborn infants of any gestational age with a genetic predisposition, antenatal exposure to chronic chorioamnionitis, lung diseases that require prolonged exposure to high oxygen concentrations, positive-pressure ventilation, inflammation, excessive pulmonary blood flow, pulmonary edema, and atelectasis may develop "classic" BPD. Classic BPD is defined pathologically by alveolar and airway destruction, inflammation, and fibrosis that result in emphysema, atelectasis, bronchial and bronchiolar mucosal hyperplasia and metaplasia, interstitial fibrosis, narrowed airways, excess mucus accumulation, interstitial edema, lymphatic dilation, pulmonary vascular smooth muscle hypertrophy, and reduction in capillary bed size. Bronchopulmonary dysplasia presents as prolonged respiratory distress associated with nonspecific clinical and radiographic findings. The course may begin with severe lung disease or mild respiratory insufficiency that is followed by progressive deterioration, often acutely exacerbated by bacterial or viral infection or increased pulmonary blood flow through a patent ductus arteriosus. Infants with severe BPD may develop pulmonary hypertension or cor pulmonale or may die from acute bronchospasm or infection.

Bronchopulmonary dysplasia has been variably defined as the need for oxygen at 28 weeks of gestation or 36 weeks postmenstrual age with or without clinical and radiographic evidence. Because physicians determine oxygen administration according to somewhat subjective, nonphysiologic criteria that often are applied inconsistently, it is a challenge to compare outcomes across

NICUs. In 2000, diagnostic criteria for BPD were developed by consensus at a workshop sponsored by the National Heart, Lung, and Blood Institute. The purpose of defining BPD was to reduce variability in reporting, improve comparability among different NICUs, and develop research priorities. The following definition was developed (Table 8–2).

A physiologic definition of BPD also has been developed to reduce subjectivity introduced by individual clinicians. The oxygen reduction test is applied to infants receiving supplemental oxygen of 0.30 FIO_2 or less at 36 weeks postmenstrual age. As in the consensus definition, infants at 36 weeks postmenstrual age or more than 56 postnatal days and receiving positive pressure ventilation, continuous positive airway pressure, or oxygen supplementation at greater than 0.30 FIO_2 are considered to have BPD and are not subject to an oxygen-reduction test.

Therapeutic Approaches—Prevention

Multiple respiratory support strategies and pharmacologic interventions have been proposed to decrease development of BPD in sick neonates. Few have

Table 8–2. Definition of Bronchopulmonary Dysplasia

	Gestational Age	
Assessment	Less Than 32 wk	32 wk or Older
Time point of assessment	36 wk PMA or discharge to home, whichever comes first Treatment with oxygen greater than 21% for at least 28 d plus:	28 d but less than 56 d postnatal age or discharge to home, whichever comes first Treatment with oxygen more than 21% for at least 28 d plus:
Mild BPD	• Breathing room air at 36 wk PMA or discharge, whichever comes first	• Breathing room air by 56 d post natal age or discharge, whichever comes first
Moderate BPD	• Need for less than 30% oxygen at 36 wk PMA or discharge, whichever comes first	• Need for less than 30% oxygen at 56 d postnatal age or discharge, whichever comes first
Severe PBD	• Need for 30% or greater oxygen or positive pressure (PPV or NCPAP), or both, at 36 wk PMA or discharge, whichever comes first	• Need for 30% or greater oxygen or positive pressure (PPV or NCPAP), or both, at 56 d postnatal age or discharge, whichever comes first

Abbreviations; BPD, bronchopulmonary dysplasia; NCPAP, nasal continuous positive airway pressure; PMA, postmenstrual age; PPV, positive-pressure ventilation
Jobe A, Bancalari E. Bronchopulmonary dysplasia. Am J Respir Crit Care Med 2001;163:1723–9.

been demonstrated adequately in controlled clinical trials of appropriate size and rigorous design to support recommendation for universal implementation. The prevention of RDS and the requirement for mechanical ventilation by the antenatal administration of corticosteroids to women at risk of preterm delivery decreases the population at risk. Surfactant replacement has increased survival without BPD but not the incidence of BPD in VLBW infants despite improved survival and fewer air leak complications. Vitamin A supplementation has been shown to be safe and to result in a small decrease in the risk of BPD in ventilated, extremely low birth weight neonates. Low-dose inhaled nitric oxide in ventilated preterm infants with RDS has not been established to increase survival or reduce BPD risk, although clinical trials are in progress. Assisted ventilation strategies to avoid deleterious hyperinflation are desirable, but strong supportive evidence for most specific, individual strategies are lacking. Aggressive use of continuous end distending pressure beginning in the delivery room has not been proved clearly to reduce the incidence of BPD; clinical trials are in progress. Permissive hypercapnia (ie, accepting higher $PaCO_2$ levels than was customary) has been suggested, but controlled studies in neonates have not demonstrated a reduction in risk for BPD. High-frequency ventilation using various modalities and strategies has not been found to be consistently efficacious. The use of synchronized ventilation, if achievable, and short inspiratory times would seem prudent to avoid ventilator-associated lung injury. High volumes of fluid intake in the first week have been shown to contribute to the persistence of a patent ductus arteriosus and perhaps to the development of BPD. However, no single fluid regimen has been shown to be safer and more efficacious; fluid restriction often means caloric restriction as well. Other modalities directed at specific antecedents of inflammatory injury have included antioxidants (vitamin E and superoxide dismutase) and erythromycin (prophylaxis or treatment for Ureaplasma colonization). None of these can be recommended at this time either because of safety issues (erythromycin) or unconfirmed efficacy (vitamin E supplementation beyond that required to prevent vitamin E deficiency is not beneficial); superoxide dismutase and other antioxidant medications have not been studied adequately.

Postnatal steroids, primarily dexamethasone, have been used in attempts to prevent and treat BPD in low birth weight infants. Randomized, controlled trials have shown that postnatal steroids have short-term benefits of earlier extubation and fewer ventilator days. However, many short-term adverse events occur, including hyperglycemia, hypertension, gastrointestinal bleeding, intestinal perforation, hypertrophic obstructive cardiomyopathy, poor weight gain, and poor head circumference growth. Mortality by the time of discharge and length of hospitalization are not reduced with postnatal steroid use. Furthermore, some studies suggest an association of postnatal steroids with an increased incidence of neurodevelopmental delay and cerebral palsy. Therefore, the routine use of systemic dexamethasone for prevention or treatment of chronic lung disease in infants with VLBW is not recommended. Rather, postnatal systemic dexamethasone use for this purpose should be limited to randomized, double-masked, controlled trials and for exceptional clinical circumstances (eg, an infant on maximal ventilatory and oxygen support). In these exceptional circumstances, parents should be fully informed about the known short- and long-term risks and agree to treatment.

Therapeutic Approaches—Treatment

Once BPD is established, current evidence and clinical experience support that diuretics and inhaled bronchodilator agents improve pulmonary function and, therefore, may facilitate reduction in ventilatory support and subsequent extubation. Oxygen supplementation is a consistent component of care, but the most efficacious therapeutic range of oxygen saturation has not been established. Episodes of spontaneous desaturation are a frequent occurrence in neonates with BPD. Oxygen supplementation has been shown to improve growth and decrease the likelihood of progression to pulmonary hypertension. Inhaled nitric oxide treatment of preterm infants receiving mechanical ventilation for severe BPD may reduce the amount of oxygen required; clinical trials to understand whether inhaled nitric oxide treatment will prevent or reduce the severity of BPD are in progress. Both inhaled and systemic corticosteroid therapy have facilitated reduction in ventilatory support and hastened extubation. However, neonates treated with systemic corticosteroids are at risk of experiencing a number of adverse effects and an increase in neurodevelopmental abnormalities. Growth failure without steroid exposure is well recognized to accompany severe BPD; energy expenditure has been shown to be significantly higher in neonates with BPD. Lung healing is impaired by inadequate nutritional intake. Therefore, although not supported by controlled trials, provision of calories, minerals, and protein to sustain a growth rate comparable with non-BPD gestational age peers seems a logical approach. Immunoprophylaxis for respiratory syncytial virus and influenza has reduced the posthospitalization morbidity of neonates with BPD.

Nutritional Needs of Preterm Neonates

Optimal nutrition is critical in the management of small, preterm neonates. There is no standard for the precise nutritional needs of preterm neonates comparable with the human milk standard for term neonates. Present recommendations are designed to provide nutrients to approximate the rate of growth and composition of weight gain for a normal fetus of the same postmenstrual age and to maintain normal concentrations of blood and tissue nutrients. However, the presence of acute neonatal illness and the immaturity of a variety of organ systems may make provision of optimal nutrition without inducing additional morbidity challenging. This is particularly true for the sickest and most immature neonates during the initial days and weeks of life, yet inadequate nutrition during this period may have life-long consequences.

Parenteral Nutrition

Parenteral administration of amino acids, glucose, and fat is an important aspect of the nutritional care of preterm neonates, particularly those who weigh less than 1,500 g. The high incidence of respiratory and other morbidities, combined with intestinal immaturity, may necessitate slow advancement of the volume of enteral feedings. Parenteral nutrition can supplement the gradually increasing enteral feedings so that total intake by both routes meets the neonate's nutritional needs.

Positive nitrogen balance, indicating an anabolic state, is achieved with amino acid intakes of 1.5 g/kg per day and with parenteral lipid and glucose energy intakes of 50–60 kcal/kg per day. With nonprotein energy intakes of 80–85 kcal/kg per day and amino acid intakes of 3 g/kg per day, nitrogen retention may occur at the fetal rate. Current evidence indicates that parenteral administration of amino acid and glucose may be safely initiated within hours of birth. Provision of amino acids at 1.5 g/kg per day, with 30–35 kcal/kg per day of nonprotein energy, will prevent negative nitrogen balance and is well tolerated in even the most immature neonates. In fact, more recently, infants given higher doses of amino acids in the first 24 hours of life demonstrated normal blood pH, plasma amino acids, and blood urea concentrations. As nonprotein energy and amino acid intake is increased, a balanced supply of glucose and intravenous lipid generally is recommended to prevent some of the metabolic complications of parenteral nutrition.

Enteral Nutrition

The method of enteral feeding chosen for each neonate should be based on gestational age, birth weight, and clinical condition. Historically, enteral feedings have been delayed in the small, preterm neonate because of extreme immaturity, perceived increased risk of necrotizing enterocolitis, or significant respiratory or other morbidity. However, evidence indicates that early introduction of "trophic" or "priming" feedings are safe, well tolerated, and associated with significant benefits. The actual route of enteral feeding (eg, nasogastric, orogastric, gastrostomy, transpyloric, or nipple) again is determined on the basis of gestational age, clinical condition, and oromotor integrity (ability to coordinate sucking, swallowing, and breathing).

Human milk from the preterm neonate's mother has a number of special features that make its use desirable in feeding preterm neonates. Fresh or properly stored refrigerated human milk contains immunologic and antimicrobial factors that are protective against infection. Fat digestion is facilitated by the lipase present and the structure of triglycerides found in human milk. However, human milk does not provide adequate protein, calcium, phosphorus, sodium, trace metals, and some vitamins to meet the tissue and bone growth needs of the VLBW neonate. Human milk fortifiers that are nutritionally balanced to correct these deficiencies when added to human milk are available commercially and can enhance growth and bone mineralization in VLBW infants.

Preterm neonates who weigh more than 2,000 g at birth generally achieve adequate growth when fed their mother's milk, postdischarge formula, or a regular 67-kcal/dL term neonate formula. However, calcium and phosphorus retention rates are slower than fetal accretion rates. They may require vitamin supplementation during the period when the volume of formula or human milk ingested does not provide the recommended daily vitamin intake, particularly of vitamin D (Table 8–3).

Special formulas for VLBW neonates (preterm formulas) contain additional protein, easily absorbed carbohydrates (glucose polymers and lactose), and easily digested and absorbed lipids (15–50% medium-chain triglycerides). The calcium and phosphorus contents are higher to achieve a bone mineralization rate equivalent to the fetal rate. The sodium content also is higher. Trace metals and vitamins have been added to meet the increased needs of the VLBW neonate. Weight gain and bone mineralization closer to that of the reference fetus and improved long-term growth and development have been shown following the use of formulas for preterm neonates as compared with that of formulas for term neonates. Also, improved neurodevelopmental outcome is seen

Table 8-3. Comparison of Enteral Intake Recommendations for Growing Preterm Neonates in Stable Clinical Condition

Nutrients per 100 kcal[†]	Consensus Recommendations*		AAPCON[‡]	ESPGAN-CON[‡]
	<1,000 g	>1,000 g		
Water, mL	125-167	125-167	–	115-154
Energy, kcal	100	100	100	100
Protein, g	3-3.16	2.5-3	2.9-3.3	2.25-3.1
Carbohydrate, g	–	–	9-13	7-14
Lactose, g	3.16-9.5	3.16-9.8	–	–
Oligomers, g	0-7	0-7	–	–
Fat, g	–	–	4.5-6	3.6-7
Linoleic acid, g	0.44-1.7	0.44-1.7	0.4+	0.5-1.4
Linolenic acid, g	0.11-0.44	0.11-0.44	–	>0.055
$C_{18:2}/C_{18:3}$	>5	>5	–	5-15
Vitamin A, USP units	583-1,250	583-1,250	75-225	270-450
With lung disease	2,250-2,333	2,250-2,333	–	–
Vitamin D, USP units	125-333	125-333	270	800-1,600/d
Vitamin E, USP units	5-10	5-10	>1.1	0.6-10
Supplement, human milk	2.9	2.9	–	–
Vitamin K, μg	6.66-8.33	6.66-8.33	4	4-15
Ascorbate, mg	15-20	15-20	35	7-40
Thiamine, μg	150-200	150-200	>40	20-250
Riboflavin, μg	200-300	200-300	>60	60-600
Pyridoxine, μg	125-175	125-175	>35	35-250
Niacin, mg	3-4	3-4	>0.25	0.8-5
Pantothenate, mg	1-15	1-15	>0.3	>0.3
Biotin, μg	3-5	3-5	>1.5	>1.5
Folate, μg	21-42	21-42	33	>60
Vitamin B_{12}, μg	0.25	0.25	>0.15	>0.15
Sodium, mg	38-58	38-58	48-67	23-53
Potassium, mg	65-100	65-100	66-98	90-152
Chloride, mg	59-89	59-89	–	57-89
Calcium, mg	100-192	100-192	175	70-140
Phosphorus, mg	50-117	50-117	91.5	50-87
Magnesium, mg	6.6-12.5	6.6-12.5	–	6-12
Iron, mg	1.67	1.67	1.7-2.5	1.5
Zinc, μg	833	833	>500	550-1,100

(continued)

Table 8–3. Comparison of Enteral Intake Recommendations for Growing Preterm Neonates in Stable Clinical Condition *(continued)*

Nutrients per 100 kcal[†]	Consensus Recommendations[*]		AAPCON[‡]	ESPGAN-CON[‡]
	<1,000 g	>1,000 g		
Copper, µg	100–125	100–125	90	90–120
Selenium, µg	1.08–2.5	1.08–2.5	–	–
Chromium, µg	0.083–0.42	0.083–0.42	–	–
Manganese, µg	6.3	6.3	>5	1.5–7.5
Molybdenum, µg	0.25	0.25	–	–
Iodine, µg	25–50	25–50	5	10–45
Taurine, mg	3.75–7.5	3.75–7.5	–	–
Carnitine, mg	2.4	2.4	–	>1.2
Inositol, mg	27–67.5	27–67.5	–	–
Choline, mg	12–23.4	12–23.4	–	–

[*]Tsang RC, Lucas A, Vany R, Zlotkin S, editors. Nutritional needs of the preterm infant: scientific basis and practical guidelines. Baltimore (MD): Williams and Wilkins; 1993.

[†]Based on a need for 120 mg/kg per day

[‡]AAPCON indicates American Academy of Pediatrics, Committee on Nutrition; ESPGAN-CON, European Society of Paediatric Gastroenterology and Nutrition, Committee on Nutrition of the Preterm Infant.

Modified from American Academy of Pediatrics. Pediatric nutrition handbook. 5th ed. Elk Grove Village (IL): AAP; 2003.

in preterm neonates fed preterm formulas or human milk versus term formula. Formulas containing long-chain polyunsaturated fatty acids may confer visual neurodevelopmental benefits.

Traditionally, VLBW preterm formula-fed neonates were changed to a standard term neonate formula in preparation for hospital discharge despite being below the tenth percentile for growth parameters at discharge. However, this practice has been reevaluated. Formulas that provide increased protein, energy, and mineral intake to meet the continuing growth needs of the small, preterm neonate have been developed. Postdischarge formulas are now available in the community at a cost slightly higher than that of standard formulas. Their use has been shown to result in greater linear growth, weight gain, and bone mineralization when compared with the use of term formula. Small, preterm neonates (born at or before 34 weeks of gestation, with a birth weight less than or equal to 1,800 g) and neonates with other morbidities (eg, BPD) may benefit from the use of such formulas for up to 9 months after hospital discharge. The enhanced growth associated with postdischarge formulas appears to reset the growth trajectory for VLBW infants even after discontinuation of postdischarge formulas at 9 months.

Surgical Procedures in the Neonatal Intensive Care Unit

Neonates in the NICU often require surgical procedures during hospitalization. These procedures range from establishing venous access to laparotomy for necrotizing enterocolitis or thoracotomy for ligation of a patent ductus arteriosus. The transport of an acutely ill neonate to the operating room may be associated with a number of risks, including hypothermia, changes in blood pressure levels, and dislodging of an intravenous catheter or endotracheal tube. For this reason, in many centers, selected surgical procedures are performed within the NICU. Studies of central venous catheter insertion, ECMO cannulation or decannulation, patent ductus arteriosus ligation, laparotomy, and other procedures have suggested that this approach can be safe and effective and may result in improved outcomes. In addition, both cryotherapy and argon laser ablation of the retina have been performed in NICUs. There are unique personnel and environmental safety precautions required when lasers are used.

With the exception of relatively minor procedures, surgery must be performed in an area of the NICU that is separate from other neonates, is equipped with adequate lighting and working space, and permits ongoing monitoring and anesthetic management. Personnel should wear appropriate operating room attire, and strict sterile techniques must be used.

Hospital policies governing all surgical procedures performed within the NICU, including management of anesthesia, should be developed in conjunction with the institutional operating room committee to ensure that appropriate guidelines are met.

Pain and Stress Management

Analgesia

Pain consists of the perception of painful stimuli (nociception) and the psychologic response to painful stimuli (anxiety). Studies measuring a variety of physiologic factors, including oxygen saturation, β-endorphin, glucose, cortisol, and epinephrine concentrations, confirm that neonates of all gestational ages have a nociceptive response to pain stimuli. Observations of neonate behavior suggest that anxiety also is a component of the infantile pain response, but its character, intensity, and duration remain undetermined. Therefore, the true significance of anxiety in the newborn remains unknown. Measures for assessing pain in the newborn have been developed and validated. Every health care facility caring for neonates should implement an effective pain-prevention and stress-reduction program that includes strategies for the following elements:

- Routine pain assessments
- Minimization of the number of painful procedures performed
- Effective use of pharmacologic and nonpharmacologic therapies for the prevention of pain associated with routine minor procedures
- Elimination of pain associated with surgery and other major procedures

Pain is managed most effectively by limiting or avoiding noxious stimuli and providing analgesia. Any unnecessary noxious stimuli (eg, acoustic, visual, tactile, and vestibular) of neonates should be avoided, if possible. Simple comfort measures such as swaddling, nonnutritive sucking, and positioning (if not contraindicated because of medical or surgical concerns) should be used whenever possible for minor procedures. Oral administration of sucrose reduces pain associated with painful procedures. The risks and benefits of pain management techniques must be considered on an individualized basis. Pharmacologic analgesia should be chosen carefully.

Intraoperative and Postoperative Pain Management

For major surgical procedures, general anesthesia by inhalation of anesthetic gases, intravenous administration of narcotic agents, or regional techniques can be safe and effective. The use of paralytic agents without analgesia during surgery is unacceptable. Anesthesia for surgical procedures for all newborns should be administered by specially trained physicians, and the choice of technique and agent should be based carefully on a comprehensive assessment of the neonate, efficacy and safety of the drug, and the technical requirements of the procedure.

The use of analgesic agents is important in the immediate postoperative period and should be continued as required. Both continuous or bolus infusions of opioids and continuous caudal or epidural blockade can be used to provide a steady course of pain relief, but both require careful management and continuous monitoring of cardiorespiratory and hemodynamic status.

Pain Management for Minor Surgical and Other Invasive Procedures

Analgesia for minor invasive procedures, such as chest tube insertion or incisional placement of central venous lines, usually can be provided by superficial infiltration of local anesthetic agents and appropriate analgesics. For circumcision, oral administration of sucrose and a regional nerve block (ring block or dorsal penile nerve block) or topical anesthetic cream is recommended. Because oral sucrose reduces but does not totally eliminate pain in neonates, it should be used with other nonpharmacologic measures to enhance its effectiveness.

Routine Medication for Prolonged Endotracheal Intubation

Use of analgesic and anxiolytic agents in newborns for amelioration of the discomfort associated with prolonged endotracheal intubation should be undertaken only after careful consideration of the observed response to pain and anxiety, as demonstrated by the individual neonate, and the side effects of the commonly used agents. The use of analgesic or sedative agents for amelioration of the discomfort associated with prolonged mechanical ventilation has not been shown to be helpful and may be harmful. Therefore, their routine use cannot be recommended.

Analgesic premedication for endotracheal intubation should be considered for all newborns, except for emergency intubation during resuscitation or in infants with suspected or proven airway anomalies. A rapid analgesic and vagolytic agent should be considered.

Concepts that must be remembered include the following list:

- Sedatives and anxiolytics do not provide analgesia.
- Chronic use of many sedatives or hypnotics may lead to tolerance, dependency, and withdrawal.
- Neurodevelopmental outcome from chronic sedation of neonates is unknown.
- Sedatives or hypnotics may cause respiratory and cardiovascular depression.
- Combined treatment with a sedative or hypnotic and an opioid requires a decreased dosage of each.
- Agitation in the chronically ventilated neonate may indicate the need to confirm airway patency and position, adjust ventilatory settings, or reduce noxious environmental stimuli.

Recommendations

The following recommendations about the use of analgesia in neonates can be made:

- Validated pain assessment tools must be used in a consistent manner and caregivers should be trained to assess newborns for pain.

- The number of routine painful or stressful events neonates are exposed to should be minimized using protocols that limit painful or stressful disruptions in care.

- Environmental and nonpharmacologic interventions should be provided as baseline measures to prevent, reduce, or eliminate stress and pain.

- Topical anesthetics can be used to reduce pain associated with vein puncture, lumbar puncture, and intravenous catheter insertion when time permits, but repeated use should be limited.

- Pharmacokinetic and pharmacodynamic properties and efficacy in neonates should be known for pharmacologic agents administered to newborns.

- Agents known to compromise cardiorespiratory function should be administered only by individuals experienced in airway management and in settings with the capacity for continuous cardiorespiratory monitoring.

Immunization

General Policy

A guideline for immunization of both preterm and term neonates who require prolonged hospital stays should be implemented in each NICU. Preterm neonates should begin the immunization series at the usual chronological age of 2 months, unless otherwise indicated for a specific vaccine or disease process. Some VLBW neonates have been found to have a reduced level of immune response when the usual timing of immunizations is followed. Additional studies are needed to define the optimal schedule for this group of infants. Vaccine doses should not be reduced for VLBW or preterm infants. Term neonates who remain in the hospital at age 2 months likewise should receive vaccines according to the recommended schedule. Thiomersal-free vaccines always should be used. Acellular pertussis and inactivated polio vaccines should be used for the initial immunization series as recommended in the *AAP Red Book*.

Vaccine-Specific Issues

The optimal time to initiate hepatitis B vaccination for preterm neonates with birth weights of less than 2,000 g whose mothers are hepatitis B surface antigen (HBsAg) negative has not been determined. Extremely preterm (born at less than 28 weeks of gestation), VLBW, and more mature preterm infants all demonstrate consistently high rates of seroconversion following the first dose of hepatitis B vaccine compared with term neonates. However, subsequent antibody levels in these neonates after the recommended three-dose hepatitis B vaccine series have been reported to be less than that found in term infants 9–12 months after initiation of the series. Nevertheless, protection appears to be conferred in preterm infants weighing less than 2,000 g who are medically stable and thriving when given hepatitis B vaccine beginning as early as 1 month after birth. Administration at 1 month rather than at 2 months may be beneficial in particularly vulnerable infants who might receive multiple blood products, undergo surgical interventions, or be exposed to hepatitis B chronic carriers. Use of combination vaccines that include hepatitis B vaccine beginning at 2 months of age has the advantage of reducing the number of injections required for comprehensive vaccination coverage. If the maternal HBsAg test result is positive, all neonates with birth weights of less than 2,000 g should receive both hepatitis B immune globulin and hepatitis B vaccine at different sites within 12 hours of birth. When born to women with unknown HBsAg status, this same group of infants who are at risk should receive the hepatitis B vaccine, and, if the mother's HBsAg status cannot be determined within the first 12 hours after delivery, hepatitis B immune globulin. The initial dose of hepatitis B vaccine given to preterm infants born to HBsAg positive women should not be counted as part of the required three-dose hepatitis B immunization series.

All infants, especially those with BPD, hemodynamically significant cardiac disease, chronic renal insufficiency or immunodeficiency, or those born preterm, should be immunized against influenza beginning at age 6 months and as soon as possible before the beginning of and during influenza season. Two doses of vaccine administered 1 month apart are recommended for infants receiving vaccine for the first time. Immunization of family members and other caretakers against influenza is recommended as well. In addition, staff of NICUs should receive influenza vaccine annually before the onset of the influenza virus season.

The heptavalent pneumococcal conjugate vaccine induces protective antibody responses in children younger than 2 years of age. Preterm infants, like term infants, should receive this 4-dose vaccine series beginning at a chronologic age of 6–8 weeks. Pneumococcal vaccine may be given at the same time as other childhood vaccines, using a separate syringe and separate site for the injection of each vaccine.

Pertussis vaccination is indicated in preterm as well as term infants beginning at a chronologic age of 2 months. Stable neurologic conditions, such as developmental delay or cerebral palsy, are not contraindications for pertussis vaccination. However, infants with progressive neurologic disorders (eg, infantile spasms and other epilepsies), history of recent seizures, and known or suspected neurologic conditions that predispose to seizures or neurologic deterioration should not receive pertussis vaccination until the diagnosis and prognosis of the primary neurologic disorder is determined.

Passive Immunization

Palivizumab for respiratory syncytial virus (RSV) prophylaxis should be administered during the local RSV season and before hospital discharge to neonates born before 35 weeks of gestation as well as those with BPD or with congenital heart disease. Preterm infants who are candidates include those born at less than 32 weeks of gestation and those born at 32–35 weeks of gestation with at least two risk factors (child care attendance, school-aged siblings, exposure to environmental air pollutants, congenital abnormalities of the airways, or severe neuromuscular disease). Infants with hemodynamically significant cyanotic and acyanotic congenital heart disease or moderate to severe pulmonary hypertension also should receive palivizumab. Immunoprophylaxis should continue on a monthly basis until the season ends locally and should resume during a second RSV season for infants with severe BPD. Passive immunization is not an effective treatment for established RSV infection. A recommendation cannot be made for prevention of nosocomial RSV infections during outbreaks of RSV in high-risk nurseries because palivizumab has not been demonstrated to prevent nosocomial disease.

The Neonate With Anticipated Early Death

Hospice care for neonates may be chosen by families whose neonate has an irreversible, fatal disease. The site for such care may vary with local community resources and family wishes. Although less well studied than for older children, the components of neonatal hospice care are not unlike those established for pediatric hospice care. These components include the following elements:

- Involvement of skilled professionals
- Control of distressing symptoms and provision of physical comfort
- Coordinated, multidisciplinary service delivery
- Social support of the family
- Follow-up and bereavement care

Enhancing the quality of the remaining life for the neonate and family is more important than the site of care delivery.

Death of a Neonate

Loss of a pregnancy or death of a neonate touches many aspects of a family's life. The intense emotions of grieving can be confusing and overwhelming. Every effort should be made to determine the cause of the loss and to understand the family's grief response and to facilitate healthy coping and adjustment. Efforts to obtain organs for donation are strongly encouraged.

In-Hospital Support and Counseling

Bereavement counseling support is important to family members' abilities to adjust to their loss and to continue with their lives. Counseling should be tailored to the specific circumstances surrounding the death; should be sensitive to specific ethical, cultural, religious, and family considerations; and should be provided by specific staff within the hospital. The period after a neonatal death always has an element of confusion because of the continuing grief, the tasks of informing relatives and friends, and the need to make final arrangements.

The time in the hospital before and after the neonate has died is the parents' only opportunity to create memories of the neonate and experience being the neonate's parent. Therefore, involvement of the parents in as much of the bedside care of even critically ill neonates as is commensurate with safety and their needs is of major importance. When a neonatal death is anticipated or after an unexpected death, specific management procedures can be useful in facilitating parental adjustment to the loss:

- Offer the parents and extended family, if desired, an opportunity to see, hold, and spend time with the neonate both before and immediately after the death.

- Facilitate involvement with the clergy or spiritual adviser of the family's choice in preparing the family for the death and supporting them afterwards.

- Encourage the family to name the neonate, if they have not done so previously, as it is easier to connect memories to a neonate if parents can refer to the neonate by name.

- Obtain pictures and remembrances (eg, identification tags, footprints, a lock of hair, birth and death certificates, height and weight records, a receiving blanket for the neonate, plaster molds of the hands and feet). Even if the parents initially say that they do not want these mementos, they frequently ask for them days, weeks, or months later.

- Provide information about options for burial, cremation, funerals, or memorial services. Encourage both parents to take an active part in making these arrangements.

- Visit the parents daily while the mother is in the hospital; listen to them sympathetically, and give them information as it becomes available.

- Provide reliable preliminary information from the appropriate medical professionals concerning the cause and circumstances of death.

- Be aware that the staff's potential reactions—a sense of guilt, failure, and uncertainty—may cause them to avoid the parents, thereby imped-ing discussion of the deceased neonate with the family. The grief of care-givers, like that of parents and family, should be addressed and supported by appropriate hospital personnel.

- Ensure that the parents have access to support from their families and friends. Anticipate with parents the difficulties they may have in sharing information about the loss with other children, family, and friends. Provide information and suggestions on how they might handle difficult situations or times and information on the availability of support groups.

- Explain the grieving process so that the parents understand the usual reactions. Parents frequently demonstrate reactions of acute grief, such as somatic disturbances, a preoccupation with the newborn's appearance or probable future appearance, guilt, hostility, and loss of ability to func-tion. Mourning should be allowed and encouraged to proceed.

- Encourage the parents to communicate their thoughts and feelings openly with one another. Help them understand and accept the differ-ences in how each of them grieves.

- Provide written materials for the parents to read in the hospital and after discharge. Although there is no substitute for a multidisciplinary group of professionals carefully organized to provide support, written materi-als can provide concrete information about specific procedures, such as autopsy and funeral arrangements, as well as guidance on long-term issues, such as grief, marital stress, explanations for young children, and consideration of another pregnancy. These materials can be designed by the individual hospital or obtained through various associations.

Finally, because families may come from a distance and may not be well acquainted with the attending physicians, it is especially important that spe-cialty and subspecialty referral centers designate a member of the team to be an advocate for the family during the hospital stay and after discharge.

The designated individual also should be responsible for documenting the management and follow-up of each death. Too often families are lost to follow-up when physicians, nurses, and families avoid sharing the sadness of bereavement.

Assessment

When a neonatal death occurs, a special effort should be made to determine the cause of death. This process is helpful for several reasons:

- It helps the family to understand the medical reasons for the death.

- It provides a basis for counseling the family about future pregnancies, including family planning, genetic counseling, and obstetric and neonatal management.

- It provides correct diagnoses for statistical reporting and analysis of perinatal care outcomes.

Requesting an autopsy after the death of a neonate must be handled with sensitivity and gentleness. Selecting the right time to introduce the idea is critical. It can be helpful when it is apparent that a neonate is dying, particularly when the underlying cause is uncertain, to introduce the idea of a postmortem examination to the parents. Its value, as a means of gaining information that will be helpful in answering their questions in the future, often is perceived as a compelling reason for consent. Involvement of the primary care physician and the mother's obstetrician in the request for autopsy consent also may facilitate the family's acceptance of the idea. If there is reluctance for consent for a complete examination of the body, consideration should be given to a limited one, to obtaining specimens of body fluids for microbial culture or other analyses as indicated, and to obtaining postmortem imaging studies if such could further elucidate the cause of death. In all neonatal deaths, every effort should be made to obtain histopathologic examination of the placenta, membranes, and umbilical cord. When an underlying genetic disorder is suspected and premortem testing is incomplete, advance planning for appropriate specimen retrieval with or without a full autopsy should occur. In every instance, the family initially should receive the final results of the autopsy and other examinations in person, if possible, and in a written report in conjunction with a verbal explanation of the findings.

Each unit should have a formal process for periodic review of all neonatal deaths. In addition, when there has been an unexpected clinical deterioration leading to a death, a contemporaneous review of the specific clinical events and decisions with all the involved staff participating can be helpful to resolve interpersonal conflicts, relieve feelings of guilt or failure, and improve both understanding and team interaction. Such sessions usually are best led by the attending neonatologist, although, on occasion, employment of an uninvolved facilitator can be useful.

Postloss Follow-up

The responsibility for ongoing bereavement counseling depends on the specific circumstances of the death and on the family's relationship to the physician. Usually a multidisciplinary approach is best. In general, such counseling should include:

- An initial session 4–6 weeks after the death
- Assessment of the grieving process
- Additional genetic services, if indicated
- Review of preliminary autopsy data
- Answers for parents' specific questions
- Education and reassurance regarding the normal grieving process
- Follow-up visits as indicated by the individual family needs
- Referral of family members to bereavement support groups or bereavement counselors

Persisting Apnea of Prematurity

Clinical Considerations

The persistence of symptomatic apnea of prematurity beyond the postmenstrual age of 36 weeks may occur in VLBW neonates. This often is associated with poor nipple feeding and is prevalent especially in extremely preterm infants. Neurologic immaturity of respiratory control is hypothesized to be a common underlying mechanism. Persistent apnea and feeding incoordination may be the only remaining issues to be resolved before discharge from the hospital. Neonates with extremely low birth weight (less than 1,000 g) and BPD are those most prone to delay in maturation of respiratory control. Although preterm neonates have been found to have a higher incidence of sudden infant death syndrome, no correlation between apnea of prematurity and sudden infant death syndrome has been established.

Use of Home Cardiorespiratory Monitors

The use of home cardiorespiratory monitors for neonates with delayed maturation of respiratory control may facilitate early hospital discharge and alleviate parental fear of recurrent apneic episodes going undetected. Studies of the predictability of cardiopulmonary polygraphic studies (polysomnography) have not found a strong correlation between documented apnea or bradycardia episodes and subsequent, serious alarm events. In the absence of objective measurements that clearly identify neonates at risk for significant cardiorespiratory instability, clinicians have used an empiric approach of requiring an event-free interval of some days before discharge. The precise number of days without apnea or bradycardia episodes that defines full maturation and diminished risk after discharge has not been determined. Therefore, the definition of cardiorespiratory stability and the decision to use home monitoring to facilitate transition to home care remain a matter of individual clinical judgment, taking into consideration the neonate's clinical course, unresolved medical problems (such as tracheostomies; airway abnormalities; neurologic and metabolic disorders that affect respiratory control; or BPD severe enough to require supplemental oxygen, continuous positive airway pressure, or mechanical ventilation after discharge), methylxanthine therapy, and parental anxiety. Programs that manage recovering neonates with home monitors should consider the following recommendations:

- Home monitoring after hospital discharge should be limited to specific clinical indications for a predetermined period.

- Home cardiorespiratory monitoring may be warranted for premature infants who are at high risk of recurrent episodes of apnea, bradycardia, and hypoxemia after hospital discharge. The use of home cardiorespiratory monitoring in this population should be limited to approximately 43 weeks of postmenstrual age or after the cessation of extreme episodes, whichever comes last.

- Home cardiorespiratory monitoring may be warranted for infants who are technology dependent (eg, tracheostomy, continuous positive airway pressure, or mechanical ventilation), have unstable airways, have rare medical conditions affecting regulation of breathing, or have symptomatic BPD.

- Home monitors should be equipped with an event recorder.

- Parents should be counseled that home monitor use does not prevent sudden, unexpected death in all circumstances.

- Use of proven prevention measures (such as supine sleep positioning, safe sleeping environment, elimination of prenatal and postnatal exposure to tobacco smoke) for sudden infant death syndrome should be encouraged.

Hospital Discharge of the High-Risk Neonate

Discharge Planning

The care of each high-risk neonate after discharge must be coordinated carefully to provide ongoing multidisciplinary support of the family. The discharge planning team should include parents, the primary care physician, the neonatologist, neonatal nurses, and a social worker. Other professionals (eg, nutritionist, physical or occupational therapist, developmental pediatrician, and pediatric medical or surgical subspecialist) may be included as needed. The initiation of discharge planning should begin soon after admission and should be escalated when it is evident that recovery is certain, although the exact date of discharge may not be predictable. The goal of the discharge plan is to ensure successful transition to home with care provided by family members. The essential elements are a physiologically stable, thriving neonate; a family that can provide the necessary care without undue strain and with appropriate support services in place within the community; and a primary care physician who provides a medical home and is prepared to assume the responsibility with appropriate backup from specialist physicians and other professionals as needed.

It is prudent that each institution establish guidelines for discharge of high-risk neonates. These should allow for individual physician judgment and flexibility. The determination of a neonate's readiness for care at home after neonatal intensive care is complex. Careful balancing of neonate safety and well-being with family needs and capabilities is required. Consideration of the availability and adequacy of community resources and support services is essential. The final decision for timing of hospital discharge, which is the responsibility of the attending physician, must be tailored for the unique constellation of issues posed by each situation. Timing of the discharge should be determined by patient, family, and medical considerations, not third party payers.

Technology-Dependent Neonates

With the increased survival rates of low birth weight neonates and the development of specialized home care services, many neonates with unresolved medical problems are being discharged from hospitals with continuing requirements for cardiorespiratory monitoring, respiratory support, or alternative feeding methods. This includes neonates with BPD; other chronic pulmonary disorders (eg, pulmonary hypoplasia, pulmonary hypertension, and neuromuscular disorders) or upper airway dysfunction with requirement for oxygen supplementation; persistent apnea of prematurity; feeding disorders;

postoperative short bowel syndrome problems; and arrhythmias. The appropriate management of these neonates requires coordination of care between the center-based subspecialty team, the primary care physician, the home health care agency, and equipment providers.

Special Considerations

Discharge planning for neonates who have been transported back to community hospitals for convalescent care should follow the same principles as planning for neonates being discharged from a subspecialty center unit. Appropriate follow-up during the most critical periods for neonates at risk for adverse sensorineural outcomes (ie, the VLBW neonate for progression of ROP and hearing screening for all high-risk neonates) needs to be coordinated between the two units before transfer of the neonate occurs.

Care coordination of follow-up after discharge between local and center-based resources is essential to improve the quality of medical and surgical care and efficiency and to prevent undue stress. When the need for services from multiple disciplines is identified before discharge, a multidisciplinary center-based clinic may be the least cumbersome option. Alternatively, care coordination service programs offered by primary care physicians, hospitals, nonprofit organizations, and third party payers may prove equally helpful. It is important in choosing home care service providers for surveillance, ancillary treatment services, and parent support to ascertain that the staff is qualified to evaluate and treat neonates. It is essential that previous performance and existing quality control programs be considered when choosing a home health care agency to provide personnel for in-home care of the technology-dependent neonate.

Readiness for Hospital Discharge

The following recommendations can be used to assess readiness for hospital discharge. They are offered as a framework for consideration as each individual neonate and caregiving situation is evaluated and the discharge decision made.

Neonate Readiness for Hospital Discharge

The responsible physician should assess the following factors when determining a neonate's readiness to be discharged from the hospital:

- A sustained pattern of weight gain of sufficient duration
- Adequate maintenance of normal body temperature with the neonate fully clothed in an open bed with normal ambient temperature (24–25°C)

- Competent suckle feeding, breast or bottle, without cardiorespiratory compromise
- Physiologically mature and stable cardiorespiratory function of sufficient duration
- Appropriate immunizations have been administered
- Appropriate metabolic screening has been performed
- Hematologic status has been assessed and indicated therapy instituted
- Nutritional risks have been assessed and indicated therapy and dietary modification instituted
- Sensorineural assessments, hearing and funduscopy, have been completed as indicated
- Review of hospital course has been completed, unresolved medical problems have been identified, and plans for treatment instituted as indicated

Home Care Plan Readiness

An individualized home care plan has been developed with input from all of the appropriate disciplines. Specific and detailed plans for neonates with complex, multiple-system problems, particularly for those requiring technological assistance, are necessary. For neonates at psychosocial risk, arranging for appropriate psychosocial surveillance and family support is essential.

Family and Home Environmental Readiness

When evaluating family and home environmental readiness, assessments of the family caregiving capabilities, resource requirements, and home physical facilities should include the following components:

- Identification of at least two family members, one of whom is an adult, and assessment of their ability, availability, and commitment
- Psychosocial assessment for parenting risks and family support systems
- A home environmental assessment that may include an on-site evaluation
- For home care of the technology-dependent neonate, an on-site assessment of the availability for 24-hour telephone access, electricity, in-house water supply, heating, and necessary modification of home facilities is recommended strongly
- Review of available financial resources and identification of adequate financial support; home care of the technology-dependent neonate cannot be achieved without this

Parents and other family members must have demonstrated the necessary capabilities to provide all components of care including:

- Feeding, whether breastfeeding, bottle-feeding, or an alternative technique, including formula preparation and vitamin and mineral supplementation as required

- Basic neonate care, including bathing; skin, umbilical cord, and genital care; temperature measurement; dressing; and comforting

- Neonate cardiopulmonary resuscitation and emergency intervention as indicated

- Assessment of clinical status, including understanding and detecting the general early signs and symptoms of illness, as well as the signs and symptoms specific to the individual neonate's condition

- Neonate safety precautions, including proper neonate positioning during sleep, use of car seats, and presence of home smoke detectors

- Special safety precautions for airway maintenance, alternative feeding methods, and other mechanical and prosthetic devices, as indicated

- Administration of medications (dosage, timing, and storage) and recognition of signs and symptoms of toxicity

- Equipment operation, maintenance, and problem solving for each mechanical support device as indicated

- Appropriate technique for each required special care procedure (eg, ostomy care, artificial airway, neonate stimulation, and reflux precautions)

Community and Health Care System Readiness

The following follow-up care needs and resources have been identified:

- Primary care physician identified, and responsibility for care of neonate accepted

- Pediatric medical and surgical subspecialty physicians and other providers (eg, nurse specialists, nutritionists, or physical therapists) identified and appropriate follow-up arrangements made

- Neurodevelopmental follow-up arranged

- Home nursing visits arranged as indicated

- Appropriate communication has been exchanged and hospital discharge summaries and home care plans provided to all involved

- Emergency intervention and transportation plans have been developed and emergency service providers identified and notified as indicated.

Follow-up of High-Risk Neonates

General Considerations

The designation of high-risk neonates indicates medical, neurologic, developmental, and psychosocial outcomes. This term encompasses the broad spectrum of outcomes experienced by vulnerable neonatal subgroups that require special care after birth (eg, extreme prematurity, congenital heart disease, multiple congenital anomalies, syndromes, and others). The organization of follow-up care will vary with the neonatal subgroup being followed, potential adverse outcomes frequently associated with individual subgroups, and the purpose for ongoing evaluation. Specific requirements for follow-up of high-risk neonatal subgroups include the following components:

- Primary care—monitoring growth and development, preventive care, and guidance
- Management of unresolved medical problems
- Early detection of abnormality or delayed developmental progress
- Early intervention and habilitation
- Neonate safety
- Parent education
- Evaluation of treatment benefit and complications
- Documentation of outcomes
- Neurosensory follow-up
- Environmental and psychosocial concerns
- Referral to other community resources

Involvement of the Primary Care Physician

The neonate's primary care physician should provide a medical home and share in the responsibility for providing continuity of care with the subspecialty or specialty care center. Frequently, the more detailed developmental and psychologic evaluations and the initial management of complex unresolved medical problems are primarily the responsibility of the care center. As the recovery progresses, medical care is shifted to the primary care physician. With recent changes in the structure of health care financing, the primary care physician may be delegated the responsibility for referral to subspecialty consultation and care. Within any format of shared patient care delivery, it is imperative that all professionals communicate information in a timely manner and share in the planning and execution of the long-term care for neonates with multidisciplinary service needs.

Surveillance and Assessment

The intervals of follow-up visits required by high-risk neonates should be determined by the needs of the individual neonate and family. It may be necessary to examine some of these neonates weekly or semimonthly at first. Neurologic, developmental, behavioral, and sensory status should be assessed more than once during the first year in high-risk neonates to ensure early identification of problems and referral for remedial care. A perinatal follow-up program with an appropriate staff of multidisciplinary personnel is useful in providing these assessments.

Children born preterm have been shown to have a greater incidence of irritability, hyperkinesis, and increased dependency. Prolonged hospitalization inevitably disrupts family relationships, particularly the parent–child relationship. Neonates and parents with such a history or with other factors associated with child abuse require closer follow-up than the family and newborn without risk factors. The interaction of the parents, especially the mother, with the neonate should be evaluated periodically. The neonate or child who fails to thrive may be a victim of neglect, if not outright abuse, and a causal relationship between neglect and failure to thrive always should be suspected. In every state, providers of health care to children are legally obligated to report suspected child abuse. Physicians and other professionals who provide follow-up care to women and neonates should be aware of and look for the physical, social, and psychologic factors associated with child abuse, as follows:

- Preterm birth
- Neonatal illness with long periods of hospitalization, especially in NICUs
- Single parenthood
- Adolescent motherhood
- Closely spaced pregnancies
- Infrequent family visits to hospitalized neonates
- Substance use

Growth parameters of the neonate should be assessed, including continued monitoring of the adequacy of weight gain, linear growth, and head growth.

Growth should be plotted on standardized, birth-weight-appropriate growth curves with the appropriate age correction for gestational age at birth. Review of nutritional intake and calculation of caloric intake are helpful in case management.

Physical examination should assess neuromotor, cardiac, pulmonary, gastrointestinal, and nutritional status, as well as any hernias, anomalies, or orthopedic deformities. Residual scars from invasive procedures during the neonatal course should be monitored for satisfactory healing. On occasion, referral for reconstructive procedures may be necessary.

Medication dosage should be reevaluated, doses increased with weight gain and age, and blood concentrations monitored as indicated. Immunization status should be reviewed, and age-appropriate administration should be maintained. Follow-up audiological and visual assessments should be obtained when indicated.

Neurologic assessment should include an appraisal of muscle tone, development, protective and deep-tendon reflexes, and visual and auditory responses. In addition, developmental progress should be monitored both by parental report of milestone acquisition and by assessment using a standard developmental screening tool, such as the Denver II Developmental Screening Test. When neurologic findings are suspect or developmental delays are suspected, neonates should be referred for more in-depth assessment, either to a neonatal follow-up program or to equivalent facilities or programs capable of providing detailed neurodevelopmental assessments. Neonates at greatest risk for adverse neurodevelopmental outcome (eg, those with a birth weight of 1,500 g or less; posthypoxic ischemic encephalopathy or neonatal seizures; hypoxic cardiorespiratory failure; or complex, multiple congenital anomalies) should have, as a minimum, formal neurodevelopmental testing with a battery of standardized tests at 1 and 2 years corrected age. This will allow for recognition of aberrant development in all domains (gross motor; fine motor and adaptive; visual perceptive and problem solving; hearing, language, and speech; and socialization). Primary care physicians should ensure that such testing is completed, irrespective of the results of developmental screening. Universal standardized testing of these populations will enhance greatly the evaluation of prenatal and neonatal interventions. The results will be useful in forming intervention strategies for those children who are identified as having functional deficits.

Early Intervention

Intervention programs for high-risk neonates have been established under federal legislation to provide early detection of developmental delay and other disabilities. Intervention services may be provided up to 3 years of age for individual neonates with confirmed neurodevelopmental delay or other disability. Programs also offer therapeutic guidelines for families, parent support groups, and respite care programs. Although no definitive data confirm the beneficial effects of infant-stimulation programs, indications are that early intervention may improve social adaptation, limit residual functional disability, and provide valuable family support.

Resources

American Academy of Pediatrics. Committee on Fetus and Newborn. Use of inhaled nitric oxide. Pediatrics 2000;106:344–5.

American Academy of Pediatrics. Pediatric Nutrition Handbook. 5th ed. Elk Grove Village (IL): AAP; 2004.

American Academy of Pediatrics. Redbook: 2006 report of the Committee on Infectious Diseases. 27th ed. Elk Grove Village (IL): AAP; 2006.

American Association of Blood Banks. Standards for blood banks and transfusion services. 24th ed. Bethesda (MD): AABB; 2006.

Antenatal corticosteroid therapy for fetal maturation. ACOG Committee Opinion No. 273. American College of Obstetricians and Gynecologists. Obstet Gynecol 2002;99:871–3.

Apnea, sudden infant death syndrome, and home monitoring. Committee on Fetus and Newborn. American Academy of Pediatrics. Pediatrics 2003;111:914–7.

Barrington KJ, Finer NN. Inhaled nitric oxide for respiratory failure in preterm infants. Cochrane Database of Systematic Reviews 2006, Issue 1. Art. No.: CD000509. DOI: 10.1002/14651858.CD000509.pub2.

The changing concept of sudden infant death syndrome: diagnostic coding shifts, controversies regarding the sleeping environment, and new variables to consider in reducing risk. American Academy of Pediatrics Task Force on Sudden Infant Death Syndrome. Pediatrics 2005;116:1245–55.

Clark RH, Yoder BA, Sell MS Prospective, randomized comparison of high-frequency oscillation and conventional ventilation in candidates for extracorporeal membrane oxygenation. J Pediatr 1994;124:447–54.

Field D, Elbourne D, Truesdale A, Grieve R, Hardy P, Fenton AC, et al. Neonatal ventilation with inhaled nitric oxide versus ventilatory support without inhaled nitric oxide for preterm infants with severe respiratory failure: the INNOVO multicentre randomised controlled trial (ISRCTN 17821339). Pediatrics 2005;115:926–36.

Finer NN, Barrington KJ. Nitric oxide for respiratory failure in infants born at or near term. Cochrane Database of Systematic Reviews 2006, Issue 4. Art. No.: CD000399. DOI: 10.1002/14651858.CD000399.pub2.

Glass P, Brown J. Outcome and follow-up of neonates treated with ECMO. In: Van Meurs K, Lally KP, Peek G, Zwischenberger JB editors, ECMO: extracorporeal cardiopulmonary support in critical care. 3rd ed. Ann Arbor (MI): Extracorporeal Life Support Organization; 2005. p. 319–28.

Hospital discharge of the high-risk neonate—proposed guidelines. American Academy of Pediatrics. Committee on Fetus and Newborn. Pediatrics 1998;102:441–7.

Inhaled nitric oxide in full term and nearly full term infants with hypoxic respiratory failure. The Neonatal Inhaled Nitric Oxide Study Group [published erratum appears in N Engl J Med 1997;337:434]. N Engl J Med 1997;336:597–604.

Inhaled nitric oxide in term and near-term infants: neurodevelopmental follow-up of The Neonatal Inhaled Nitric Oxide Study Group (NINOS). The Neonatal Inhaled Nitric Oxide Study Group. J Pediatr 2000;136:611–7.

Jobe A, Bancalari E. Bronchopulmonary dysplasia. Am J Respir Crit Care Med 2001;163: 1723–9.

Kinsella JP, Truog WE, Walsh WF, Goldberg RN, Bancalari E, Mayock DE, et al. Randomized, multicenter trial of inhaled nitric oxide and high frequency oscillatory ventilation in severe, persistent pulmonary hypertension of the newborn. J Pediatr 1997;131:55–62.

Konduri GG, Solimano A, Sokol GM, Singer J, Ehrenkranz RA, Singhal N, et al. A randomized trial of early versus standard inhaled nitric oxide therapy in term and near-term infants with hypoxic respiratory failure. Neonatal Inhaled Nitric Oxide Study Group. Pediatrics 2004;113:559–64.

Management of hyperbilirubinemia in the newborn infant 35 or more weeks of gestation. American Academy of Pediatrics. Subcommittee on Hyperbilirubinemia [published erratum appears in Pediatrics 2004;114:1138]. Pediatrics 2004;114:297–316.

Mestan KK, Marks JD, Hecox K, Huo D, Schreiber MD. Neurodevelopmental outcomes of premature infants treated with inhaled nitric oxide. N Engl J Med 2005;353:23–32.

National Fetal and Infant Mortality Review Program. Fetal and infant mortality review manual: a guide for communities. Washington, DC: NFIMR; 1998.

Postnatal corticosteroids to treat or prevent chronic lung disease in preterm infants. American Academy of Pediatrics Committee on Fetus and Newborn and Canadian Paediatric Society, Fetus and Newborn Committee. Pediatrics 2002;109:330–8.

Prevention and management of pain and stress in the neonate. American Academy of Pediatrics. Committee on Fetus and Newborn. Committee on Drugs. Section on Anesthesiology. Section on Surgery. Canadian Paediatric Society. Fetus and Newborn Committee. Pediatrics 2000;105:454–61.

Revised indications for the use of palivizumab and respiratory syncytial virus immune globulin intravenous for the prevention of respiratory syncytial virus infections. American Academy of Pediatrics Committee on Infectious Disease and Committee on Fetus and Newborn. Pediatrics 2003;112:1442–6.

Saari TN. Immunization of preterm and low birth weight infants. American Academy of Pediatrics Committee on Infectious Diseases. Pediatrics 2003;112:193–8.

Schreiber MD, Gin-Mestan K, Marks JD, Huo D, Lee G, Srisuparp P. Inhaled nitric oxide in premature infants with the respiratory distress syndrome. N Engl J Med 2003;349:2099–107.

Screening examination of premature infants for retinopathy of prematurity. Section on Ophthalmology, American Academy of Pediatrics; American Academy of Ophthalmology; American Association for Pediatric Ophthalmology and Strabismus. Pediatrics 2006;117:572–6.

Supplemental Therapeutic Oxygen for Prethreshold Retinopathy of Prematurity (STOP-ROP), a randomized, controlled trial. I: primary outcomes. Pediatrics 2000;105:295–310.

Surfactant replacement therapy for respiratory distress syndrome. American Academy of Pediatrics. Committee on Fetus and Newborn. Pediatrics 1999;103:684–5.

Van Meurs KP, Wright LL, Ehrenkranz RA, Lemons JA, Ball MB, Poole WK, et al. Inhaled nitric oxide for premature infants with severe respiratory failure. Preemie Inhaled Nitric Oxide Study. N Engl J Med 2005;353:13–22.

Walsh MC, Wilson-Costello D, Zadell A, Newman N, Fanaroff A. Safety, reliability, and validity of a physiologic definition of bronchopulmonary dysplasia. J Perinatol 2003;23:451–6.

chapter 9

Perinatal Infections

Certain infections that occur in the antepartum or intrapartum period may have a significant effect on the fetus and newborn. Appropriate antepartum and intrapartum care of the mother and subsequent care of the newborn soon after birth can reduce the frequency of or ameliorate many serious problems and can minimize the risk of subsequent transmission in the nursery. In addition, some infections, such as varicella, may have more severe outcomes in pregnant women than in other adults. Communication and cooperation among all perinatal care personnel are essential to obtain the best results. The infections discussed in this chapter have been selected on the basis of new and evolving information that affects management.

Viral Infections

Cytomegalovirus

Approximately 1% of all newborns are infected with cytomegalovirus (CMV) in utero and excrete CMV after birth. Although the majority of congenital CMV infections are asymptomatic, approximately 5% of infected neonates are symptomatic at birth.

Transmission occurs via transplacental passage of the virus, contact of the fetus with infectious secretions at the time of birth, ingestion of infected breast milk, or transfusion of blood from seropositive donors. Transmission via transfusion has been virtually eliminated by the use of blood from CMV-negative donors, the use of frozen deglycerolized red blood cells, and filtration to remove white blood cells. Newborns of women who are seronegative and who receive milk from human milk banks are at risk of developing CMV disease. This can be minimized by limiting donor milk to CMV-negative donors or by ensuring appropriate pasteurization. Both primary CMV infection and reactivation of a latent infection can occur in the mother and result in congenital CMV infection. Symptomatic CMV infection in a congenitally infected infant is more likely to occur in an infant born to a mother with primary CMV infection. Although ganciclovir and CMV hyperimmune globulin have been used to treat some congenitally infected infants, these are not recommended routinely because of insufficient efficacy data.

Because there is neither a vaccine for prevention of infection nor effective therapy for acute maternal infection, routine serologic screening of women or neonates is of little benefit. Testing generally is limited to pregnant women in whom CMV exposure is suspected. Routine serologic testing of personnel in newborn nurseries is not recommended.

Although the presence of immunoglobulin M (IgM) CMV antibody is highly suggestive of primary maternal infection, false-positive and false-negative test results occur. Positive IgM test results should be confirmed by viral culture or viral DNA quantitation assays on maternal blood. Establishing that seroconversion has occurred is the most accurate method for documenting primary maternal infection. Isolation of the virus or detection of CMV genome by polymerase chain reaction (PCR) from amniotic fluid is the most sensitive test for detecting fetal infection. Fetal blood obtained by cordocentesis may be tested for CMV-specific IgM, but this test is less sensitive than culture or PCR of amniotic fluid. For an infected fetus, ultrasound abnormalities or cordocentesis to detect elevated hepatic enzymes, anemia, and thrombocytopenia may be prognostic of severe infection.

Unequivocal evidence of CMV infection in the neonate who has not been diagnosed in utero requires recovery of the virus within 3 weeks of birth. Later in infancy, differentiation between intrauterine and perinatal infection is difficult to determine. For breastfeeding guidelines, see Chapter 7.

Enteroviruses

Wild-type poliovirus infection has been eliminated from the Western Hemisphere. Other enteroviral infections (coxsackieviruses, echoviruses, and polioviruses) are common and are spread by fecal–oral and respiratory routes. Infection in the third trimester can trigger labor. Signs of maternal infection often are mild and nonspecific.

Maternal enterovirus infections rarely cross the placenta and cause disease in the fetus. Vertical transmission of enteroviruses may occur at birth following exposure to virus-containing maternal blood or cervical secretions. Symptoms in an enterovirus-infected neonate generally begin between 3 days and 7 days after birth. Neonates who acquire infection without maternal antibody are at risk for severe disease. Manifestations can include pneumonia, exanthems, aseptic meningitis, encephalitis, paralysis, hepatitis, conjunctivitis, myocarditis, and pericarditis.

Diagnosis is confirmed by recovery of the virus from swabs of the throat or the anus and samples of stool, spinal fluid, or blood. Polymerase chain reaction testing of spinal fluid is more sensitive than a culture.

No specific therapy is commercially available. Hospitalized newborns should be managed with contact as well as standard precautions.

Hepatitis A Virus

Hepatitis A virus (HAV) has little effect on pregnancy and rarely is transmitted perinatally. The risk of transplacental transmission to the fetus is negligible, and there is no evidence that the virus is a teratogen. The most common mode of transmission is by the fecal–oral route. Diagnosis is confirmed by the demonstration of anti-HAV IgM antibodies.

Vaccines for hepatitis A are highly effective and approved for use. Although vaccine safety in pregnancy has not been established, the risk to the developing fetus is minimal because the vaccine contains inactivated, purified viral proteins. Pregnant women with the following risk factors are candidates for vaccination: intravenous drug users, travelers to endemic regions, those living in communities with a high prevalence of hepatitis A, women who work with HAV-infected primates, women with either chronic liver disease or a liver transplant, and women with clotting disorders who receive clotting factor concentrate. Immunoglobulin is effective for both preexposure and postexposure prophylaxis and can be used during pregnancy.

Nosocomial outbreaks have been reported in neonatal intensive care units, but these are infrequent. Prevention of the spread of the virus is based on contact precautions, with emphasis on careful handwashing. With appropriate hygienic precautions, breastfeeding by a mother with HAV infection is permissible. Although immunoglobulin has been administered to newborns in specific situations, the efficacy of this practice has not been established.

Hepatitis B Virus

Perinatal transmission of Hepatitis B virus (HBV) infection generally occurs from exposure to maternal blood during labor and delivery. Perinatal infection occurs in 70–90% of infants born to mothers who are both hepatitis B surface antigen (HBsAg) and hepatitis B e antigen (HBeAg) positive if appropriate and timely treatment is not instituted. Transplacental passage of HBV is rare. More than 90% of infants who are infected perinatally will develop chronic HBV infection.

Maternal Infection

Because historical information about risk factors identifies less than one half of chronic carriers, serologic testing for HBsAg is recommended for all pregnant women as part of routine prenatal care. A copy of the original laboratory report should be transferred to the patient's medical record at the delivery hospital. Women who have not been screened during prenatal care, those who are at high risk for infection (eg, intravenous drug users and women with recurrent sexually transmitted diseases [STDs]), and those with clinical hepatitis should be tested at admission in labor or for complications of pregnancy.

Pregnant women with chronic HBV should be informed about transmission risks and ways to prevent newborn infection. Newborns of HBsAg positive women should receive timely postexposure prophylaxis and follow-up.

Women who are HBsAg negative but who have risk factors for HBV infection should be offered vaccination during pregnancy. The adult dose of HBV vaccine is 10–20 μg (1 mL) injected into the deltoid muscle; intramuscular injection in the buttocks may not be as effective and is not recommended. A series of three doses is required; the second and third doses are given 1 and 6 months after the first dose. A two-dose schedule, administered at time zero and again 4–6 months later, is available for adolescents aged 11–15 years using the adult dose of a hepatitis B recombinant vaccine.

Hepatitis B vaccine is recommended for household contacts and sexual partners of chronic carriers of HBV (ie, those who are positive for HBsAg) unless immunity has previously been demonstrated. Nonimmunized sexual partners of persons with acute HBV infection should receive a single dose of hepatitis B immune globulin (HBIG) and should begin an HBV vaccine series if their test results are serologically negative.

Newborn Immunization

Universal HBV immunization is recommended for all neonates. Delivery hospitals should develop policies and procedures that ensure administration of a birth dose of the vaccine as part of the routine care of all medically stable infants weighing at least 2,000 g at birth, unless there is a physician's order to defer immunization and the serologic status of the mother is in the infant's medical record. Three intramuscular doses are required to provide effective protection (Table 9–1). For neonates born to women who are known to be HBsAg

Table 9–1. Hepatitis B Immunoprophylaxis Schedule by Infant Birth Weight*

Maternal Status	Infant ≥2,000 g	Infant <2,000 g
HBsAg positive	Hepatitis B vaccine plus HBIG (within 12 h of birth)	Hepatitis B vaccine plus HBIG (within 12 h of birth)
	Continue vaccine series beginning at 1–2 mo of age according to recommended schedule for infants born to HBsAg-positive mothers.	Continue vaccine series beginning at 1–2 mo of age according to recommended schedule for infants born to HBsAg-positive mothers.
		Immunize with 4 vaccine doses; do not count birth dose as part of vaccine series.
	Check anti-HBs and HBsAg after completion of vaccine series.†	Check anti-HBs and HBsAg after completion of vaccine series.†
	HBsAg-negative infants with anti-HBs levels ≥10 mIU/mL are protected and need no further medical management.	HBsAg-negative infants with anti-HBs levels ≥10 mIU/mL are protected and need no further medical management.
	HBsAg-negative infants with anti-HBs levels <10 mIU/mL should be reimmunized with three doses at 2-mo intervals and retested.	HBsAg-negative infants with anti-HBs levels <10 mIU/mL should be reimmunized with three doses at 2-mo intervals and retested.
	Infants who are HBsAg positive should receive appropriate follow-up, including medical evaluation for chronic liver disease.	Infants who are HBsAg positive should receive appropriate follow-up, including medical evaluation for chronic liver disease.
HBsAg status unknown	Test mother for HBsAg immediately after admission for delivery.	Test mother for HBsAg immediately after admission for delivery.
	Hepatitis B vaccine (by 12 h)	Hepatitis B vaccine (by 12 h)
	Administer HBIG (within 7 days) if mother tests HBsAg positive.	Administer HBIG if mother tests HBsAg positive or if mother's HBsAg result is not available within 12 h of birth.
	Continue vaccine series beginning at 1–2 mo of age according to recommended schedule based on mother's HBsAg result.	Continue vaccine series beginning at 1–2 mo of age according to recommended schedule based on mother's HBsAg result.
		Immunize with four vaccine doses; do not count birth dose as part of vaccine series.

(continued)

Table 9–1. Hepatitis B Immunoprophylaxis Schedule by Infant Birth Weight* *(continued)*

Maternal Status	Infant ≥2,000 g	Infant <2,000 g
HBsAg negative	Hepatitis B vaccine at birth†	Hepatitis B vaccine dose 1–30 days of chronologic age if medically stable, or at hospital discharge if before 30 days of chronologic age
	Continue vaccine series beginning at 1–2 mo of age.	Continue vaccine series, beginning at 1–2 mo of age.
	Follow-up anti-HBs and HBsAg testing is not needed.	Follow-up anti-HBs and HBsAg testing is not needed.

Abbreviations: anti-HBs, antibody for hepatitis B surface antigen; HBsAg, hepatitis B surface antigen; HBIG; hepatitis B immune globulin

*Extremes of gestational age and birth weight no longer are a consideration for timing of hepatitis B vaccine doses.

†Test at 9–18 months of age, generally at the next well-child visit after completion of the primary series. Use testing method that allows determination of a protective concentration of anti-HBs (≥10 mIU/mL).

‡The first dose may be delayed until after hospital discharge for an infant who weighs ≥2,000 g and whose mother is HBsAg negative but only if a physician's order to withhold the birth dose and a copy of the mother's original HBsAg-negative laboratory report are documented in the infant's medical record.

American Academy of Pediatrics. Red Book: 2006 Report of the Committee on Infectious Diseases. 27th ed. Elk Grove Village (IL): AAP; 2006.

negative, the first dose of vaccine should be administered during the newborn period or by 2 months of age, although administration of the first dose before hospital discharge is preferred; the second dose 1–2 months later; and the third dose by 6–18 months of age. Alternatively, vaccines may be administered at 2-month intervals, concurrent with other childhood vaccines, at 2, 4, and 6 months of age. Because of suboptimal immune response in some preterm neonates, the current American Academy of Pediatrics (AAP) recommendation is to delay the start of hepatitis B immunization in low-risk preterm neonates who weigh less than 2,000 g at birth until they reach the chronologic age of 1 month, regardless of initial birth weight or gestational age. The appropriate dose (Table 9–2) can be given into the anterolateral thigh muscle of neonates.

Both term and preterm neonates born to women known to be HBsAg positive should receive both hepatitis B vaccine and one dose of HBIG within 12 hours of birth. Prophylaxis for exposed newborns can prevent perinatal HBV infection in approximately 95% of neonates when the three-dose immunization series is completed and HBIG is given within 12 hours after birth. The initial

Table 9–2. Recommended Dosages of Hepatitis B Vaccines

| | Vaccine* | |
Patients	Recombivax HB[†] Dose, μg (mL)	Engerix-B[‡] Dose, μg (mL)
Infants of HBsAg-negative mothers and children and adolescents younger than 20 years of age	5 (0.5)	10 (0.5)
Infants of HBsAg-positive mothers (HBIG [0.5 mL] also is recommended)	5 (0.5)	10 (0.5)
Adults 20 years of age or older	10 (1)	20 (1)
Adults undergoing dialysis and other immunosuppressed adults	40 (1)[§]	40 (2)[‖]

Abbreviations: HBsAg, hepatitis B surface antigen; HBIG, hepatitis B immune globulin

*Both vaccines are administered in a three- or four-dose schedule; four doses may be administered if a birth dose is given and a combination vaccine is used to complete the series. Only single-antigen hepatitis B vaccine can be used for the birth dose. Single-antigen or combination vaccine containing hepatitis B vaccine may be used to complete the series.

[†]Available from Merck & Co Inc. A two-dose schedule, administered at 0 months and then 4–6 months later, is available for adolescents 11–15 years of age using the adult formulation of Recombivax HB (10 μg). A combination of hepatitis B (Recombivax, 5 μg) and *Haemophilus influenzae* type b (PRP-OMP) vaccine is recommended for use at 2, 4, and 12–15 months of age (Comvax). This vaccine cannot be administered at birth, before 6 weeks of age, or after 71 months of age.

[‡]Available from GlaxoSmithKline Biologicals. The U.S. Food and Drug Administration has licensed this vaccine for use in an optional four-dose schedule at 0, 1, 2, and 12 months of age. A combination of hepatitis B (Engerix-B, 20 μg) and hepatitis A (Havrix, 720 ELU) vaccine (Twinrix) is licensed for use in people 18 years of age and older in a three-dose schedule administered at 0, 1, and 6 or more months later. A combination of diphtheria and tetanus toxoids and acellular pertussis (DTaP), inactivated poliovirus (IPV), and hepatitis B (Engerix-B 10 μg) is recommended for use at 2, 4, and 6 months of age (Pediarix). This vaccine cannot be administered at birth, before 6 weeks of age, or at ≥7 years of age or older.

[§]Special formulation for dialysis patients

[‖]Two 1-mL doses given in one site in a four-dose schedule at 0, 1, 2, and 6 months of age.

American Academy of Pediatrics. Red Book: 2006 Report of the Committee on Infectious Diseases. 27th ed. Elk Grove Village (IL): AAP; 2006.

dose of HBV vaccine can be administered concurrently with HBIG but should be given at a different site. No special care of the neonate is indicated other than removal of maternal blood to avoid the virus contaminating the skin. The second dose of vaccine should be administered at 1–2 months of chronologic age, regardless of the neonate's gestational age or birth weight. The third dose should be given at 6 months of age. For preterm neonates who weigh less than 2,000 g at birth, the initial vaccine dose is given at birth but is not counted in the required three-dose schedule; therefore, these infants receive four doses: 1) at birth, 2) when their weight reaches 2,000 g or at 2 months of age, 3) 1–2 months later, and 4) at 6 months of age.

At 1–3 months after completion of the immunization schedule for newborns of HBsAg positive women, testing is indicated to ensure response or to identify neonates who have become chronically infected. Breastfeeding of newborns by HBsAg positive women poses no additional risk for the transmission of HBV.

Newborns of women whose HBsAg status is unknown should receive HBV vaccine within 12 hours of birth in a dose appropriate for neonates born to HBsAg positive women. The woman's blood should be obtained for testing on admission. If the woman subsequently is found to be HBsAg positive, the neonate should receive HBIG as soon as possible (within 7 days of birth) and should receive the second and third doses of vaccine as recommended for neonates of HBsAg positive women. Both maternal HBsAg test results and the infant's immunization should be documented in the infant's medical record.

Hepatitis C Virus

Hepatitis C virus (HCV) is the principal cause of non-A, non-B hepatitis. The prevalence of HCV infection in the general population of the United States is estimated to be 1.8% but varies in different populations in proportion to risk factors. The primary known route of transmission is parenteral exposure to blood and blood products from individuals who are infected with HCV. Sexual transmission among monogamous couples is uncommon, as is transmission among family contacts. In most cases, no source can be identified.

Infection with HCV is diagnosed serologically by the presence of HCV antibodies or by detection of HCV RNA. Positive enzyme immunoassay antibody test results should be confirmed by additional testing with a more specific assay, such as recombinant immunoblot assay, particularly when individuals at low risk are being tested. As many as 70% of patients with HCV infection develop chronic liver disease, and cirrhosis ultimately develops in 20–25% of these patients. Therefore, liver enzyme and function tests should be performed in patients who test positive for the antibodies.

Routine serologic testing during pregnancy for HCV infection is not recommended. Testing should be reserved for those whose histories suggest an increased risk of infection, such as blood transfusions before 1990, intravenous drug use, or occupational or recreational percutaneous or mucosal surface blood exposure.

Women who are infected with HCV should be advised that transmission of HCV by breastfeeding is possible but has not been documented. According to current guidelines of the U.S. Public Health Service, maternal HCV infection is not a contraindication to breastfeeding. The decision to do so should be based on an informed discussion between the woman and her health care provider.

The risk of maternal–fetal (vertical) transmission of HCV ranges from 2% to 12%. The risk of transmission, which correlates with maternal HCV RNA levels, appears to be increased for women infected with human immunodeficiency virus (HIV). Immune globulin manufactured in the United States does not contain antibodies to HCV and has no role in postexposure prophylaxis. Immunoglobulin G and antiviral agents are not recommended for postexposure prophylaxis of neonates born to women with HCV. The natural history of perinatally acquired hepatitis C infection is the subject of ongoing studies. Children born to HCV positive women should be tested for HCV infection. However, antibody testing should be deferred until at least 18 months of age, when passively transferred maternal HCV antibodies have decreased below detectable levels. If earlier diagnosis of HCV infection is desired, the presence of two or more PCR-RNA measurements after 1 month of age will identify infants infected through vertical transmission.

Herpes Simplex Virus

Treatment and Counseling During Pregnancy

Genital herpes may be caused by herpes simplex virus (HSV) type 2 (HSV-2) (in approximately 80–85% of cases) or by HSV type 1 (HSV-1). The prevalence of infection with HSV-2 has increased 30% in the past few decades, so that overall seroprevalence for HSV-2 is approximately 30% in females in the United States. Most adults with unequivocal serologic evidence of HSV-2 infection have not been diagnosed clinically, indicating that most primary infections are asymptomatic. Nevertheless, all women and their partners should be asked about a history of genital HSV infection. A genital herpes infection is classified as primary when it occurs in a woman with no evidence of prior HSV infection (ie, seronegative to both HSV-1 and HSV-2), nonprimary first episode when it occurs in a woman with a history of heterologous infection (eg, first HSV-2 infection in a woman with prior HSV-1 infection), and recurrent when it occurs in a woman with clinical or serologic evidence of prior genital herpes (of the same serotype).

Women who have primary genital HSV infection in late pregnancy (whether symptomatic or asymptomatic) and who give birth vaginally have a high risk (30–60%) of transmitting the infection to their neonates. Similarly, nonprimary first-episode HSV infection occurring late in pregnancy also has a high risk of vertical transmission to the neonate. The risk of transmission during a vaginal delivery is much lower with recurrent disease (less than 2–5%). Distinguishing between primary, nonprimary first episode, and recurrent HSV infection in women on the basis of clinical findings is not accurate. A combination of positive viral detection and negative serologic test results or evidence of seroconversion is necessary to diagnose HSV infection. To correctly classify the type of HSV infection, the HSV type and type-specific maternal antibodies are needed. Valid type-specific assays for HSV antibodies must be based upon HSV-specific glycoprotein G. The U. S. Food and Drug Administration has approved several such assays (refer to www.fda.gov for a current list). Currently, most newborns infected with HSV are delivered to women who have asymptomatic or unrecognized infections.

In a meta-analysis of acyclovir use among pregnant women near term, it was concluded that acyclovir treatment orally reduces the risk of clinical HSV recurrence at delivery, cesarean delivery for recurrent genital herpes, and the risk of HSV shedding at delivery. Acyclovir is indicated intravenously to treat severe maternal genital HSV infection (eg, disseminated infection that includes encephalitis, pneumonitis, and hepatitis). Although long-term safety and efficacy of administering acyclovir systemically have not been established, no evidence has been found of any adverse effects to the fetus.

Couples should be educated about the natural history of genital HSV infection and should be advised that, if either partner is infected, they should abstain from sexual contact while lesions or prodromes are present. To minimize the risk of sexual transmission, use of condoms is recommended for HSV-infected individuals when asymptomatic. However, protection provided by condoms is incomplete (estimated to be approximately 50% effective). Susceptible pregnant women should avoid sexual contact during the last 6–8 weeks of gestation if their partners have active genital HSV infections. In addition, oral–genital sexual contact should be avoided in the latter weeks of pregnancy to avoid acquisition of HSV-1 in susceptible individuals.

Obstetric Management

Women with a history of genital HSV infection should be questioned about recent symptoms and should undergo careful examination of the perineum before delivery. If no lesions are observed, neonates may be delivered vaginally. A detailed examination of the cervix is not required because recurrent infections rarely cause isolated cervical lesions.

Cesarean delivery is indicated for all women with active genital HSV lesions or with a typical herpetic prodrome at the time of delivery. In patients with active HSV infection and ruptured membranes at or near term, a cesarean delivery should be performed as soon as the necessary personnel and equipment can be readied. In the rare case of active HSV infection and premature rupture of membranes remote from term, the risks of potential intrauterine infection versus those of prematurity must be individualized. Local neonatal infection may result from the use of fetal scalp electrode monitoring in patients with a history of herpes, even when maternal lesions are not present. However, if there are indications for fetal scalp monitoring, it may be appropriate in a woman who has a history of recurrent HSV and no active lesions.

Contact precautions, use of gown or gloves, and covering of all lesions (in addition to standard precautions), should be used for women with clinically evident or serologically confirmed primary genital HSV infection or nongenital HSV infection in the labor, delivery, and postpartum care areas. For recurrent mucocutaneous lesions, standard precautions are sufficient. Infected family members and others in contact with the infant also should use contact precautions. Health care personnel and the woman herself should use gloves for direct contact with the infected area or with contaminated dressings, and meticulous handwashing is essential. The labor and delivery rooms require only routine, careful cleaning and disinfection before using the rooms for other patients.

Management of Infection in Exposed Newborns

Most neonatal infections are caused by HSV-2, although infection with HSV-1 also can occur. Most neonates who develop HSV infection acquire the infection during passage through the infected maternal lower genital tract or by ascending infection to the fetus, sometimes even though membranes apparently are intact. Less common sources of neonatal infection include postnatal transmission from the parents, hospital personnel, or other close contact, most often from a nongenital infection (eg, mouth, hands, or around the breasts); and postnatal transmission in the nursery from another infected neonate, probably from the hands of personnel attending the neonates.

Neonates born vaginally through infected birth canals with active lesions (or viral shedding) require close observation because, as noted, the transmission rate of HSV is as high as 50% for neonates of women with active primary or nonprimary first episode genital herpes at or near term. Specimens for herpes cultures should be obtained at 24–48 hours after birth from urine, stool or rectum, mouth, eye, and nasopharynx. Some experts recommend empiric treatment with acyclovir (20 mg/kg intravenously every 8 hours) for infants born vaginally to a mother with symptomatic primary herpes infection, pending results of cultures and clinical course, although no data exist to support the efficacy of this approach. Other experts recommend awaiting positive culture results or clinical manifestations of infection before starting acyclovir therapy. Parents and providers should be educated about the signs and symptoms of neonatal HSV infection, which include vesicular lesions of the skin, respiratory distress, seizures, or signs of sepsis. A neonate with any of these manifestations should be evaluated immediately for possible HSV infection. Specimens for HSV culture should be obtained from skin lesions, conjunctiva, nasopharynx, mouth, rectum, urine, blood buffy coat, and cerebrospinal fluid. Cerebrospinal fluid also should be studied by PCR. Acyclovir therapy should be initiated if the cultures or PCR test results are positive or if HSV infection is otherwise strongly suspected.

Neonates born vaginally (or by cesarean delivery if membranes have ruptured) to women with active HSV lesions should be physically separated from other neonates and managed with contact precautions if they remain in the nursery during the incubation period; an isolation room is not essential. Alternatively, the neonate may stay with the woman in a private room after the woman has been instructed on proper preventive care to reduce postpartum transmission.

The risk of HSV infection is extremely low in neonates born vaginally to asymptomatic women with a history of recurrent genital herpes and in those born to symptomatic women by cesarean delivery before rupture of membranes. Special isolation precautions are not needed for these neonates. Neonates born by cesarean delivery to women with herpetic lesions with intact membranes should be cultured for HSV as recommended previously for neonates exposed by vaginal delivery, and they should be observed. The length of in-hospital observation is empirical and is based on risk factors, local resources, and access to adequate follow-up. Parents should be instructed to report early signs of infection. Antiviral therapy should be initiated if culture results from the neonate are positive or if HSV infection is strongly suspected for other reasons.

Early Diagnosis and Management of Disease in Neonates

Cultures obtained from the eye, mouth, or rectum of neonates born to women who are known or who are strongly suspected of being infected with HSV can assist in management decisions. A positive culture obtained 24–48 hours or more after delivery suggests HSV infection and is an indication for immediate institution of antiviral therapy, even in the absence of symptoms. Direct fluorescent antibody staining of scrapings of skin, eye, or mucus membrane lesions can provide a rapid diagnosis. Polymerase chain reaction is a sensitive method for detecting HSV DNA; it is useful for examining spinal fluid samples.

The neonate should be physically segregated and managed with contact precautions for the duration of the illness; an isolation room is desirable. Personnel having contact with skin lesions or potentially infectious secretions should use gowns and gloves. Antiviral therapy is effective in the treatment of neonatal HSV infection and should be initiated promptly if HSV is suspected. Neonates with HSV disease should be managed in a facility that provides level III subspecialty care and consultation. Of treated neonates, 5–10% will develop recurrences requiring retreatment in the first month of life. The value of long-term suppressive or intermittent acyclovir therapy for neonates with disease of the skin, eyes, or mouth is being evaluated.

Although HSV infection is more likely to occur at a site of skin trauma, no data indicate that the circumcision of male neonates who may have been exposed to HSV at birth should be postponed. It may be prudent, however, to delay circumcision for approximately 1 month in neonates at the highest risk of disease (eg, neonates delivered vaginally to women with active genital lesions).

Contact of Neonates With Infected Mothers

A woman with HSV infection should be taught about her infection and about hygienic measures to prevent postpartum transmission of the infection to her neonate. Before touching her newborn, the woman should wash her hands carefully and use a clean barrier to ensure that the neonate does not come into contact with lesions or potentially infectious material. If the woman has genital HSV infection, her newborn may room with her after she has been instructed in protective measures. Breastfeeding is permissible if the woman has no vesicular herpetic lesions in the breast area and all active cutaneous lesions are covered.

A woman with herpes labialis (cold sore) or stomatitis should not kiss or nuzzle her newborn until the lesions have cleared. Careful handwashing is important. She should wear a disposable surgical mask when she touches her newborn until the lesions have crusted and dried. Herpetic lesions on other skin sites should be covered. Direct contact of a newborn with other family members or friends who have active HSV infection should be avoided.

Prevention

In a meta-analysis, significant benefits with use of acyclovir beginning at 36 weeks of gestation were shown in women with a history of HSV infection. Some authorities have recommended routine serological screening for HSV infection among all pregnant women. However, the cost-effectiveness of this approach has not been established and currently neither the American College of Obstetricians and Gynecologists (ACOG) or the Centers for Disease Control and Prevention (CDC) recommend this seroscreening.

Human Immunodeficiency Virus

Etiology

Acquired immunodeficiency syndrome (AIDS) is caused by HIV type 1 (HIV-1) and, less commonly, HIV type 2 (HIV-2), a related virus. Human immunodeficiency virus type 2 is extremely uncommon in the United States but is more common in West Africa and South America.

Epidemiology

Human immunodeficiency virus has been isolated from blood (including lymphocytes, macrophages, and plasma), cerebrospinal fluid, pleural fluid, human milk, semen, cervical secretions, saliva, urine, and tears. However, only blood, semen, cervical secretions, and human milk have been implicated epidemiologically in the transmission of infection.

Well-documented modes of HIV transmission in the United States are sexual contact (both heterosexual and homosexual), skin penetration by contaminated needles or other sharp instruments, transfusion of contaminated blood products, and mother-to-fetus transmission before or near the time of birth and from breastfeeding. Infection with HIV continues to spread among women of childbearing age and is occurring increasingly in rural, as well as urban, areas. The predominant risk behavior is unprotected sexual intercourse. Before effective perinatal HIV interventions, the incidence of perinatal HIV infection mirrored increases in STDs in women.

Before the introduction of antiretroviral therapy in pregnancy, the risk of infection for a neonate born to an HIV seropositive mother was approximately

25% (range, 13–39%). All pregnant women who are infected with HIV should be offered antiretroviral drug regimens, which will likely decrease the HIV viral load to undetectable levels, thereby decreasing the maternal-to-child transmission rate to less than 2%.

The exact timing of transmission from an infected mother to her neonate is uncertain. Evidence suggests that in the absence of breastfeeding, 30% of transmission occurs before birth and 70% occurs around the time of delivery. Most prenatal transmission probably occurs close to delivery. Breastfeeding has been documented to be a mechanism of maternal-to-child transmission.

Management

Clear medical benefits are derived from pregnant women knowing their HIV serostatus. Demonstrated benefits include early diagnosis and treatment to delay active disease in women and significant reduction in perinatal transmission through early treatment.

Pregnant women universally should be tested for HIV infection with patient notification as part of the routine battery of prenatal blood tests unless they decline the test (ie, opt-out approach) as permitted by local and state regulations. Refusal of testing should be documented. In some states, it is necessary to obtain the woman's written authorization before disclosing her HIV status to health care providers who are not members of her health care team. Women at high risk for HIV infection should be retested during the third trimester, ideally before 36 weeks of gestation. Repeat testing in areas with a high HIV prevalence also should be considered.

If a woman's HIV status is unknown during labor and delivery, she should be given a rapid HIV test unless she declines. A rapid HIV test is an HIV screening test with results available within hours. A negative rapid HIV test result is definitive. A positive HIV test result is not definitive and must be confirmed with a supplemental test, such as a Western blot test or immunofluorescence assay; however, antiretroviral prophylaxis should be initiated (with consent) without waiting for the results of the confirmatory test to reduce further the risk of possible transmission to the infant. According to CDC guidelines, if a mother's HIV status is still unknown after delivery, the newborn should be tested using the rapid HIV test as soon as possible so that appropriate antiretroviral prophylaxis can be given, if necessary. Neonatal antiretroviral prophylaxis is most beneficial when begun no more than 12 hours after birth.

The individual providing health care for the newborn should be informed of the mother's HIV serostatus to ensure appropriate care and testing. In some states, physicians are required to obtain the mother's written authorization before disclosing her HIV status to other health care providers who are not members of the woman's health care team, such as her neonate's health care provider. Health care providers who are not experienced in the care of pregnant, HIV-infected women may want to refer to providers who are knowledgeable in this area for specialty care.

Prenatal and intrapartum administration of zidovudine (ZDV) to pregnant women who are infected with HIV has been shown to reduce the rate of HIV transmission to newborns by 68% (from 25.5% to 8.3%). No significant short-term side effects were observed from ZDV use other than mild, self-limited anemia in the neonates. Neonates have been monitored for several years and no untoward effects of ZDV have been observed. Thus, it is recommended that ZDV chemoprophylaxis be included in the antiretroviral combination regimen.

Substantial advances have been made in the understanding of the pathogenesis of HIV-1 infection and in the treatment and monitoring of HIV-1 disease. Accordingly, these have resulted in changes in standard antiretroviral therapy for HIV-1 infected adults. More aggressive combination drug regimens that maximally suppress viral replication are now recommended. Pregnancy should not preclude the use of optimal therapy. Offering antiretroviral therapy to HIV-1 infected women during pregnancy, either to treat HIV-1 infection or to reduce perinatal transmission or both, should be accompanied by discussion of the known and unknown short-term and long-term benefits and risks of such therapy for infected women and their neonates. Standard antiretroviral therapy should be discussed with and offered to pregnant women infected with HIV-1. Additionally, to prevent perinatal transmission, ZDV chemoprophylaxis should be incorporated into the antiretroviral regimen.

As noted, a substantial proportion of HIV cases occur as a result of exposure to the virus during labor and delivery. Consistent results indicating a significant relationship between route of delivery and vertical transmission of HIV have been published. This body of evidence indicates that cesarean delivery performed before the onset of labor and before the rupture of membranes (scheduled cesarean delivery) reduces the likelihood of vertical transmission of HIV (to approximately 2%) compared with either unscheduled cesarean delivery or vaginal delivery. This is true whether or not the patient is receiving ZDV. There are not enough data to address the question of how long after the onset of labor or rupture of the membranes the benefit is lost. It is clear that the rate of maternal morbidity is higher with cesarean delivery than with vaginal delivery. There is a gradient of benefit for the neonate to be gained from cesarean delivery, with the greatest benefit to be gained from scheduled procedures in women at highest risk for vertical transmission with relatively high plasma viral loads. Women infected with HIV whose viral loads are greater than 1,000 copies/mL should be offered scheduled cesarean delivery at 38 weeks of gestation without an amniocentesis for lung maturity to further reduce the risk of vertical transmission of HIV beyond that achievable with ZDV prophylaxis alone. There are insufficient data to demonstrate a benefit of cesarean delivery performed after the onset of labor or rupture of membranes.

Women with very low plasma viral loads (less than 1,000 copies/mL) were found to have a low risk of vertical transmission (less than 2%), even without routine use of scheduled cesarean delivery. There are not enough data to demonstrate a benefit of scheduled cesarean delivery for women with plasma viral loads of less than 1,000 copies/mL. The decision regarding route of delivery in these circumstances must be individualized. The patient's autonomy in making the decision regarding route of delivery must be respected.

Current recommendations for adults are that plasma viral load determinations should be done at baseline and every 3 months or following changes in therapy. Additionally, CD4+ T-lymphocyte counts should be followed during pregnancy. Because of the rapid advances in this area, refer to the CDC (www.cdc.gov) and the HIV/AIDS Treatment Information Service (www.hivatis.org) for treatment recommendations.

Human immunodeficiency virus RNA has been detected in both the cellular and cell-free fractions of human breast milk, and breastfeeding has been implicated in the transmission of HIV infection. Women infected with HIV should be counseled not to breastfeed their babies, and they should not donate to milk banks.

Serial testing for HIV should be performed on neonates born to seropositive mothers. Infants born to HIV infected women should be tested by HIV DNA PCR during the first 48 hours of life. Because of possible contamination with maternal blood, umbilical cord blood should not be used for this determination. A second test should be performed at 1–2 months of age. A third test is recommended at 2–4 months of age. Any time an infant has test results that are positive for HIV, testing should be repeated on a second blood sample as soon as possible to confirm the diagnosis. An infant is considered infected if two separate samples are positive.

Early identification of infected neonates is essential for adequate medical management. Antiretroviral therapy is indicated for most children who are infected with HIV. Whenever possible, enrollment into clinical trials should be encouraged. Therapeutic strategies are changing rapidly, so primary care physicians are encouraged to participate in the care of children infected with HIV in consultation with specialists. Several web sites provide information regarding diagnosis and therapy (www.hivatis.org, www.atis.org).

If a neonate is found to be HIV seropositive when the maternal serostatus is unknown, the health care provider for the child should ensure that this information and its significance are relayed to the mother. With her consent, and possibly written authorization as required by state law, it also should be communicated to her health care provider.

Because HIV (as well as other viral agents, such as HBV) may be present in blood, vaginal secretions, amniotic fluid, and other fluids, standard precautions (previously known as universal precautions) should be followed strictly during all vaginal and cesarean deliveries. Gloves should be used when handling the placenta or the neonate until blood and amniotic fluid have been removed from the neonate's skin.

After delivery, HIV infected women can receive care in the postpartum care unit, with the use of standard precautions. Obstetric providers may need to refer women who are infected with HIV to another health care provider for continuing medical care after pregnancy. Few neonates with HIV infection show clinical evidence of infection in the first weeks after delivery. To minimize risk to health care personnel, routine standard precautions should be used. Prompt and careful removal of blood from the neonate's skin is important. There is no need for other special precautions or for isolation of the neonate from an HIV-infected mother; rooming-in is acceptable. Gloves should be worn for contact with blood or blood-containing fluids and for procedures that entail exposure to blood. Gloving for all infant diaper changes is now considered part of standard precautions for hospital personnel.

Human Papillomavirus

Infections by human papillomaviruses (HPV) are common. Infection with certain types of HPVs (such as HPV 16, 18, 31, 33, and 35) cause genital warts as well as cervical and anogenital carcinomas. Approximately 90% of cervical HPV infections are transient. Persistent infection is more likely with oncogenic types. Cervical or vaginal HPV infections usually are asymptomatic. Studies using DNA diagnostic techniques detect the virus in up to 40% of sexually active young women. Pap tests are less useful for the diagnosis of subclinical cervical infection. Most genital HPV infections are sexually transmitted.

Genital HPV infections may be exacerbated during pregnancy. Papillary lesions (condylomata acuminata) may proliferate on the vulva and in the vagina, and lesions may become increasingly friable during pregnancy. Cryotherapy, laser therapy, and trichloroacetic acid may be used safely to treat genital HPV infection in pregnancy. Podophyllin, 5-fluorouracil, and interferon generally are not recommended during pregnancy because of concern that they may be toxic to the fetus. Fetal death has been reported following large topical doses of podophyllin to the mother. Conclusive data is not available on the use of imiquimod topical immune response modulators. While the HPV vaccine has not been shown to have a harmful effect on pregnancy, it is not recommended that pregnant women be vaccinated. If a woman discovers she is pregnant during the vaccine schedule, she should delay finishing the series until after she gives birth. Women who are breastfeeding can receive the vaccine.

The risk that a neonate born to a mother who has a genital HPV infection will develop subsequent respiratory papillomatosis is very small. These lesions are thought to result from aspiration of infectious secretions during passage through the birth canal. The latent period may be several years before HPV lesions become clinically significant in children. Because the risk of respiratory papillomatosis is low, cesarean delivery is not recommended solely to protect the neonate from HPV infection. In women with extensive condylomata, however, cesarean delivery rarely may be necessary because of poor vaginal or vulvar distensibility and the related increased likelihood of extensive vulvovaginal lacerations. Neonates born to mothers with HPV infection do not need to be managed with special precautions in the nursery.

Human Parvovirus

Parvovirus B19 is the cause of erythema infectiosum. Most public attention has focused on parvovirus B19 infection (fifth disease) because of its ability to cause fetal death. More than one half of pregnant women are immune to parvovirus B19. In most cases of B19 infection during pregnancy, the fetus is not affected. Fetal death or miscarriage occurs in less than 10% of infected pregnancies. Parvovirus B19 can infect fetal erythroid precursors and cause anemia, which can lead to nonimmune hydrops and death. Most reported maternal infections that have resulted in fetal death occur between the 10th and 20th week of pregnancy, and fetal death and spontaneous abortion usually have occurred 4–6 weeks after infection. Third-trimester maternal infections causing hydrops fetalis and death have been described. Congenital anomalies caused by parvovirus have been reported in small series and rare case reports. However, the determination that parvovirus is a teratogen remains unproven at this time.

Because of widespread asymptomatic parvovirus infection in both adults and children, all women are at some risk of exposure, particularly those with school-aged children. Pregnant women who learn that they have been in contact with children who were either in the incubation period of erythema infectiosum or in an aplastic crisis should be counseled about the potential risk to the fetus and should be offered serologic testing for parvovirus IgG and IgM. Fetal ultrasound examination will detect hydrops, but the frequency with which serial measurements should be performed is not known. In some cases, maternal serum alpha-fetoprotein levels may be elevated by the presence of fetal hydrops. A hydropic fetus can be treated by intrauterine transfusion when severe anemia has been documented by cordocentesis, although spontaneous resolution may occur.

In view of the high prevalence of parvovirus B19, the low risk of ill effects to the fetus, and the fact that avoidance of child care or teaching can reduce but not eliminate the risk of infection, pregnant women should not be excluded routinely from workplaces where B19 is present. Pregnant health care workers should be aware that otherwise healthy patients with erythema infectiosum are contagious during the week before the onset of rash and are not contagious after the onset of rash. In contrast, patients who are immunocompromised or who have a hemoglobinopathy remain contagious from before the onset of symptoms through the time of the rash. Routine infection control practices such as handwashing, standard precautions, and droplet precautions reduce transmission.

Respiratory Syncytial Virus

Respiratory syncytial virus (RSV) is a common cause of respiratory infection in infancy and the most common cause of hospitalization for lower respiratory illness in newborns. Preterm newborns and those with chronic lung disease of prematurity or congenital heart disease are at increased risk for severe RSV disease. Prophylaxis to prevent RSV in newborns at increased risk for severe disease, particularly those with chronic lung disease receiving medical management on a long-term basis, is available using RSV intravenous immune globulin or an intramuscular monoclonal antibody, palivizumab. Prophylaxis with palivizumab will decrease the risk of severe RSV disease and hospitalization by approximately 50%. Palivizumab is administered as 5 monthly intramuscular injections (15 mg/kg per dose) during RRV season, with the first dose typically administered in November. The current AAP recommendations are as follows:

1. Respiratory syncytial virus prophylaxis should be considered for newborns and children younger than 24 months of age with chronic lung disease of prematurity who require ongoing medical management within 6 months before the RSV season, including supplemental oxygen, diuretics, corticosteroids, or bronchodilator therapy. Those with more severe chronic lung disease may benefit from prophylaxis for two RSV seasons.

2. Newborns without chronic lung disease of prematurity born at less than 32 weeks of gestation also may benefit from RSV prophylaxis. Newborns born at 28 weeks of gestation or younger may benefit from prophylaxis up to 12 months of age, whereas those born at 29–32 weeks of gestation may benefit from prophylaxis up to 6 months of age.

3. Given the large number of patients born between 32 weeks and 35 weeks of gestation and the cost of the drug, palivizumab use in this population should be reserved for newborns with at least two additional risk factors (see "Passive Immunization" in Chapter 8 for a list of risk factors).

4. Children who are 24 months of age or younger with hemodynamically significant cyanotic or acyanotic congenital heart disease will benefit from 5 monthly intramuscular injections of palivizumab (15 mg/kg per dose).

5. Respiratory syncytial virus may be transmitted in the hospital setting and may cause serious disease in higher-risk newborns. The major means to prevent RSV disease is strict observance of infection control practices, including identifying and cohorting RSV-infected patients.

A critical aspect of RSV prevention is parent education about the importance of avoiding exposure to and transmission of the virus. Preventive measures include limiting, when feasible, exposure to contagious settings, such as child-care centers. The importance of handwashing should be emphasized in all settings, including the home, particularly during periods when contact with high risk children who have a respiratory infection can occur.

Rubella

Prevention and Management During Pregnancy

Between 2001 and 2004, there were fewer than 25 cases of rubella each year and a total of 4 cases of congenital rubella syndrome reported in the United

States. At the present time, most cases of rubella and congenital rubella syndrome in this country occur in persons who were born outside the United States.

Surveillance for susceptibility to rubella infection is essential in prenatal care. Each patient should be screened serologically at the first prenatal visit unless she is known to be immune by a previous serologic test. Seropositive women do not need further testing, regardless of their subsequent history of exposure. If a seronegative pregnant woman is exposed to rubella or develops symptoms that suggest infection, she should be retested for antibody titers to establish whether infection has occurred. Specimens should be obtained as soon as possible after exposure, again 2 weeks later, and, if necessary, 4 weeks after exposure. Serum specimens from both acute and convalescent periods should be tested on the same day in the same laboratory; a negative test result in all samples indicates infection has not occurred, whereas a positive test result in the second sample, but not the first (seroconversion), indicates recent infection. Detection of rubella-specific IgM antibodies usually indicates recent infection, but false–positive results occur. Isolation of the virus from throat swabs establishes a diagnosis of acute rubella.

If rubella is diagnosed in a pregnant woman, the patient should be advised of the risks of fetal infection; the choice of pregnancy termination should be discussed. Structural malformation may be caused by infection during embryogenesis, and while fetal infection may occur throughout pregnancy, defects are rare when infection occurs after the 20th week of gestation. The overall risk of defects during the third trimester is probably no greater than that associated with uncomplicated pregnancies. If a woman chooses not to terminate her pregnancy, administration of immune globulin as soon as possible after exposure may be considered. However, no data demonstrate that immune globulin prevents fetal infection. The absence of clinical signs in a woman who has received immune globulin does not guarantee that infection has been prevented.

The rubella vaccine is a live attenuated virus and is highly effective with few side effects in women of reproductive age who are susceptible to rubella. Women found to be susceptible during pregnancy should be offered vaccination postpartum and before discharge from the hospital. Breastfeeding is not a contradiction to receiving the rubella vaccine.

Rubella vaccination is not recommended during pregnancy. Following immunization, women should be advised to avoid conception for 1 month. However, a woman who conceives within 1 month of rubella vaccination or who is inadvertently vaccinated in early pregnancy should be counseled that the teratogenic risk to the fetus is theoretic. Although asymptomatic infection can occur, no case of congenital rubella syndrome has arisen from a woman given the current rubella vaccine (human diploid vaccine RA 27/3) during pregnancy. Therefore, receipt of the rubella vaccine during pregnancy is not an indication for termination of pregnancy. However, all suspected cases of congenital rubella syndrome, whether caused by wild-type virus or vaccine virus infection, should be reported to local and state health departments. A pregnant household member is not a contraindication to vaccination of a child.

Neonatal Management

Neonates who show signs of congenital rubella infection or who were born to women known to have had rubella during pregnancy, including neonates with few or no obvious clinical manifestations at birth, should be managed with contact isolation, preferably in a private room. Care of the neonate should be provided only by personnel known to be immune to rubella. Efforts should be made to obtain viral cultures from the neonate and to document the infection. Neonates with congenital rubella should be considered contagious until 1 year of age unless nasopharyngeal and urine cultures (after 3 months of age) are repeatedly negative for the rubella virus.

Varicella–Zoster Virus

Women with varicella–zoster virus (VZV) infection (chickenpox) during pregnancy are no more likely to develop varicella pneumonia than are other adults, but varicella pneumonia is more severe during pregnancy. Therefore, pregnant women with VZV infection should be observed closely for pulmonary symptoms. Although no evidence indicates that maternal administration of VZV immune globulin (VZIG) after exposure reduces the rare occurrence of congenital varicella syndrome, postexposure prophylaxis with VZIG may prevent or ameliorate the illness in nonimmune pregnant women, as it does in other adults. However, VZIG is no longer available, but VariZIG has become available under an investigational new drug application submitted to the U.S. Food and Drug Administration. It is a purified human immune globulin preparation made from plasma containing high levels of antivaricella antibodies and is administered intramuscularly. Most women (70–90%) with a negative or uncertain history of varicella are immune. A positive history of varicella is highly predictive of serologic immunity (greater than 95%), and it is unnecessary to perform serologic testing in such women. A pregnant woman who has been exposed to VZV (through intimate or household contact) and who has no history of prior infection should be tested for immunity. If she is not immune, administration of VariZIG should be considered within 96 hours of exposure. If chickenpox is diagnosed during pregnancy, antiviral therapy with acyclovir is another consideration.

Fetal infection after maternal varicella during the first half of pregnancy occasionally results in varicella embryopathy, which may include limb atrophy and scarring of the skin of the extremities as well as central nervous system and ocular manifestations. The incidence of congenital varicella syndrome among infants born to mothers with varicella is approximately 2% when infection occurs before 20 weeks of gestation.

Varicella infection can be fatal for an infant if the mother develops varicella within 5 days before to 2 days after delivery. All infants with this type of exposure should receive VariZIG.

Extremely low birth weight neonates (born at less than 28 weeks of gestation or less than 1,000 g) who are exposed to VZV postnatally are at increased risk of severe varicella, regardless of maternal history, because of the poor transfer of antibodies across the placenta early in pregnancy. Hospitalized, preterm neonates born at 28 weeks of gestation or later who are exposed postnatally to chickenpox and whose mothers have no history of chickenpox also should receive VariZIG.

Hospitalized women with VZV infection must be kept under airborne and contact precautions. Hospitalized neonates born to women with active VZV infection should be isolated until 21 days of age (if IVIG is not given) or until 28 days of age (if IVIG is given). Hospitalized neonates who are exposed postnatally should be isolated from 8 days to 21 days after onset of the rash in the index case. Neonates with VZV infection should be isolated in a private room, and airborne and contact precautions should be maintained for the duration of the illness. Neonates with congenital VZV infection acquired earlier in gestation do not require special precautions or isolation unless vesicular lesions are present. Mothers with zoster should not be in the nursery, and both mother and baby should be isolated.

Live-attenuated VZV vaccine, licensed in 1995, routinely is recommended for susceptible children, beginning at 12 months of age, and adolescents. Susceptible adults, particularly those in high-risk categories, also should be offered immunization. For adolescents and adults, the primary vaccination series consists of two doses, administered subcutaneously, 4–8 weeks apart.

Pregnant women should not be vaccinated, and vaccinated women should be advised to avoid pregnancy for 1 month after each dose because of concern about possible fetal effects. Women who do not have varicella immunity should receive the first dose of VZV vaccine in the postpartum period before hospital or birth center discharge. Surveillance data to date on fetal outcomes after inadvertent vaccine exposures, however, have not found any cases of fetal varicella syndrome. A pregnant household member is not a contraindication to vaccination of a child.

West Nile Virus

West Nile virus is associated with fever, rash, arthritis, myalgias, weakness, lymphadenopathy, and meningoencephalitis. This virus is carried by mosquitoes and birds and can be transmitted through blood transfusion or organ transplant. To date, outcomes of 72 pregnancies have been published, and there has been only one fetus with proven intrauterine infection and subsequent bilateral chorioretinitis. It is unclear whether pregnant women are more susceptible to West Nile virus and whether the disease is more severe. Transmission through breast milk also is possible, but most infants infected by this route are asymptomatic or have mild symptoms. Women with symptoms should not be discouraged from breastfeeding. Pregnant and breastfeeding mothers should be encouraged to wear protective clothing, minimize their outdoor exposure at dawn and dusk when mosquitoes are most active, and use insect repellant containing N,N-diethyl-3-methylbenzamide (DEET) as a preventative measure.

Bacterial Infections

Group B Streptococci

The proportion of pregnant women colonized with group B streptococci (GBS) ranges from approximately 10–30%, but colonization may be transient. Although antepartum rectal or genital colonization usually is asymptomatic, GBS may account for significant peripartum infection (eg, endometritis, amnionitis, and urinary tract infections).

Before adoption of national prevention guidelines, an estimated 7,600 episodes of GBS sepsis occurred annually in newborns (a rate of 1.8 per 1,000 live births) in the United States, with more than 300 deaths annually among neonates younger than 90 days. Invasive GBS disease in the newborn primarily is characterized by sepsis, pneumonia, and meningitis. Vertical transmission of GBS during labor or delivery may result in invasive infection in the newborn during the first week of life. Known as early-onset GBS infection, this now constitutes approximately 50% of GBS disease in newborns. Late-onset GBS disease in the newborn also may occur as a result of vertical transmission or of nosocomial or community-acquired infection. In recent years, there have been reports of invasive GBS disease occurring beyond 3 months of age (late, late-onset disease), usually in very low birth weight preterm neonates.

The risk of early-onset disease is increased by preterm birth (birth at less than 37 weeks of gestation), a prolonged interval (18 hours or more) between rupture of amniotic membranes and delivery, and intraamniotic infection (maternal temperature at or above 38°C [100.4°F]). Other factors associated with a higher risk of early-onset disease include GBS bacteriuria during pregnancy and previous delivery of a neonate with GBS disease. However, up to 40% of cases of early-onset disease occur in neonates with no risk factors.

In 1996, the CDC, ACOG, and AAP recommended the first national GBS prevention guidelines. In 2002, these were revised to recommend the culture-based prevention strategy only (Fig. 9-1). The culture-based approach requires obtaining a single swab from the lower vagina (introitus) and perianal area, placing the swab in transport media, and culturing in selective broth media. Use of prenatal cultures remote from term to identify women who are colonized with GBS at delivery may not be accurate, and the CDC, ACOG, and AAP recommend obtaining rectovaginal cultures at 35–37 weeks of gestation. All women with positive culture of GBS should be treated with intrapartum antibiotic prophylaxis. If the culture status is unknown when a patient presents with labor or premature rupture of membranes (PROM), then prophylaxis should be given if any of the following conditions exist:

- Women with preterm labor (less than 37 weeks of gestation)
- Preterm PROM (less than 37 weeks of gestation)
- Rupture of membranes 18 hours or longer
- Maternal fever during labor (at or above 38°C [100.4°F]).

Women with GBS bacteriuria during their current pregnancy or women who previously gave birth to an infant with early-onset GBS disease are candidates for intrapartum antibiotic prophylaxis. When culture results are not available, intrapartum prophylaxis should be offered only on the basis of the presence of intrapartum risk factors for early-onset GBS disease.

Other key points provided in the 2002 guidelines include changes in recommended antibiotics for patients who cannot take penicillin. Recommended antibiotics for intrapartum prophylaxis are given in the table showing recommended regimens (Table 9–3). As described previously, emerging resistance to erythromycin and clindamycin have shaped these recommendations. A key change for obstetricians is the need to get a detailed history from colonized

Vaginal and rectal GBS screening cultures at 35–37 weeks of gestation for ALL pregnant women (unless patient had GBS bacteriuria during the current pregnancy or a previous infant with invasive GBS disease)

Intrapartum prophylaxis indicated

- Previous infant with invasive GBS disease
- GBS bacteriuria during current pregnancy
- Positive GBS screening culture during current pregnancy (unless a planned cesarean delivery, in the absence of labor or amniotic membrane rupture, is performed)
- Unknown GBS status (culture not done, incomplete, or results unknown) and any of the following:
  –Delivery at less than 37 weeks of gestation*
  –Amniotic membrane rupture at 18 hours or greater
  –Intrapartum temperature at100.4°F or greater (38.0°C or greater)[†]

Intrapartum prophylaxis not indicated

- Previous pregnancy with a positive GBS screening culture (unless a culture was also positive during the current pregnancy)
- Planned cesarean delivery performed in the absence of labor or membrane rupture (regardless of maternal GBS culture status)
- Negative vaginal and rectal GBS screening culture result in late gestation during the current pregnancy, regardless of intrapartum risk factors

Fig. 9–1. Indications for intrapartum antibiotic prophylaxis to prevent perinatal group B streptococcal disease under a universal prenatal screening strategy based on combined vaginal and rectal cultures collected at 35–37 weeks of gestation from all pregnant women. Abbreviation: GBS, group B streptococci. *If onset of labor or rupture of amniotic membranes occurs earlier than 37 weeks of gestation and there is a significant risk for preterm delivery (as assessed by the clinician), follow the suggested algorithm for GBS prophylaxis as indicated by the Centers for Disease Control and Prevention. [†]If amnionitis is suspected, broad-spectrum antibiotic therapy that includes an agent known to be active against GBS should replace GBS prophylaxis. (Schrag S, Gorwitz R, Fultz-Butts K, Schuchat A. Prevention of perinatal group B streptococcal disease. Revised guidelines from CDC. MMWR Recomm Rep 2002;51(RR-11):1–22.

women who report penicillin allergy to determine whether they are at high risk for anaphylaxis. Among penicillin-allergic patients, women at high risk for anaphylaxis are defined as those who have experienced immediate hypersensitivity to penicillin, including a history of penicillin-related anaphylaxis, and those with other conditions, such as asthma or treatment with β-adrenergic blocking agents, that would make anaphylaxis more dangerous or difficult to treat. Women undergoing a planned cesarean delivery in the absence of labor or membrane rupture do not require GBS prophylaxis even if their rectovaginal culture is positive. This recommendation is based on evidence that the risk of neonatal early-onset disease was sufficiently low in this circumstance and that the potential risks associated with intrapartum antibiotics outweighed the benefits. The guidelines also propose an algorithm for GBS testing and prophylaxis for women with preterm labor or PROM. (Please refer to the CDC web

Table 9–3. Recommended Regimens for Intrapartum Antimicrobial Prophylaxis for Perinatal Group B Streptococcal Disease Prevention*

Regimens	Antimicrobial
Recommended	Penicillin G, 5 million units IV initial dose, then 2.5 million units IV every 4 hours until delivery
Alternative	Ampicillin, 2 g IV initial dose, then 1 g IV every 4 hours until delivery
If penicillin allergic[†]	
• Patients not at high risk for anaphylaxis	Cefazolin, 2 g IV initial dose, then 1 g IV every 8 hours until delivery
• Patients at high risk for anaphylaxis[‡]	
—GBS susceptible to clindamycin and erythromycin[§]	Clindamycin, 900 mg IV every 8 hours until delivery
	or
	Erythromycin, 500 mg IV every 6 hours until delivery
—GBS resistant to clindamycin or erythromycin or susceptibility unknown	Vancomycin,[‖] 1 g IV every 12 hours until delivery

Abbreviations: GBS, group B streptococci; IV, intravenously

*Broader-spectrum agents, including an agent active against GBS, may be necessary for treatment of chorioamnionitis.

[†]History of penicillin allergy should be assessed to determine whether a high risk for anaphylaxis is present. Penicillin-allergic patients at high risk for anaphylaxis are those who have experienced immediate hypersensitivity to penicillin including a history of penicillin-related anaphylaxis; other high-risk patients are those with asthma or other diseases that would make anaphylaxis more dangerous or difficult to treat, such as persons being treated with beta-adrenergic–blocking agents.

[‡]If laboratory facilities are adequate, clindamycin and erythromycin susceptibility testing should be performed on prenatal GBS isolates from penicillin-allergic women at high risk for anaphylaxis.

[§]Resistance to erythromycin often but not always is associated with clindamycin resistance. If a strain is resistant to erythromycin but appears susceptible to clindamycin, it may still have inducible resistance to clindamycin.

[‖]Cefazolin is preferred over vancomycin for women with a history of penicillin allergy other than immediate hypersensitivity reactions, and pharmacologic data suggest it achieves effective intraamniotic concentrations. Vancomycin should be reserved for penicillin-allergic women at high risk for anaphylaxis.

Schrag S, Gorwitz R, Fultz-Butts K, Schuchat A. Prevention of perinatal group B streptococcal disease. Revised guidelines from CDC. MMWR Recomm Rep 2002;51(RR-11):1–22.

site, www.cdc.gov/groupbstrep, for the latest recommendations on strategies to help prevent early onset GBS infection in newborns.)

Listeriosis

The major cause of epidemic and sporadic listeriosis infection is food-borne transmission. Incriminated foods include unpasteurized milk, cheese, and other dairy products; undercooked poultry; and prepared meats, such as hot dogs, deli meats, and pâté. Asymptomatic fecal and vaginal carriage can result in sporadic neonatal disease, which can cause early-onset neonatal infections from transplacental or ascending intrauterine infection or from exposure during delivery. Maternal infection has been associated with preterm delivery and other obstetric complications. Late-onset neonatal infection results from acquisition of the organism during passage through the birth canal or possibly from environmental sources. To prevent pregnancy-related listeria infections, pregnant women are advised not to eat hot dogs or luncheon meats unless they are steaming hot and to avoid unpasteurized soft cheeses.

Listeria monocytogenes can be recovered on blood agar media from cultures of usually sterile body sites (eg, blood, cerebrospinal fluid). Special techniques may be needed to recover *L monocytogenes* from sites with mixed flora (eg, vagina, rectum). Because of morphologic similarity to diphtheroids and streptococci, a culture isolate of *L monocytogenes* mistakenly can be considered a contaminant or saprophyte.

Prompt diagnosis and antibiotic treatment of maternal listeriosis may prevent fetal or perinatal infection. *Listeria monocytogenes* is highly sensitive to ampicillin, but there may be a synergistic benefit from ampicillin plus gentamicin. Signs of listeriosis in the newborn vary widely and often are nonspecific. The clinical picture may be similar to that of GBS infection with early- and late-onset syndromes. Therapy with intravenous ampicillin and an aminoglycoside is recommended for neonatal infections. (Resources from the CDC include an information sheet at: www.fsis.usda.gov/fact_sheets/Listeriosis_and_pregnancy_ what_is_your_risk/index.asp.)

Pertussis

Pertussis, commonly known as whooping cough, is a respiratory disease commonly causing paroxysms of cough. Complications in adults include pneumonia, sleep disturbance, rib fracture, and incontinence. In the first six months of life, symptoms are more severe, and infant complications include pneumonia, seizures, encephalopathy, and death.

Infants younger than 6 months of age frequently require hospitalization for supportive care and to manage complications. Antimicrobial agents given during the catarrhal stage may lessen the severity of the disease. Azithromycin is the drug of choice for treatment of pertussis in infants younger than 1 month of age. Although there is a risk of developing infantile hypertrophic pyloric stenosis associated with erythromycin use, that risk is outweighed by the risk of severe pertussis and life-threatening complications from the disease in infants younger than 1 month of age. All infants younger than 1 month of age should be monitored for infantile hypertrophic pyloric stenosis after treatment with any macrolide.

In addition to standard precautions, droplet precautions are recommended for 5 days after initiating effective therapy, or if appropriate antimicrobial therapy is not given in older individuals, until 3 weeks after the onset of paroxysms.

Universal immunization is recommended to prevent transmission of pertussis. The diphtheria and tetanus toxoids and acellular pertussis (DTaP) vaccine is given to children at 2, 4, 6, and 12–18 months of age and 4–6 years of age. The adolescent and adult tetanus and reduced diphtheria toxoids and acellular pertussis (Tdap) vaccines are approved as a booster dose for those who were vaccinated for pertussis in childhood. The Tdap vaccine is offered routinely to adolescents and adults between the ages of 11–64 years, including immediate postpartum women who have not previously received Tdap. The Tdap vaccine may be offered if a tetanus and diphtheria vaccine was given at age 5 years or older.

The Tdap vaccine is not contraindicated in pregnancy. It can be given to pregnant women in place of a tetanus and diphtheria vaccine and should be given if there is an outbreak of pertussis. Because there is little data on the safety of Tdap in pregnancy, health care providers are encouraged to report Tdap vaccination during pregnancy, regardless of trimester (sanofi pasteur [800] 822-2463).

Gonorrhea

Management in Pregnant Women

Gonorrhea occurs most commonly in individuals aged 15–29 years, and the highest reported incidence occurs in young men aged 20–24 years. In females, the highest rates are in adolescents aged 15–19 years. Risk factors include lower socioeconomic status, single status, early onset of sexual activity, multiple sexual partners, and substance use.

Pregnant women with risk factors for or symptoms of gonorrhea should be tested for *Neisseria gonorrhoeae* at an early prenatal visit. A repeat test should be obtained in the third trimester for women at increased risk for gonorrhea and other STDs. Polymerase chain reaction tests for detecting *N gonorrhoeae* have generally replaced cultures.

Because of the prevalence of penicillin-resistant *N gonorrhoeae*, an extended spectrum (third-generation) cephalosporin (ceftriaxone 125 mg intramuscularly or cefixime 400 mg orally) is recommended for treatment. Tetracyclines and fluoroquinolones are contraindicated in pregnancy. Women who cannot tolerate a cephalosporin should be administered a single 2-g dose of spectinomycin intramuscularly. Because concurrent infection with *Chlamydia trachomatis* is common, patients with gonococcal infections also should be treated for chlamydial infection (unless it has been ruled out) and should be evaluated for coinfection with syphilis, HIV, and other STDs. Either erythromycin or amoxicillin is recommended for the treatment of presumptive or diagnosed *C trachomatis* infection during pregnancy. Azithromycin in a single dose (1 g) is a recommended regimen for the treatment of *C trachomatis* infection in nonpregnant individuals, but because well-controlled, adequate studies in pregnant women have not been performed, it is an alternate regimen for pregnant women. A test-of-cure is not recommended routinely in persons with uncomplicated gonorrhea, provided that symptoms resolve. All cases of gonorrhea must be reported to public health officials.

Neonatal Clinical Manifestations

Infection in the newborn usually involves the eyes. Antimicrobial prophylaxis soon after delivery is recommended for all neonates. If a woman with ruptured membranes has known gonorrheal infection, the newborn must be treated immediately. Applications of a 1 cm ribbon of sterile ophthalmic ointment containing tetracycline (1%) or erythromycin (0.5%) in each lower conjunctival sac are considered equally effective in preventing gonococcal ophthalmia. An occasional case of gonococcal ophthalmia or disseminated gonococcal infection can occur in neonates born to women with gonococcal disease. Neonates born to women with active gonorrhea should receive a single dose of ceftriaxone, 125 mg, intravenously or intramuscularly; for low birth weight neonates, the dose is 25–50 mg/kg of body weight. Cefotaxime in a single dose (100 mg/kg given intravenously or intramuscularly) is an alternative. Single-dose systemic antibiotic therapy is effective treatment for gonococcal ophthalmia and prophylaxis for disseminated disease.

In addition to ophthalmia, neonatal disease may include scalp abscess, vaginitis, and systemic disease with bacteremia, arthritis, meningitis, or endocarditis. Neonates with clinical gonococcal disease should be hospitalized, and cultures of blood, cerebrospinal fluid, eye discharge, or other sites of infection should be obtained. For neonates with positive cultures (ie, disseminated infection), the recommended antimicrobial therapy is ceftriaxone (25–50 mg/kg per day, intravenously or intramuscularly, not to exceed 125 mg given in a single daily dose) or cefotaxime (50–100 mg/kg per day, divided into two doses given every 12 hours). Cefotaxime is preferred for neonates with hyperbilirubinemia. The duration of antibiotic treatment depends on the site of infection; a single dose is adequate for conjunctivitis, whereas 7 days is recommended for disseminated infection; 10–14 days is recommended for meningitis. Infected neonates should be managed with standard precautions.

Chlamydia

Chlamydia trachomatis has been detected in the cervix of 2–13% of pregnant women and generally is found in 5% or more of women in all populations. Prevalence is highest (about 37%) in sexually active adolescent females. Unrecognized infection is common. Important risk factors for chlamydial infection include unmarried status, recent change in sexual partner, multiple concurrent partners, age younger than 25 years, inner-city residence, history or presence of other STDs, and little or no prenatal care. Pregnant women should be screened for chlamydia infection during the first prenatal care visit, and women at increased risk (women aged 25 years or younger or women who have a new, or more than one, sexual partner) may be tested again in the third trimester.

Most infected women have few symptoms, but *C trachomatis* may cause urethritis and mucopurulent (nongonococcal) cervicitis. Chlamydial infection also is associated with postpartum endometritis and infertility. Infection may be transmitted from the genital tract of infected women to their neonates during birth; approximately 50% of neonates born to infected women become colonized with *C trachomatis*. Purulent conjunctivitis develops a few days to several weeks after delivery in 25–50% of neonates who acquire *C trachomatis* infection, and neonatal pneumonia occurs in 5–20%. The diagnosis of *C trachomatis* infection is based on a cell culture, direct fluorescent antibody staining, enzyme immunoassay, DNA probe, or PCR. Nucleic acid amplification tests are the most sensitive diagnostic measure.

Treatment should be administered to women who have known *C trachomatis* infection (ie, with mucopurulent cervicitis) or whose neonates are infected. Women whose sexual partners have nongonococcal urethritis or epididymitis are presumed to be infected and also should be treated. Simultaneous treatment of partners is an important component of the therapeutic regimen. Doxycycline and ofloxacin are contraindicated in pregnancy. Limited data on azithromycin in pregnant women suggests that it is safe and efficacious. Recommended regimens for treating *C trachomatis* infection in pregnant women include 1 g azithromycin in a single dose or amoxicillin 500 mg, orally, three times daily for 7 days. Alternative regimens in pregnant women include erythromycin base, 250 mg orally, four times daily for 14 days; erythromycin ethylsuccinate, 800 mg orally, four times daily for 7 days; erythromycin ethylsuccinate, 400 mg orally, four times daily for 14 days; or erythromycin base, 500 mg orally, 4 times daily for 14 days. Note that erythromycin estolate is contraindicated during pregnancy because of drug-related hepatotoxicity. Repeat testing, preferably by culture, should be done 3 weeks after completion of treatment regimens to confirm successful treatment.

Neonates born to women known to have untreated chlamydial infection should be evaluated and monitored for development of disease. Chlamydial infections in the neonate generally are mild and responsive to antimicrobial therapy. Prophylactic cesarean delivery is not warranted. Routine instillation of topical erythromycin or tetracycline into the conjunctival sac of the neonate shortly after birth has not been proved to prevent neonatal conjunctivitis or other infections caused by *C trachomatis*. Neonates with chlamydial conjunctivitis or chlamydial pneumonia should be treated with oral erythromycin for 14 days. If hospitalized, patients should be managed with standard precautions. Recent evidence shows an association between infantile hypertrophic pyloric stenosis and orally administered erythromycin in infants younger than 6 weeks of age.

Tuberculosis

Screening

Once considered rare in the United States, the incidence of tuberculosis has increased considerably in women of childbearing age. In endemic areas, the incidence of tuberculosis may approach 0.1% of pregnant women. All pregnant women who are at high risk for tuberculosis should be screened with a Mantoux test with purified protein derivative (PPD) when they begin receiving prenatal care. High-risk factors for tuberculosis include:

- Human immunodeficiency virus infection
- Close contact with individuals known or suspected to have tuberculosis
- Medical risk factors known to increase risk of disease (eg, lymphoma, diabetes mellitus, chronic renal failure, immunosuppression)
- Birth in a country with a high prevalence of tuberculosis

- Medically underserved status
- Low socioeconomic status
- Alcohol addiction
- Intravenous drug use
- Residence in a long-term care facility (eg, correctional institutions, mental institutions, nursing homes and facilities)
- Health care professionals working in facilities where the risk of exposure to *Mycobacterium tuberculosis* is increased

Definitions and Diagnosis

Latent tuberculosis infection is defined by a positive tuberculin skin test in an individual with no physical findings of disease and either a normal chest X-ray or only granuloma or calcification in the lung parenchyma or regional lymph nodes or both. The purpose of treating latent tuberculosis infection is to prevent progression to disease. Tuberculosis disease is diagnosed in an individual with infection who also has signs, symptoms, positive cultures, or radiographic manifestations of *M tuberculosis*.

Isolation of *M tuberculosis* by culture from early morning gastric aspirate, sputum, pleural fluid, or other body fluids establishes the diagnosis of active disease. *Mycobacterium tuberculosis* is slow growing, usually requiring 2–10 weeks for isolation from cultured materials. Smears to demonstrate acid-fast bacilli should be performed on sputum and body fluids.

Management During Pregnancy

Treatment regimens for tuberculosis are based on the presence or absence of active disease, primarily determined by chest X-ray findings and sputum culture and, in the absence of active disease, the likelihood of progressing to disease. The risk of progression to active disease is highest in the 2 years after conversion to positive PPD. For this reason, the recommended medication in women known to have converted within the previous 2 years but with no evidence of active disease is isoniazid (300 mg per day) starting after the first trimester and continuing for 9 months. For women who are infected with HIV, the duration of isoniazid therapy is 12 months.

Pregnant women should be skin tested if they have a specific risk factor for latent tuberculosis infection or active tuberculosis. When the skin test is positive, the time of conversion usually is not known. If a chest X-ray is normal, some experts prefer to delay treatment until after delivery because pregnancy itself does not increase the risk for progression to disease and because of an increased risk of drug-induced hepatotoxicity during pregnancy and immediately postpartum. Other experts recommend treatment with monthly monitoring for hepatotoxicity. All pregnant women receiving isoniazid also should take pyridoxine.

If a pregnant woman is diagnosed with active disease (by positive cultures or by compatible clinical or X-ray findings), prompt, multidrug therapy is recommended to protect both the woman and the fetus. Isoniazid and rifampin, supplemented by ethambutol if isoniazid drug resistance is suspected, currently are recommended drugs. Pyrazinamide frequently is used in a three- or four-drug regimen, but safety data in pregnancy have not been published. Therapy is continued for at least 6 months for drug-susceptible disease.

Neonatal Management

Because tuberculosis usually is transmitted by inhalation of droplet nuclei produced by an adult or adolescent with infectious primary tuberculosis, acquisition of *M tuberculosis* by newborns generally occurs only after delivery. Infection can occur before birth as a result of hematogenous dissemination, which seeds the placenta; as a result of infected amniotic fluid in utero; or at the time of delivery as a result of fetal aspiration of tubercle bacilli in women with tuberculosis endometritis. On the rare occasions in which congenital tuberculosis is suspected, diagnostic evaluations and treatment of the neonate and the mother should be initiated promptly.

Management of a newborn whose mother (or other household contact) is suspected of having tuberculosis is based on individual considerations. Whenever possible, separation of the mother (or contact) and the neonate should be minimized. Differing circumstances and resulting recommendations are listed as follows:

- The mother (or household contact) has a negative X-ray result—If the mother is asymptomatic, no separation of the mother and the neonate is required. The mother usually is a candidate for treatment of latent tuberculosis infection. The newborn needs no special evaluation or therapy. Because the positive tuberculin test result could be a marker of an unrecognized case of contagious tuberculosis within the household, other household members should have Mantoux tests with PPD and further evaluation.

- The mother (or household contact) has an abnormal chest X-ray result—If the X-ray result is abnormal, the mother and the neonate should be separated until the mother has been evaluated and, if active tuberculosis disease is found, until she is receiving antituberculosis therapy and sputum AFB smears are negative. Other household members should have Mantoux tests with PPD and further evaluation.

- The mother (or household contact) has an abnormal chest roentgenogram but no evidence of active disease—If the mother's chest roentgenogram is abnormal but the history, physical examination, sputum smear, and roentgenogram indicate no evidence of active disease, the neonate can be assumed to be at low risk of *M tuberculosis* infection. The radiographic abnormality in this circumstance probably is because of another cause or because of a quiescent focus of tuberculosis. In the latter case, the mother may develop contagious, active tuberculosis, if untreated, and should receive appropriate therapy if not treated previously. She and her neonate should receive follow-up care. Other household members should have Mantoux tests with PPD and further evaluation.

- The mother (or household contact) has clinical or radiographic evidence of active, possibly contagious tuberculosis—The mother (or household contact) should be reported immediately to the public health department so that investigation of all household members can be performed within several days. All contacts should have a tuberculin skin test, chest roentgenogram, and physical examination. The neonate should be evaluated for congenital tuberculosis and should be tested for HIV infection. The mother and the neonate should be separated until both are receiving appropriate therapy and the mother is deemed to be noncontagious. If the infant is receiving isoniazid, separation is not necessary. Other household members should have skin testing and further evaluation.

If congenital tuberculosis is excluded, isoniazid is given until the neonate is 3–4 months of age, at which time the Mantoux test with PPD should be repeated. If the skin test result is positive, the child should be reassessed for tuberculosis. If disease is not present, isoniazid should be continued for a total of at least 9 months for skin conversion; children infected with HIV should be treated for 12 months. If the skin test result is negative and the mother and other family members with tuberculosis have good adherence and response to treatment and are no longer infectious, isoniazid may be discontinued. The neonate should be evaluated at monthly intervals during treatment.

If the mother (or household contact) has disease caused by multiple-drug-resistant *M tuberculosis* or has poor adherence to treatment and directly observed therapy is not possible, the neonate should be separated from the ill family member and bacille Calmette–Guérin (BCG) vaccination may be considered for the neonate. Because the response to the vaccine in neonates may be delayed and inadequate for prevention of tuberculosis, directly observed therapy of the affected household contact is preferred.

Untoward effects of isoniazid therapy in newborns are rare. The incidence of hepatitis during isoniazid therapy is so low in otherwise healthy neonates that routine determination of serum aminotransferase concentrations is not recommended. The maternal use of isoniazid is considered to be compatible with breastfeeding. Breastfeeding is considered safe during maternal antituberculosis therapy as long as the neonate is not concurrently taking oral antituberculosis therapy. (If both the mother and the neonate are taking antituberculosis therapy, excessive drug concentrations may occur in the neonate.) Breastfed neonates of women taking isoniazid therapy should receive a multivitamin supplement, including pyridoxine. Drugs in breast milk should not be considered effective treatment or prophylaxis of the neonate.

Bacille Calmette–Guérin vaccine is a live vaccine prepared from attenuated strains of *Mycobacterium bovis*. Although BCG vaccination is recommended by the Expanded Programme on Immunization of the World Health Organization and is widely used throughout the world, BCG vaccination use in the United States is limited to selected circumstances. Bacille Calmette–Guérin vaccine should be considered only for uninfected neonates and children who are at high risk of intimate and prolonged exposure to patients with persistently infectious pulmonary tuberculosis, who cannot be removed from the source of exposure, and who cannot be placed on long-term preventive therapy. The vaccine also should be considered for neonates who are continuously exposed to patients infected with *M tuberculosis* that is resistant to isoniazid and rifampin and who cannot be removed from the source of exposure.

Spirochetal Infections

Syphilis

Syphilis persists in the United States; rates of infection are highest in urban areas and the rural South. All pregnant women should be serologically screened for syphilis as early as possible in pregnancy and again at delivery (as well as after exposure to an infected partner). Because false-negative serologic tests results may occur in early primary infection and infection after the first prenatal visit is possible, patients who are considered to be at high risk for syphilis or who are from areas of high prevalence should be retested at the beginning of the third trimester.

The specificity of serologic testing is high if both a nontreponemal screening test (Venereal Disease Research Laboratories [VDRL] or Rapid Plasma Reagin [RPR] test result) and a subsequent treponemal serologic test result are reactive. Microscopic dark-field and histologic examinations for spirochetes are most reliable when lesions are present.

Congenital syphilis most often is acquired through hematogenous transplacental infection of the fetus, although direct contact of the neonate with infectious lesions during or after delivery also can result in infection. Transplacental infection can occur throughout pregnancy and at any stage of maternal infection.

Treatment for Pregnant Women

Pregnant women with syphilis should be treated with a penicillin regimen appropriate to the stage of infection. Women who are allergic to penicillin should be desensitized and then treated with the drug. Tetracycline and doxycycline are contraindicated during pregnancy. Erythromycin is suboptimal because poor transplacental passage or poor patient compliance may result in failure to cure infection in the fetus.

Women with syphilis should be queried about substance use, especially cocaine. Results of the maternal serologic tests and treatment, if given, should be recorded in the neonate's medical record or be made available to the neonate's pediatrician.

Evaluation of Newborns for Congenital Infection

No newborn should leave any hospital without determination of the syphilis serologic status of his or her mother. A neonate should be evaluated for congenital syphilis if he or she is born to a mother with a positive treponemal test result who has one or more of the following conditions:

- Syphilis and HIV infection
- Untreated or inadequately treated syphilis
- Syphilis during pregnancy treated with a nonpenicillin regimen and inadequate regimen, such as erythromycin
- Syphilis during pregnancy treated with an appropriate penicillin regimen that failed to produce the expected decrease in nontreponemal antibody titer after therapy
- Syphilis treated less than 1 month before delivery (because treatment failures occur and the efficacy of treatment cannot be assumed)

- Syphilis treatment not documented
- Syphilis treated before pregnancy but with insufficient serologic follow-up during pregnancy to assess the response to treatment and current infection status

Neonates born to women with any of the preceding conditions should be evaluated for syphilis. This evaluation should include the following components:

- Physical examination
- Quantitative nontreponemal and a treponemal serologic test for syphilis on the infant's serum sample
- Cerebrospinal fluid evaluation, including a VDRL test, cell count, and protein evaluation
- Long-bone X-ray (unless the diagnosis has been otherwise established)
- Complete blood cell and platelet counts
- Other clinically indicated tests (eg, chest X-ray)
- Pathologic examination of the placenta or umbilical cord, if available, also is recommended

The VDRL or RPR test commonly is used to evaluate newborns for congenital infection with *Treponema pallidum*. For testing, serum from the neonate is preferred to umbilical cord blood because the latter can produce false-positive and false-negative results.

A diagnosis of congenital syphilis is frequently difficult to establish because clinical evidence of infection may not be apparent at birth and serologic test results may be equivocal or difficult to interpret. A reactive serologic test result for syphilis (eg, VDRL, RPR, or fluorescent treponemal antibody absorption test) on neonatal blood does not necessarily indicate that the neonate is infected. If the reaction is caused only by passively transferred maternal antibody, the neonate's VDRL titer usually is lower than the mother's and usually reverts to negative in 4–6 months. A positive fluorescent treponemal antibody absorption test result caused by passively transferred antibody may take up to 1 year to become negative. A persistently reactive serologic test result for syphilis suggests infection, and an increasing titer is almost diagnostic.

Clinical symptoms of early congenital syphilis frequently are absent or nonspecific. Long-bone X-rays may be useful in establishing a diagnosis in neonates with suspected congenital syphilis.

Moist, open syphilitic lesions are infectious. Standard precautions are sufficient for neonates with suspected or proven congenital syphilis. Health care personnel and parents should wear gloves when handling the neonate until antibiotic therapy has been administered for at least 24 hours. Individuals in intimate contact with the neonate before isolation precautions and treatment were instituted should be examined for the presence of lesions 2–3 weeks later and tested serologically for infection.

Parenteral penicillin G remains the preferred therapy for syphilis at any stage. Treatment of neonates with congenital syphilis is summarized in Table 9–4. Cases of syphilis must be reported to the public health authorities.

Table 9–4. Recommended Treatment of Neonates (≤4 Weeks of Age) With Proven or Possible Congenital Syphilis

Clinical Status	Evaluation	Antimicrobial Therapy*
Proven or highly probable disease[†]	CSF analysis for VDRL, cell count, and protein CBC and platelet count Other tests as clinically indicated (eg, long-bone radiography, liver function tests, ophthalmologic examination)	Aqueous crystalline penicillin G, 100,000–150,000 units/kg per day, administered as 50,000 unit/kg per dose, IV, every 12 h during the first 7 days of life and every 8 h thereafter for a total of 10 days or Penicillin G procaine,[‡] 50,000 units/kg per day, IM, in a single dose for 10 days
Normal physical examination and serum quantitative nontreponemal titer the same or less than fourfold the maternal titer:		
(a) (i) Mother was not treated or inadequately treated or has no documented treatment; (ii) mother was treated with erythromycin or other nonpenicillin regimen; (iii) mother received treatment ≤4 weeks before delivery	CSF analysis for VDRL, cell count, and protein CBC and platelet count Long-bone radiography	Aqueous crystalline penicillin G, IV, for 10 days[§] or Penicillin G procaine,[‡] 50,000 units/kg, IM, in a single dose for 10 days[§] or Penicillin G benzathine,[‡] 50,000 units/kg, IM, in a single dose[§]

(continued)

Table 9–4. Recommended Treatment of Neonates (≤4 Weeks of Age) With Proven or Possible Congenital Syphilis *(continued)*

Clinical Status	Evaluation	Antimicrobial Therapy*
(b) (i) Adequate maternal therapy given >4 wk before delivery; (ii) mother has no evidence of reinfection or relapse	None	Clinical, serologic follow-up, and penicillin G benzathine, 50,000 units/kg, IM, in a single dose‖
(c) Adequate therapy before pregnancy and mother's nontreponemal serologic titer remained low and stable during pregnancy and at delivery	None	None¶

Abbreviations: CBC, complete blood count; CSF, cerebrospinal fluid; IM, intramuscularly; IV, intravenously; VDRL, Venereal Disease Research Laboratories

*If more than 1 day of therapy is missed, the entire course should be restarted.

†Abnormal physical examination, serum quantitative nontreponemal titer that is fourfold greater than the mother's titer, or positive result of dark-field or fluorescent antibody test of body fluid(s)

‡Penicillin G benzathine and penicillin G procaine are approved for IM administration only.

§A complete evaluation (CSF analysis, bone radiography, CBC) is not necessary if 10 days of parenteral therapy is administered but may be useful to support a diagnosis of congenital syphilis. If a single dose of penicillin G benzathine is used, then the infant must be evaluated fully, the full evaluation must be normal, and follow-up must be certain. If any part of the infant's evaluation is abnormal or not performed or if the CSF analysis is uninterpretable, the 10-day course of penicillin is required.

‖Some experts would not treat the infant but would provide close serologic follow-up.

¶Some experts would treat with penicillin G benzathine, 50,000 units/kg, as a single IM injection if follow-up is uncertain.

American Academy of Pediatrics. Red Book: 2006 Report of the Committee on Infectious Diseases. 27th ed. Elk Grove Village (IL): AAP; 2006.

Lyme Disease

Lyme disease is caused by a spirochete (*Borrelia burgdorferi*) transmitted by the bite of a deer tick. Early stages of the disease are characterized by a distinctive "bull's-eye" skin lesion (erythema migrans) that occurs in 60–80% of patients and nonspecific, flulike symptoms. Untreated disease can result in neurologic or cardiac manifestations within 4–6 weeks after the onset of early signs and symptoms. A late manifestation of Lyme disease is arthritis, usually intermittent inflammatory arthritis of a large joint. Untreated patients can develop joint involvement ranging from mild to moderate arthralgia to chronic destructive joint disease. No definitive early diagnostic tests, including serology, are commercially available. Patients in the later stages of Lyme disease usually will be seropositive, but false-positive and false-negative test results are common.

Suspicion of early maternal infection is based on a history of exposure to tick bites, the presence of the distinctive skin lesion, and nonspecific, flulike symptoms. Adequately treated patients may never develop antibodies to spirochetes.

Because congenital infection occurs with other spirochetal infections, there has been concern that an infected pregnant woman could transmit *B burgdorferi* to her fetus. No causal relationship between maternal Lyme disease and congenital abnormalities caused by *B burgdorferi* has been documented. No evidence shows that Lyme disease can be transmitted via breast milk. The neonate's health care provider should be informed when maternal disease is suspected.

Recommended treatment of suspected early disease in pregnant women is amoxicillin, 500 mg three times per day, for 2–3 weeks. For women who are allergic to penicillin, erythromycin is recommended for 2–3 weeks. For patients who are unable to tolerate erythromycin, cefuroxime axetil is an alternative for patients with immediate and anaphylactic hypersensitivity to penicillin who have undergone penicillin desensitization.

The best preventive measure is to avoid heavily wooded areas. If entrance into such areas is necessary, long-sleeved shirts and long pants tucked in at the ankle are helpful. Prophylactic antibiotic therapy for deer tick bites is not recommended routinely.

Parasitic Infections

Malaria

Although malaria mainly is confined to tropical areas of Africa, Asia, and Latin America, international travel and migration have made malaria a disease to consider in developed countries. The classic symptoms are high fever with chills, rigors, sweats, and headache.

Malaria infection may be more severe in pregnant women and also may increase the risk of adverse outcomes of pregnancy, including spontaneous abortion, stillbirth, preterm birth, and low birth weight. Because of the risk to both the woman and the fetus, and because no chemoprophylactic regimen is completely effective, pregnant women (or women likely to become pregnant) should avoid travel to malaria-endemic areas. If travel to a malaria-endemic area is necessary, appropriate consultation should be sought for chemoprophylaxis recommendations based on the malaria species and drug-resistance patterns prevalent in that area. (For current information and recommendations from the CDC, visit www.cdc.gov/travel.)

Congenital malaria is rare. Signs and symptoms resemble those of neonatal sepsis. Definitive diagnosis (of the mother and the neonate) relies on identification of the parasite on stained blood films. Both thick and thin films should be examined. Treatment of infection is based on the infecting species, possible drug resistance, and severity of disease. If malaria is a diagnostic consideration in a pregnant woman or newborn, consultation with appropriate specialists is recommended for optimal patient management.

Toxoplasmosis

Toxoplasmosis is a protozoan infection caused by *Toxoplasma gondii*. Approximately 15% of women in the United States have antibodies to this organism. Infection is acquired from eating infected raw or poorly cooked meat and from exposure to oocysts in the stools of infected members of the cat family. Infected women generally are asymptomatic.

Although congenital infection is more common after maternal infection in the third trimester, the sequelae from first-trimester fetal infection are more severe. Signs of congenital infection at birth may include chorioretinitis, hydrocephaly, microcephaly, and intracranial calcifications; however, most affected neonates are asymptomatic. Neonates of women who are infected with both HIV and *T gondii* should be evaluated for congenital toxoplasmosis.

The diagnosis of maternal infection is based on serologic test results. Routine screening of pregnant women is not indicated, except in the presence of HIV infection. Because the presence of antibodies before pregnancy indicates immunity, the appropriate time to test for immunity to toxoplasmosis in women at risk is before conception. Demonstration of seroconversion is the best method of confirming the diagnosis of acute infection. A significant increase in IgG titer in paired samples taken 2–4 weeks apart (tested simultaneously) or the presence of *T gondii*-specific IgM most often indicates recent or current infection.

Although the presence of antitoxoplasma IgM antibodies is suggestive of acute infection, such IgM antibodies may persist for several months. In addition, false-positive test results are common with commercially available kits. Before making treatment recommendations, confirmation of increased antitoxoplasma IgM antibodies should be obtained in a reference laboratory.

A definitive diagnosis of congenital toxoplasmosis can be made prenatally by: 1) detecting the parasite in amniotic fluid by PCR, or 2) documenting antitoxoplasma IgM and IgA antibodies in fetal blood. If the diagnosis is suspected (but unconfirmed) at the time of birth, ophthalmologic, auditory, and neurologic examinations should be performed. Congenital toxoplasmosis can be diagnosed serologically by the detection of antitoxoplasma-specific IgM or IgA antibodies soon after birth or by the persistence of antitoxoplasma IgG beyond 12 months of age.

Therapy of infected mothers with spiramycin (available through the U.S. Food and Drug Administration) may reduce the incidence of fetal infection but will not prevent sequelae in the fetus if congenital infection does occur. The combination of pyrimethamine and sulfadiazine should be considered if the mother acquires infection during the third trimester, although the efficacy of such therapy has not been proved. In one study, routine neonatal screening for toxoplasmosis with early treatment of infected neonates decreased the frequency of long-term sequelae. However, in the United States, routine screening during pregnancy currently is not recommended, except in women infected with HIV.

For neonates with both symptomatic and asymptomatic congenital toxoplasmosis, pyrimethamine and sulfadiazine (supplemented with folinic acid) are recommended. The duration of therapy is prolonged (1 year) and has been shown to improve outcome. Neonates with congenital toxoplasmosis should be managed in consultation with infectious disease specialists. (Please refer to the CDC web site for further professional and patient information: www.cdc.gov/ncidod/dpd/parasites/toxoplasmosis.)

Resources

American Academy of Pediatrics. Red book 2006: report of the Committee on Infectious Diseases. 27th ed. Elk Grove Village (IL): AAP; 2006.

American Academy of Pediatrics, American College of Obstetricians and Gynecologists. Joint statement on human immunodeficiency virus screening. ACOG Statement of Policy. Elk Grove Village (IL): AAP; Washington, DC: ACOG; 1999.

American College of Obstetricians and Gynecologists. Management of herpes in pregnancy. ACOG Practice Bulletin 8. Washington, DC: ACOG; 1999.

American College of Obstetricians and Gynecologists. Perinatal viral and parasitic infections. ACOG Practice Bulletin 20. Washington, DC: ACOG; 2000.

American College of Obstetricians and Gynecologists. Scheduled cesarean delivery and the prevention of vertical transmission of HIV infection. ACOG Committee Opinion 234. Washington, DC: ACOG; 2000.

American College of Obstetricians and Gynecologists. Viral hepatitis in pregnancy. ACOG Educational Bulletin 248. Washington, DC: ACOG, 1998.

Centers for Disease Control and Prevention. Parasitic disease information. Toxoplasmosis. Atlanta (GA): CDC; 2004. Available at: http://www.cdc.gov/ncidod/dpd/parasites/toxoplasmosis. Retrieved January 3, 2007.

Centers for Disease Control and Prevention. Rubella. In: Epidemiology and prevention of vaccine-preventable diseases. 9th ed. Washington, DC: Public Health Foundation; 2006. p. 155–70.

Gibbs RS, Schrag S, Schuchat A. Perinatal infections due to group B streptococci. Obstet Gynecol 2004;104:1062–76.

Human papillomavirus vaccination. ACOG Committee Opinion No. 344. American College of Obstetricians and Gynecologists. Obstet Gynecol 2006;108:699–705.

Human milk, breastfeeding, and transmission of human immunodeficiency virus in the United States. American Academy of Pediatrics Committee on Pediatric AIDS. Pediatrics 1995;96:977–9. Reaffirmed 1999, 2003.

Management of herpes in pregnancy. ACOG Practice Bulletin No. 81. American College of Obstetricians and Gynecologists. Obstet Gynecol 2007;109:1233–48.

Meningococcal vaccination for adolescents. ACOG Committee Opinion No. 314. American College of Obstetricians and Gynecologists. Obstet Gynecol 2005;106: 667–9.

Perinatal human immunodeficiency virus testing. Provisional Committee on Pediatric AIDS, American Academy of Pediatrics. Pediatrics 1995;95:303–7.

Prevention of early-onset group B streptococcal disease in newborns. ACOG Committee Opinion No. 279. American College of Obstetricians and Gynecologists. Obstet Gynecol 2002;100:1405–12.

Public Health Service Task Force recommendations for the use of antiretroviral drugs in pregnant women infected with HIV-1 for maternal health and for reducing perinatal HIV-1 transmission in the United States. Centers for Disease Control and Prevention [published errata appear in MMWR Morb Mortal Wkly Rep 1998;47:287; MMWR Morb Mortal Wkly Rep 1998;47:315]. MMWR Recomm Rep 1998;47(RR-2):1–20.

Recommendations of the U.S. Public Health Service Task Force on the use of zidovudine to reduce perinatal transmission of human immunodeficiency virus. Centers for Disease Control and Prevention. MMWR Recomm Rep 1994;43(RR-11):1–20.

Revised guidelines for prevention of early-onset group B streptococcal (GBS) infection. American Academy of Pediatrics Committee on Infectious Diseases and Committee on Fetus and Newborn. Pediatrics 1997;99:489–96.

Revised indications for the use of palivizumab and respiratory syncytial virus immune globulin intravenous for the prevention of respiratory syncytial virus infections. American Academy of Pediatrics. Committee on Infectious Diseases and Committee on Fetus and Newborn. Pediatrics 2003;112:1442–6.

Schrag S, Gorwitz R, Fultz-Butts K, Schuchat A. Prevention of perinatal group B strep-tococcal disease. Revised guidelines from CDC. MMWR Recomm Rep 2002;51 (RR-11):1–22.

Sexually transmitted diseases in adolescents. ACOG Committee Opinion No. 301. American College of Obstetricians and Gynecologists. Obstet Gynecol 2004;104: 891–8.

Sexually transmitted diseases treatment guidelines, 2006. Centers for Disease Control and Prevention [published erratum appears in MMWR Recomm Rep 2006;55:997]. MMWR Recomm Rep 2006;55(RR11):1–94.

Sheffield JS, Hollier LM, Hill JB, Stuart GS, Wendel GD. Acyclovir prophylaxis to prevent herpes simplex virus recurrence at delivery: a systematic review. Obstet Gynecol 2003; 102:1396–403.

Sweet RL, Gibbs RS. Infectious diseases of the female genital tract. 4th ed. Philadelphia (PA): Lippincott Williams and Wilkins; 2002.

Targeted tuberculin testing and treatment of latent tuberculosis infection. The official state-ment of the American Thoracic Society was adopted by the ATS Board of Directors, July 1999. This is a Joint Statement of the American Thoracic Society (ATS) and the Centers for Disease Control and Prevention (CDC). This statement was endorsed by the Council of the Infectious Diseases Society of America. (ISDA), September 1999, and the sections of this statement. Am J Respir Crit Care Med 2000;161:S221–47.

United States Department of Agriculture, Food Safety and Inspection Service. Listeriosis and pregnancy: what is your risk? Safe food handling for a healthy pregnancy. Washington, DC: USDA; 2001. Available at: http://www.fsis.usda.gov/Fact_Sheets/ Listeriosis_and_Pregnancy_What_is_Your_Risk/index.asp. Retrieved January 3, 2007.

chapter 10

Infection Control

The mother–newborn dyad usually is free of significant infectious processes. However, colonization of the neonate by organisms acquired during the delivery can occur. When exposed to certain organisms, the outcome may be devastating for the neonate, the mother, or both. Many neonatal infections that occur in intensive care units are caused by pathogens acquired from the hospital environment (ie, health care-associated infections).

Surveillance for Health Care-Associated Infection

The infection-control committee of each hospital should work with perinatal care personnel to establish workable definitions of health care-associated infection for surveillance purposes. For obstetric patients, a health care-associated infection can be defined broadly as one that is neither present nor incubating when the patient is admitted to the hospital. Many cases of endometritis or urinary tract infection that occur postpartum are health care-associated, even though the causative organisms may be endogenous to the female genital tract.

Health care-associated infection in the neonate is defined as an infection that develops more than 48 hours after delivery, although many of these are caused by organisms acquired from the mother rather than from the hospital environment. This definition should be applied consistently to allow uniform reporting and analysis of health care-associated infections.

Obstetric and nursery personnel should cooperate with hospital infection-control personnel in conducting and reviewing the results of surveillance programs for health care-associated infections. This type of monitoring provides information about any unusual problems or clusters of infection, the risks associated with certain procedures or techniques, and the success of specific preventive measures. It also can reveal temporal trends, allow comparison with other nurseries using this standard definition, and provide feedback to responsible personnel in the nursery.

Prevention of infections requires a multifaceted approach. This includes meticulous patient care techniques, hand hygiene, and the judicious use of antibiotics to reduce the potential for disrupting the balance of colonizing flora and promoting antimicrobial-resistant organisms.

Prevention and Control of Infections

Nursery Admission Policies

Newborns transferred from a nursery at another hospital usually are not admitted to the normal newborn nursery but to intensive care nursery areas. Neonates should be approached as though they harbor colonies of unique flora that should not be transmitted to any other neonate. To promote appropriate continuity of care, some neonates may need to be readmitted to the nursery a few days after being discharged. Newborns with suspected infectious diseases should not be readmitted to the normal newborn nursery but can be admitted to specialized areas where additional precautions (airborne, contact, droplet) can be provided to control the risks to other newborns.

In the last several years, cobedding multiple gestation infants in a single incubator or crib has become popular. There are many reported benefits to this practice; however, there are few data documenting safety and efficacy. Nursery policies should be clear on the indications and contraindications for cobedding.

Routine culturing of neonates' respiratory or gastrointestinal tract or skin for surveillance purposes is not recommended, but cultures from lesions or sites of infection should be taken to identify the etiology. When clusters of infections caused by a single strain of bacteria are noted, appropriate personnel should be notified. Routine surveillance cultures of infants and nursery staff can be useful to characterize and to control an outbreak of infection with a common organism.

During an outbreak of infection, it is important to document organisms colonizing all neonates so that appropriate isolation and cohorting procedures can be undertaken.

Both obstetric and nursery personnel are involved in providing perinatal care. Therefore, precise communication between these groups about infectious diseases is essential. Nursery personnel should be notified in advance of the birth of a neonate who may have a congenital or perinatal infection or a mother who is known to be infected with, or be a chronic carrier of, a potentially infectious organism (eg, *Salmonella* species, human immunodeficiency virus [HIV], hepatitis B virus [HBV], hepatitis C virus, or herpes simplex virus).

Labor and Delivery Admission Policy

The pediatrician or neonatologist should be notified of all mothers admitted to the antepartum obstetrics unit who are colonized with known pathogens that may be transmitted vertically to the neonate. For example, both group A streptococci and group B streptococci (GBS) are pathogens that may be indigenous to the female genital tract, and both may cause serious, life-threatening infection in the mother and newborn. Although there are national guidelines for the management of GBS colonization in the mother, there is no consensus for the management of maternal group A streptococci colonization. However, it may be reasonable to use antibiotic prophylaxis in mothers with known group A streptococci colonization given the potential for serious maternal and newborn infection and outbreaks of group A streptococcal infection in maternity units.

Standard Precautions

The Centers for Disease Control and Prevention (CDC) recommend that standard precautions be used for all patients. Standard precautions are intended to prevent transmission of bloodborne pathogens, recognizing the importance of all body fluids, secretions, excretions, and contaminated items in the transmission of health care-associated pathogens. These precautions apply to: 1) blood, semen, vaginal secretions, cerebrospinal fluid, synovial fluid, pleural fluid, pericardial fluid, peritoneal fluid, amniotic fluid, saliva in dental procedures, any body fluid that is visibly contaminated with blood, and all body fluids in situations in which it is difficult or impossible to differentiate between body fluids, except sweat; 2) nonintact skin; and 3) mucous membranes. Standard precautions include handwashing, using gloves (in addition to handwashing), using masks, using eye protection, using face shields, and wearing nonsterile gowns.

Disposal of contaminated equipment or materials always should be accomplished using standard precautions and careful handwashing. Instruments should not be shared, and each newborn's bedside should be considered a separate, clean environment.

The federal Occupational Safety and Health Administration (OSHA) has issued regulations designed to minimize the transmission of HIV, HBV, and other potentially infectious organisms in the workplace. The OSHA guidelines are discussed extensively in Appendix H. The regulations apply to all employees in physicians' offices, hospitals, medical laboratories, and other health care facilities where workers reasonably could be anticipated to come into contact with blood and other potentially infectious material. The OSHA regulations require employers to implement an exposure-control plan to minimize employees' exposure to bloodborne and infectious pathogens. The plan must contain the following components:

- Personal protective equipment for employees exposed to blood and other body fluids
- Housekeeping requirements
- Provision of HBV vaccination to employees
- Postexposure evaluation and follow-up procedures
- Employee training
- Use of warning labels
- Record-keeping requirements
- Adoption of certain work practice controls (eg, handwashing facilities, safer medical devices such as needleless systems and sharps with engineered sharps protection)

These requirements are enforced by OSHA or, in the case of states with OSHA-approved comparable job safety and health plans, by state agencies. Violations are punishable by fines.

Health Standards for Personnel

Obstetric and nursery personnel, as well as others who have significant contact with newborns, should be as free of transmissible infectious diseases as possible. Each hospital should establish written policies and procedures for assessing the health of personnel assigned to perinatal care services, restricting their contact with patients when necessary, maintaining their health records, and requiring staff to report any illness they may have. These policies and procedures should address screening for immunity to measles, rubella, mumps, varicella–zoster virus, HBV, pertussis, tetanus, diphtheria, and tuberculosis. The frequency of and need for screening employees should be determined by local epidemiologic data. Personnel with active tuberculosis should be restricted from patient contact until adequate treatment has occurred and noninfective status has been verified. All susceptible, nonpregnant hospital personnel should be offered immunization against rubella, varicella–zoster virus, and HBV. Offering annual influenza immunization to all health care providers is encouraged strongly, as they care for patients at high risk for developing influenza-related complications. Vaccinations protect both staff and patients and may reduce health care costs.

Ideally, individuals with a respiratory, cutaneous, mucocutaneous, or gastrointestinal infection should not have direct contact with neonates. Personnel with exudative skin lesions or weeping dermatitis should refrain from all direct patient care and should not handle patient care equipment until the condition resolves. Personnel in contact with neonates should report personal infections, inability to perform adequate hand hygiene (eg, because of casts or braces), and other conditions to their immediate supervisors and should be medically examined to determine suitability for patient contact. Decisions regarding the exclusion of staff members from obstetric and nursery areas should be made on an individual basis. Employee health policies should be worded and applied in a way to ensure that personnel feel free to report infectious problems without fear of income loss.

Transmission of herpes simplex virus from infected personnel to neonates in newborn nurseries is rare. Personnel (including patients' family members) with cold sores who have direct contact with newborns should cover their lesions and carefully observe hand hygiene policies. Family members with proven or suspected oral herpes simplex infection should be advised not to kiss their infants. Transmission of herpes simplex virus infection from personnel with genital lesions is not likely. Personnel with herpetic hand infections (herpetic whitlow) should not participate in patient care until the lesions have healed.

Personnel in neonatal units are likely to be exposed to infants excreting cytomegalovirus. Acquisition of cytomegalovirus infection from infants is prevented by compliance with standard precautions. Women of childbearing age who work in neonatal units should be counseled about the relatively low risk of exposure should they become pregnant. A routine program of serologic testing of obstetric and nursery hospital employees for immunity to cytomegalovirus is not recommended.

When possible, personnel assigned to obstetric or newborn areas should not be moved to or from other assigned areas of the hospital. Employee education regarding standard precautions and other proper infection control techniques should occur regularly. All personnel should be required to follow strictly established infection-control procedures.

Hand Hygiene

Health care personnel should be alert to the potential for contamination and practice meticulous techniques to prevent acquisition of pathogens from infected patients. Proper hand hygiene before and after each patient contact remains the single most important routine practice in the control of health care-associated infections in both mother and neonate. Additional policies and procedures are required for critically ill neonates (see the CDC web site, www.cdc.gov).

Before handling neonates for the first time on a work shift, personnel should scrub their hands and arms to a point above the elbow with an antiseptic soap. Disposable sponges are as effective as brushes and are less damaging to the skin. After washing, the hands should be rinsed thoroughly and dried with paper towels.

A 10-second wash without a brush, but with soap and vigorous rubbing, is required before and after handling each neonate and after touching objects, whether or not gloves are worn. Handwashing facilities and materials must be easily accessible. Handwashing is required even when gloves have been worn. Handwashing should occur before and immediately following removal of gloves. Personnel should remove rings, watches, and bracelets before washing their hands and entering the obstetric or nursery areas. Fingernails should be trimmed short, and artificial fingernails or extenders should not be permitted. Clear nail polish on natural nails appears to have no detrimental effect, but dark colors may obscure the subungual space and reduce the likelihood of careful cleaning. Antiseptic preparations can be used for scrubbing before entering the nursery, before and after providing care, before performing invasive procedures, and after touching secretions, blood, or equipment.

For routine handwashing, bactericidal soap and water may be sufficient. The bactericidal agents most useful for handwashing in the nursery are chlorhexidine gluconate (4%) and iodophor preparations; both are active against a broad spectrum of gram-positive and gram-negative organisms. Iodophor preparations often are more drying to the skin. Hexachlorophene-based preparations may be useful during nursery outbreaks of *Staphylococcus aureus* infection, but they are not recommended for routine handwashing.

All antiseptic or bactericidal soaps are sensitizing or irritating to the skin, and some individuals may need to use plain soap or mild detergents. Liquid soap dispensers and their contents can become contaminated. This problem can be avoided by using disposable brushes or pads that contain an antiseptic hand cleanser. Alcohol-containing foams and gel satisfactorily kill bacteria when applied to clean hands and require 15 seconds to 2 minutes of contact (in accordance with manufacturers' recommendations). However, alcohol-containing products are not appropriate for cleaning physically soiled hands. When hands are visibly contaminated with proteinaceous material or soiled with blood or other body fluids, they should first be washed well with soap and water.

Exposure of Health Care Professionals to Human Immunodeficiency Virus

Health care workers who have had percutaneous or mucous membrane exposure to blood or bloody secretions from an HIV-infected woman or an HIV-exposed or HIV-infected newborn must be given medical evaluation and follow-up as prescribed in the OSHA regulations on occupational exposure to bloodborne pathogens. Human immunodeficiency virus infection and evaluation is discussed in Chapter 9.

Dress Codes

Each hospital should establish dress codes for regular and part-time personnel who enter the labor, delivery, and nursery areas. Sterile, long-sleeved gowns should be worn by all personnel who have direct contact with the sterile field during vaginal deliveries, obstetric surgical procedures, and surgical procedures in the nursery. When personnel leave the operative room and while they are in the hospital, surgical scrub suits should be covered. Hospital policies regarding sterile areas should be established and maintained. It has become commonplace for medical care providers to wear surgical scrubs to and from work. This has engendered recent controversy regarding the efficacy and safety of laundering surgical scrubs at home versus the hospital. According to the CDC, "the risk of actual disease transmission from soiled linen is negligible." It is further stated by the CDC that, "in the home, normal washing and drying cycles including 'hot' and 'cold' cycles are adequate to ensure patient safety." To date, there are no data indicating that there is any significant difference between home and hospital laundering of scrubs.

Some hospitals have approved more flexible dress codes for personnel who work in birthing rooms; however, the CDC recommends that all health care workers who perform or assist in deliveries wear gloves, gowns, surgical masks, caps, shoe covers, and eye protection during the procedure. Wearing aprons or gowns made of impervious material during cesarean delivery may provide additional protection. Gloves should be worn when handling the placenta or the neonate until blood and amniotic fluid have been removed from the neonate's skin. Hands should be washed immediately before gloving and after gloves are removed or when skin surfaces are contaminated with blood.

Recent studies have demonstrated that cover gowns are not necessary for regular personnel in the nursery or neonatal intensive care unit, as long as proper hand hygiene is enforced strictly. When a neonate is held outside the bassinet by nursing or other neonatal intensive care unit personnel, a long-sleeved gown should be worn over the clothing and either discarded after use or maintained for use exclusively in the care of that neonate. If one gown is used for each neonate, the gowns should be changed regularly.

Caps, beard bags, and masks should be worn during certain surgical procedures, including umbilical vessel catheterization. Long hair should be restrained so that it does not touch the neonate or equipment during patient examinations or treatments. High-efficiency, disposable masks should be used, but even these masks remain effective only for a few hours. Masks should be worn so that they cover both the nose and the mouth, and they should be discarded as soon as they are removed from the nose and mouth.

Sterile gloves should be used during deliveries and all invasive procedures performed in either the obstetric or the nursery area. Disposable, nonsterile gloves may be useful in the care of patients in isolation or in the performance of procedures that may result in contamination of the hands.

Obstetric Considerations

The areas where cesarean deliveries and tubal ligations are performed are operating rooms and are subject to all policies pertaining to such facilities. Therefore, all persons present should wear appropriate operating room attire. For those close to the sterile surgical field, this attire includes clean scrub clothing, sterile operating room gowns, caps, masks, eye protection, gloves, and shoe covers. For those not involved with the surgical field, a sterile operating room gown is not required, but caps, masks, and shoe covers should be worn. The surgical field should be prepared and draped according to standard recommendations. Preoperative clipping of hair very close to the skin is preferred to shaving.

Intrauterine pressure catheters (for monitoring contractions or for amnioinfusion) or internal fetal electrodes (for fetal heart rate monitoring) should be inserted and maintained in accordance with standard sterile techniques. Fluids used with pressure catheters should be sterile. To minimize the chance of contamination, the packages containing the devices should be opened only at the time of their use, and proper sterile techniques should be followed during their handling and insertion. Disposable items should be used whenever possible.

Neonatal Considerations

Invasive Procedures

Percutaneous placement of arterial or venous cannulas or catheters is associated with a lower risk of infection in neonates than is surgical placement. The cannulas should be removed promptly if signs of device-associated infection occur. A safe maximal duration of cannulation for intravascular catheters has not been established; the risks and benefits should be assessed daily for each neonate. Intravascular catheters should not be used or left in place unless they are clearly indicated for medical management. Each unit should have a written policy on the procedures governing the use of these catheters.

Arterial cannulas and catheters present a risk of acquired infection, especially when used for obtaining blood samples. Samples should be obtained aseptically, with precautions to avoid contamination of the system and with the realization that the risk of infection is increased when using the cannula or catheter.

Maximum sterile barrier precautions (ie, cap, mask, sterile gown, sterile gloves, and sterile drapes) during the insertion of central venous catheters, including all umbilical catheters, substantially reduce the incidence of catheter-related bloodstream infections compared with standard precautions (ie, sterile gloves and small drapes). Although the efficacy of such precautions for insertion of peripherally inserted central catheters and midline catheters has not been studied, the use of maximum barrier precautions probably is applicable.

Total parenteral nutrition generally is safe, but it has been associated with infection, including bacteremia and fungemia. A multidisciplinary team approach involving pharmacists, nurses, and physicians strongly is recommended to reduce the incidence of infections and other complications. Meticulous attention should be given to aseptic insertion and maintenance of the cannula and to aseptic techniques of fluid administration. All parenteral nutrition fluids should be mixed in a central pharmacy under a laminar flow hood. Because lipid emulsions especially are susceptible to contamination with a wide variety of bacteria and fungi that can proliferate to high concentrations within hours, particular caution must be taken in the storage and administration of these emulsions. Unit-dose amounts may be delivered from the pharmacy. Opened bottles must be discarded no later than 24 hours after the seal has been broken. Intravenous tubing, stopcocks, and flush syringes should be changed (using sterile technique) on a regular basis no less frequently than every 72 hours. If an increased incidence of infection is noted, tubing should be changed more frequently.

Intravascular Solutions

The hospital pharmacy should establish a system to ensure a satisfactory and safe means of providing sterile, unpreserved fluids to the nursery areas. The CDC has no recommendations for the duration of infusion (hang time) of intravenous fluids, including lipid-free parenteral-nutrition fluids. Infusion of lipid-containing parenteral nutrition fluids should be completed within 24 hours of hanging the fluid. Infusion of lipid emulsions alone should be completed within 12 hours of hanging the fluid. Infusions of blood products should be completed within 4 hours of hanging the product.

Solutions with benzyl alcohol are contraindicated in neonates because their use may lead to severe metabolic acidosis, encephalopathy, and death. All solutions intended for parenteral infusion should be compounded in the hospital pharmacy, including those containing heparin. Flush solutions should be kept at room temperature no longer than 8 hours before being used or discarded. They should be labeled clearly with the time of opening or preparation. Single-use prefilled saline or heparin flushes also may be used.

Antibiotics

The efficacy of prophylactic antibiotic therapy for the prevention of infection in newborns has not been documented. Antibiotic prophylaxis in newborns is strongly discouraged except for specific indications (eg, ophthalmic antibiotics for prevention of ophthalmia neonatorum). The relative frequencies of documented infections in neonates, etiologic agents, and patterns of antimicrobial susceptibility should be monitored by the infection-control committee in collaboration with the unit's medical director. These data should guide the selection of antibiotics to be used for treating suspected infection while awaiting the results of body fluid cultures. The best tolerated, narrowest spectrum, and most effective antibiotic regimen should be selected for this purpose based on the accumulated data on the antibiotic sensitivity patterns of microbial isolates. The indiscriminate and injudicious use of either systemic or topical antibiotics promotes the emergence of resistant strains of bacteria, making subsequent therapy for clinical infections more difficult and dangerous.

Women with Postpartum Infections

The neonate need not be isolated from a mother with a postpartum infection in most circumstances. Women with abscesses or infected or draining wounds should have appropriate cover dressings. If it is not possible to cover the infected or draining wound completely, the infant should be placed in a separate room. Gloves and, if necessary, gowns should be worn by staff during all contact with infected patients.

Mothers with communicable diseases (eg, group A streptococci, active tuberculosis, or varicella) that are likely to be transmitted to the newborn should be separated from the newborn until the infection is no longer communicable, based on the natural history of the infection and the effectiveness of therapy in eliminating the contagion. A mother with postpartum fever that does not have a specific, communicable cause can be allowed to feed and care for her newborn. With the exception of certain infections (see "Contraindications to Breastfeeding" in Chapter 7), breastfeeding rarely is contraindicated because of maternal infection. Criteria for allowing a mother to handle her infant include the following factors:

- She feels well enough to handle the infant.
- She washes her hands thoroughly under supervision.
- She wears a clean gown.
- She avoids contact of the neonate with contaminated clothes, linen, dressings, or pads.

A woman with a respiratory tract infection should be made aware that the infection can be transmitted not only by droplets but also by hands and fomites. Therefore, she should practice strict handwashing technique and appropriately handle or dispose of contaminated tissues and any other items that may have come in contact with infectious secretions. If needed, she can wear a surgical mask to reduce the chance of droplet spread to her neonate.

Postpartum women who are infected with nonobstetric-related communicable diseases should be treated according to the precautions and isolation techniques required by the specific disease. If the required guidelines cannot be followed safely in the obstetric unit, the patient should be transferred to the appropriate unit where such care can be provided.

Cohorts

During epidemics, a comprehensive program of infection control is required. Even if an intensive investigation is not indicated, the results of the control measures should be evaluated to ensure that they have been effective and that the problem has been resolved. Because many infections become apparent only after neonates leave the hospital, each hospital should establish procedures to be used during a suspected or confirmed epidemic for disease surveillance of recently discharged neonates. Hospital infection-control personnel and appropriate public health officials should be notified promptly about suspected or confirmed epidemics.

In an epidemic, neonates with overt infection and those who are colonized should be identified rapidly and placed in cohorts—separate areas where newborns with similar exposure or illness receive care. If rapid identification of these neonates is not possible, separate cohorts should be established for neonates with disease, those who have been exposed, those who have not been exposed, and those who are newly admitted. The success of cohort programs depends largely on the willingness and ability of nursery and ancillary personnel to adhere strictly to the cohort system and to follow established infection-control practices.

Neonates With Infections

The housing of an infected neonate or one suspected of being infected depends on the type of infection, the condition of the neonate, the type of care required, the available space and facilities, the ratio of available nurses to patients, and the size and type of the clinical service. Other factors to be considered include the clinical manifestations of the infection, the source and possible modes of its transmission, and the number of colonized or infected neonates.

Isolation. In many instances (notable exceptions are neonatal varicella–zoster virus infection or epidemics of bacterial infection), it is unnecessary to isolate infected neonates if certain criteria are met:

- Sufficient nursing and medical staff are on duty to provide comprehensive care.
- Adequate sinks for handwashing are available in each nursery room or area.
- Continuing instruction is provided about the ways in which infections spread.
- If multiple infants are kept in a single room, a 4–6-foot aisle is open between infant stations.

Physical separation with assignment of separate health care personnel for each area is best. In 1996, the CDC recommended new isolation guidelines for hospitalized patients. These guidelines suggest standard precautions for all patients regardless of diagnosis and transmission-based precautions for patients who are infected or colonized with pathogens that are spread by airborne, droplet, or contact routes. Isolation categories, with examples, are listed in Table 10–1.

Forced-air incubators filter incoming air, but they do not filter the air that is discharged from the incubator into the nursery. Therefore, they are satisfactory for limited protective isolation of neonates, but they should not be relied on to prevent transmission of microorganisms from infected neonates to others.

When an isolation room is deemed necessary (eg, for patients with highly contagious infections), blinds, windows, and other structural items must allow for ease of regular room cleaning. An intercom should be provided. Air from this room should be exhausted to the outside and not to the rest of the nursery.

Gastroenteritis, Abscess, Viral Respiratory Infection, or Cutaneous Infection. Contact precautions should be observed when treating patients with viral respiratory infection, gastroenteritis, cutaneous infections, or draining lesions or abscesses that cannot be contained adequately by a dressing. All personnel

Table 10–1. Transmission-Based Precautions for Hospitalized Patients*

Category of Precautions	Single-Patient Room	Respiratory Tract and Mucous Membrane Protection	Gowns	Gloves
Airborne	Yes, with negative air-pressure ventilation, 6–12 air exchanges per hour, and HEPA filtration	Respirators: N95 or higher level	No[†]	No[†]
Droplet	Yes[‡]	Surgical masks[§]	No[†]	No[†]
Contact	Yes[‡]	No	Yes	Yes

Abbreviation: HEPA, high-efficiency particulate air

*These recommendations are in addition to those for standard precautions for all patients.

[†]Gowns and gloves may be required as a component of standard precautions (eg, for blood collection or during procedures likely to cause blood splashes or if there are skin lesions containing transmissible infectious agents).

[‡]Preferred. Cohorting of children infected with the same pathogen is acceptable if a single-patient room is not available, a distance of more than 3 feet between patients can be maintained, and precautions are observed between all contacts with different patients in the room.

[§]Masks should be donned on entry into the room.

American Academy of Pediatrics. Red book: 2006 Report of the Committee on Infectious Diseases. 27th ed. Elk Grove Village (IL): AAP; 2006.

should use gowns and disposable gloves when providing direct patient care. Contaminated items should be properly discarded, and gowns and gloves should be discarded before leaving the room. The environment may be heavily contaminated with the infecting microorganism, and these organisms often are transmitted on the hands of personnel to other neonates. If more than one neonate is infected, a cohort approach should be taken.

Congenital Infections. Standard precautions provide adequate isolation for most congenital infections, with two exceptions: congenital rubella, which requires droplet isolation, and suspected herpetic infection, which requires contact isolation.

Viral Infections. Many viruses, such as respiratory syncytial virus, coxsackieviruses, or echoviruses, spread rapidly among neonates and personnel in a nursery. Such viral infections can be serious in neonates, sometimes resulting in death. Because neonates may shed selected viruses after their clinical illness has been resolved, they become reservoirs of infection. It is believed that the enteroviruses and respiratory syncytial virus are transmitted predominantly by direct or indirect contact by the hands of personnel that become contaminated with virus-containing secretions or with contaminated environmental surfaces or fomites. Contact isolation is required to prevent this type of spread.

Neonates usually are ineffective disseminators of infectious bacterial or viral aerosols. Neonates with confirmed or possible infections caused by a viral agent that could be transmitted by the airborne route should be separated from other neonates by: 1) transfer from the nursery area, 2) rooming-in with the mother, or 3) enclosure of all other neonates in the area in incubators.

Multi-Drug-Resistant Organisms. During the past few years, the prevalence of multi-drug-resistant organisms in hospitals has increased. In the acute care setting, most multi-drug-resistant organisms are transmitted via the hands of health care workers. In addition, the prevalence of methicillin-resistant *Staphylococcus aureus* also has increased. Nursery patients with multi-drug-resistant organisms or methicillin-resistant *Staphylococcus aureus* should be isolated, and contact precautions should be observed.

Environmental Control

The responsible physicians and the nurse managers of the obstetric and nursery areas should work with infection-control personnel and other appropriate groups (eg, representatives of the respiratory therapy service, central supply, and housekeeping) to establish an environmental control program for the labor, delivery, and nursery areas. This program should include specific procedures in a written policy manual for cleaning and disinfection or sterilization of patient-care areas, equipment, and supplies. Consultation for specific details and problems should be encouraged. Nursing supervisors should ensure that these procedures are carried out correctly.

Methods of Sterilization and Disinfection

All medical and hospital personnel should understand the difference between sterilization and disinfection. Sterilization is the destruction of all microorganisms, including spores. Disinfection is a reduction in the number of contaminating microorganisms. High-level disinfection is the elimination or destruction of all microorganisms except spores. Cleaning is the physical removal of organic material or soil, including microorganisms, from objects.

Devices that enter tissue or the vascular system should be sterile. For neonates, devices that come into contact with mucous membranes or that have prolonged or intimate contact with skin also should be sterile. Much of the equipment required in perinatal care areas, however, can be used safely if it is satisfactorily cleaned and disinfected; clean, dry surfaces do not support the growth of microorganisms.

Sometimes it is necessary to decontaminate equipment before it is cleaned and sterilized or disinfected to allow processing without exposing personnel to hazardous microbes. The equipment must be cleaned thoroughly to remove all blood, tissue, secretions, food, and other residue. Without thorough cleaning, no method of sterilization or disinfection can be effective. Furthermore, some chemical disinfectants are inactivated by organic materials.

Sterilization

Methods of sterilization include steam autoclaving, dry heat, and gaseous (ethylene oxide) or liquid chemical (eg, 2% glutaraldehyde) techniques. The preferred method of sterilization is steam autoclaving because it is the least expensive method and provides the greatest margin of safety. Some equipment may be damaged by steam, however, and must be sterilized by another method. The best method for sterilization must be established for each piece of equipment.

Equipment made of material that absorbs ethylene oxide usually requires 8–12 hours of aeration after sterilization with ethylene oxide before it can be used again. Ethylene oxide sterilization of supplies or equipment should be preceded by a comprehensive review of data on the aeration time required for each material to be processed and the extent to which toxicity standards have been established. An ethylene oxide sterilization plan requires the presence of sufficient backup equipment to allow time for aeration.

Equipment that cannot be sterilized with steam or ethylene oxide may be satisfactorily sterilized after cleaning by immersion for 10 hours in acetic acid liquid sterilant or 2% glutaraldehyde or other acceptable liquid sporicide. This immersion should be followed by three rinses with sterile water (or tap water with at least 10 mg of hypochlorite per liter), thorough drying, and packaging in sterile wrappers.

High-Level Disinfection

Equipment that does not need to be sterilized may be subjected to high-level disinfection. Both hot-water pasteurization and chemical disinfection are satisfactory. Pasteurization of equipment requires immersing it in water at 80–85°C (176–185°F) for 15 minutes or 75°C (167°F) for 30 minutes. After air drying (preferably in a cabinet with heated, filtered air), disinfected items should be wrapped aseptically and stored until needed. Although spores are not eradicated by this method, bacterial and viral decontamination is adequate. The recommendations of the equipment manufacturer should be consulted for a list of any parts or materials that may be warped or damaged at these temperatures.

The choice of liquid chemicals for high-level disinfection depends on the type of equipment to be disinfected. In many instances, immersion of the equipment for 20 minutes in 2% glutaraldehyde, followed by three rinses with sterile water (or tap water with at least 10 mg of hypochlorite per liter) and thorough drying is satisfactory.

Cleaning and Disinfecting Noncritical Surfaces

Selection of Disinfectants

Although numerous disinfectants are available, no single agent or preparation is ideal for all purposes. Consideration should be given to the agent and its special use, as well as to the types of organisms likely to be contaminating the object that is to be disinfected. Special attention should be given to the recommended concentration of each disinfectant and to its time of exposure. Unnecessary exposure of neonates to disinfectants should be avoided, and strict adherence to manufacturers' recommendations is essential.

Quaternary ammonias, chlorine compounds, and phenolic compounds are satisfactory disinfectants, although neonatal exposure to phenolic compounds has been associated with hyperbilirubinemia. Sodium hypochlorite has been suggested for disinfection of HIV-exposed surfaces. Use of any of these substances should be limited to disinfectant–detergent products registered with the U.S. Environmental Protection Agency and recommended by the manufacturer for nursery surfaces with which neonates have contact. Information about specific label claims of commercial germicides can be obtained from the U.S. Environmental Protection Agency (www.epa.gov/pesticides/factsheets/antimic. htm) or from the Association for Professionals in Infection Control and Epidemiology (www.apic.org).

General Housekeeping

Cleaning should be conducted in the following time sequence:

1. Patient areas

2. Accessory areas

3. Adjacent halls

It is not known whether floor bacteria are a source of health care-associated infection, but regular cleaning prevents the accumulation of pathogenic bacteria. Disinfectant–detergents have been shown to be more effective than soap and water alone in cleaning floors, although hospital floors are recontaminated rapidly after disinfection. Available disinfectant–detergents may differ in effectiveness.

During the cleaning process, dust should not be dispersed into the air. Removal of dust by a dry vacuum machine followed by wet vacuuming is effective in cleaning and disinfecting hospital floors. Once dust has been removed, scrubbing with a mop and a disinfectant–detergent solution should be sufficient to clean and disinfect floors. Mop heads should be machine laundered and thoroughly dried daily. In the past, the selection of surface finishes was not given much attention, but as carpets have become more durable and cleanable, their use has increased.

Cabinet counters, work surfaces, and similar horizontal areas may be subject to heavy contamination during routine use. These areas should be cleaned once per day and between patient use with a disinfectant–detergent and clean cloths; application of friction during cleaning is important to ensure physical removal of dirt and contaminating microorganisms. Surfaces that are contaminated by patient specimens or accidental spills should be cleaned carefully and disinfected.

Walls, windows, and storage shelves may be reservoirs of pathogenic microorganisms if visibly soiled or if dust and dirt are allowed to accumulate. These areas and similar noncritical surfaces should be scrubbed periodically with a disinfectant–detergent solution as part of the general housekeeping program.

Faucet aerators may be useful to reduce water splashing in sinks, but they are extremely susceptible to contamination with a variety of hydrophilic bacteria. For this reason, removing aerators permanently may be preferred. Sinks should be sufficiently deep and have backsplashes to prevent splashing of hands with water pooled in the sink drain, a source of bacterial growth. Sinks should be scrubbed clean daily with a disinfectant–detergent; drain traps should not need routine cleaning or disinfection. The walls and floor surrounding the sinks should be covered with easily cleanable surfaces.

Written policies should be established for the removal and disposal of solid waste. Sturdy plastic liners should be used in trash receptacles; these liners should be sealed before they are removed from the trash receptacles. In patient care areas, trash receptacles should be cleaned and disinfected regularly. Potentially infectious material requires special handling and disposal.

Dedicated housekeeping personnel should be assigned to clean the nursery. If the nursery is small, they also may be assigned to work in the obstetric areas or other clean areas of the hospital. The nursery should be cleaned daily at an appropriate time. Intensive care nurseries ideally should be cleaned when traffic is minimal.

Cleaning and Disinfecting Patient Care Equipment

Incubators, Open Care Units, and Bassinets

After a neonate has been discharged, the care unit used by that neonate should be thoroughly cleaned and disinfected. A disinfectant–detergent registered by the U.S. Environmental Protection Agency should be used for this purpose. Manufacturers' directions for use of a disinfectant–detergent should be followed carefully. A bassinet or incubator should never be cleaned when occupied. Newborns who remain in the nursery for an extended period should be transferred periodically to a different, disinfected unit.

When a care unit is being cleaned and disinfected, all detachable parts should be removed and scrubbed meticulously. If the incubator has a fan, it should be cleaned and disinfected; the manufacturer's instructions should be followed to avoid equipment damage. The air filter should be maintained as recommended by the manufacturer. Mattresses should be replaced when the surface covering is broken; such a break precludes effective disinfection or sterilization. Mattresses may be sterilized by heat or gas. Incubator portholes and porthole cuffs and sleeves are contaminated easily and often heavily; cuffs should be replaced on a regular schedule or cleaned and disinfected frequently with freshly prepared mild soap or quaternary ammonium disinfectant–detergent solution. Incubators not in use should be dried thoroughly by running the incubator hot without water in the reservoir for 24 hours after disinfection.

Evaporative humidifiers in incubators usually do not produce contaminated aerosols, but contaminated water reservoirs may be responsible for direct, rather than airborne, transmission of infection. Reservoirs should be filled with sterile water only, and they should be drained and refilled with sterile water every 24 hours. In many areas of the United States and in hospitals with a central ventilation system, environmental humidity levels may be sufficiently high to eliminate the need for additional humidification in most cases, and water reservoirs may be left dry. If humidification is necessary, a source of humidity external to the incubator may be preferable to incubator humidifiers. An external humidifier can be changed daily and the equipment can then be sent for cleaning and sterilization or disinfection.

Nebulizers, Water Traps, and Respiratory Support Equipment

Nebulizers and attached tubing should be replaced by clean, sterile equipment (or equipment that has been subjected to high-level disinfection) in accordance with established hospital policy. Failure to replace tubing may result in contamination of freshly cleaned equipment. Water traps also should be replaced regularly by autoclaved or disinfected equipment. Only sterile water should be used for nebulizers or water traps; residual water should be discarded when these containers are refilled. Water condensed in tubing loops should be removed and discarded and should not be allowed to reflux into the container.

Other Equipment

Cleaning and disinfection or sterilization of equipment should be performed between patients. Equipment that is used for only one patient should be replaced, cleaned, and disinfected or sterilized according to an established schedule. Disposable equipment should be replaced with approximately the same frequency as reusable equipment is recycled. Disposable equipment never should be reused.

Resuscitators, face masks, laryngoscopes, eye speculums, and other items used in direct contact with neonates should be dismantled, thoroughly cleaned, and sterilized, if possible. Alternately, the equipment may be subjected to high-level disinfection with liquid chemicals or by pasteurization. Equipment such as tubing for respiratory or oxygen therapy should be sterilized or discarded after use. In-line, closed suctioning systems are thought to reduce the risk of spreading potential pathogens from the airway of intubated patients. Stethoscopes and similar types of diagnostic instruments should be wiped with iodophor or alcohol before use. Mouth-controlled suctioning should not be used. Standard precautions should be used when any type of suctioning is performed.

Nursery Linen

Procedures for laundering, making up linen packs, and delivering linen to the nursery should be established by the medical, nursing, laundry, and administrative staffs of the hospital. Each delivery of clean linen should contain sufficient linen for at least one 8-hour shift. Linen should be cleaned and transported in covered carts to the nursery areas. Autoclaving linen has not been shown to be effective in preventing infections in normal newborn nurseries or intensive care areas. New garments and linen for neonates should be laundered before use.

An established procedure for the disposal of soiled linen should be followed strictly. Chutes for the transfer of soiled linen from patient care areas to the laundry are not acceptable unless they are under negative air pressure. Soiled linen should be discarded into impervious plastic bags placed in hampers that are easy to clean and disinfect. Soiled diapers should be placed in special diaper receptacles immediately after removal from the neonate. All personnel should be aware that handling dirty diapers with bare hands can result in heavy contamination and transient colonization of the hands with microorganisms that cannot be eliminated easily with hand hygiene and are transmitted readily to the next neonate.

Plastic bags of soiled diapers and other linen should be sealed and removed from the nursery at least every 8 hours. Individuals who collect the bags of soiled diapers or linen need not enter the nursery if all bags are placed outside the nursery. Sealed bags of reusable, soiled nursery linens should be taken to the laundry at least twice each day; sealed bags of soiled diapers also should be removed from the unit at least twice per day.

Laundering

Diapers and other nursery linens should be washed separately from other hospital linen and with products used to retain softness. Acidification neutralizes the alkalis used in the washing process and is responsible for the greatest bacterial destruction. Standard precautions should be taken in handling linen soiled with blood. Chlorine bleach should be used for any items that are contaminated with blood.

Trichlorocarbanilide and the sodium salt of pentachlorophenol should not be used in hospital laundering because they may be harmful. Therefore, caution should be exercised when new laundry or cleaning agents are introduced into the nursery or when procedures are changed.

Resources

American Academy of Pediatrics. Red book: 2006 report of the Committee on Infectious Diseases. 27th ed. Elk Grove Village (IL): AAP; 2006.

Belkin N. Home laundering of soiled surgical scrubs: surgical site infections and the home environment. Am J Infect Control 2001;29:58–64.

Boyce JM, Pittet D. Guideline for hand hygiene in health-care settings. Recommendations of the Healthcare Infection Control Practices Advisory Committee and the HICPAC/SHEA/APIC/IDSA Hand Hygiene Task Force. Society for Healthcare Epidemiology of America/Association for Professionals in Infection Control/Infectious Diseases Society of America. MMWR Recomm Rep 2002;51(RR-16):1–45;quiz CE1–4.

Centers for Disease Control and Prevention. Guidelines for environmental infection control in health-care facilities. Recommendations of CDC and the Healthcare Infection Control Practices Advisory Committee (HICPAC). Atlanta (GA): CDC; 2003.

Centers for Disease Control and Prevention. Laundry: washing infected materials. Atlanta (GA): CDC; 2000. Available at: http://www.cdc.gov/ncidod/dhqp/bp_laundry.html. Retrieved December 15, 2006.

Environmental Protection Agency. Antimicrobial pesticide products. Washington, DC: EPA; 2004. Available at http://www.epa.gov/pesticides/factsheets/antimic.htm. Retrieved January 3, 2007.

Garner JS. Guideline for isolation precautions in hospitals. Part I. Evolution of isolation practices, Hospital Infection Control Practices Advisory Committee. Am J Infect Control 1996;24:24–31.

Garner JS. Guideline for isolation precautions in hospitals. The Hospital Infection Control Practices Advisory Committee [published erratum appears in Infect Control Hosp Epidemiol 1996;17:214]. Infect Control Hosp Epidemiol 1996;17:53–80.

Hinson P. The infection control professional as a learner. In: Association of Professionals in Infection Control and Epidemiology. APIC infection control and applied epidemiology. St. Louis (MO): Mosby; 1996. p.32-1–32-2.

Jurkovich P. Home- versus hospital-laundered scrubs: a pilot study. MCN Am J Matern Child Nurs 2004;29:106–10.

Moolenaar RL, Crutcher JM, San Joaquin VH, Sewell LV, Hutwagner LC, Carson LA, et al. A prolonged outbreak of Pseudomonas aeruginosa in a neonatal intensive care unit: did staff fingernails play a role in disease transmission? Infect Control Hosp Epidemiol 2000;21:80–5.

Needlestick Safety and Prevention Act, Pub L. No. 106–430, 114 Stat. 1901, 2000.

O'Grady NP, Alexander M, Dellinger EP, Gerberding JL, Heard SO, Maki DG, et al. Guidelines for the prevention of intravascular-catheter related infections. Centers for Disease Control and Prevention. MMWR Recomm Rep 2002;51(RR-10):1–29.

Polizzi J, Byers JF, Kiehl E. Co-bedding versus traditional bedding of multiple-gestation infants in NICU. J Health Qual 2003;25:5–10; quiz 10–1.

Updated U.S. Public Health Service guidelines for occupational exposure to HIV. MMWR Morb Mortal Wkly Rep 1996;45:468–80.

appendix A

ACOG Antepartum Record and Postpartum Form

DATE _____

NAME _____
    LAST   FIRST   MIDDLE

ID # _____ HOSPITAL OF DELIVERY _____

NEWBORN'S PHYSICIAN _____ REFERRED BY _____

PRIMARY PROVIDER/GROUP _____

FINAL EDD _____

ADDRESS _____

BIRTH DATE	AGE	RACE	MARITAL STATUS S M W D SEP	ADDRESS
MONTH DAY YEAR				
OCCUPATION			EDUCATION (LAST GRADE COMPLETED)	ZIP / PHONE / (H) / (O)
LANGUAGE			ETHNICITY	INSURANCE CARRIER/MEDICAID #
HUSBAND/DOMESTIC PARTNER		PHONE		POLICY #
FATHER OF BABY		PHONE		EMERGENCY CONTACT / PHONE

TOTAL PREG	FULL TERM	PREMATURE	AB. INDUCED	AB. SPONTANEOUS	ECTOPICS	MULTIPLE BIRTHS	LIVING

MENSTRUAL HISTORY

LMP: ☐ DEFINITE ☐ APPROXIMATE (MONTH KNOWN)   MENSES MONTHLY ☐ YES ☐ NO   FREQUENCY: Q _____ DAYS   MENARCHE _____ (AGE ONSET)
    ☐ UNKNOWN ☐ NORMAL AMOUNT/DURATION   PRIOR MENSES _____ DATE   ON BCP AT CONCEPT ☐ YES ☐ NO   hCG + ___/___/___
    ☐ FINAL _____

PAST PREGNANCIES (LAST SIX)

DATE MONTH/YEAR	GA WEEKS	LENGTH OF LABOR	BIRTH WEIGHT	SEX M/F	TYPE DELIVERY	ANES.	PLACE OF DELIVERY	PRETERM LABOR YES/NO	COMMENTS/ COMPLICATIONS

MEDICAL HISTORY

	O Neg. + Pos.	DETAIL POSITIVE REMARKS INCLUDE DATE & TREATMENT		O Neg. + Pos.	DETAIL POSITIVE REMARKS INCLUDE DATE & TREATMENT
1. DIABETES			17. D (Rh) SENSITIZED		
2. HYPERTENSION			18. PULMONARY (TB, ASTHMA)		
3. HEART DISEASE			19. SEASONAL ALLERGIES		
4. AUTOIMMUNE DISORDER			20. DRUG/LATEX ALLERGIES/ REACTIONS		
5. KIDNEY DISEASE/UTI					
6. NEUROLOGIC/EPILEPSY			21. BREAST		
7. PSYCHIATRIC			22. GYN SURGERY		
8. DEPRESSION/POSTPARTUM DEPRESSION			23. OPERATIONS/ HOSPITALIZATIONS (YEAR & REASON)		
9. HEPATITIS/LIVER DISEASE					
10. VARICOSITIES/PHLEBITIS			24. ANESTHETIC COMPLICATIONS		
11. THYROID DYSFUNCTION			25. HISTORY OF ABNORMAL PAP		
12. TRAUMA/VIOLENCE			26. UTERINE ANOMALY/DES		
13. HISTORY OF BLOOD TRANSFUS.			27. INFERTILITY		

	AMT/DAY PREPREG	AMT/DAY PREG	# YEARS USE			
14. TOBACCO				28. ART TREATMENT		
15. ALCOHOL				29. RELEVANT FAMILY HISTORY		
16. ILLICIT/RECREATIONAL DRUGS				30. OTHER		

COMMENTS _____

ACOG ANTEPARTUM RECORD (FORM A)

Patient Addressograph

SYMPTOMS SINCE LMP

GENETIC SCREENING/TERATOLOGY COUNSELING
INCLUDES PATIENT, BABY'S FATHER, OR ANYONE IN EITHER FAMILY WITH:

	YES	NO		YES	NO
1. PATIENT'S AGE 35 YEARS OR OLDER AS OF ESTIMATED DATE OF DELIVERY			13. HUNTINGTON'S CHOREA		
			14. MENTAL RETARDATION/AUTISM		
2. THALASSEMIA (ITALIAN, GREEK, MEDITERRANEAN, OR ASIAN BACKGROUND): MCV LESS THAN 80			IF YES, WAS PERSON TESTED FOR FRAGILE X?		
3. NEURAL TUBE DEFECT (MENINGOMYELOCELE, SPINA BIFIDA, OR ANENCEPHALY)			15. OTHER INHERITED GENETIC OR CHROMOSOMAL DISORDER		
			16. MATERNAL METABOLIC DISORDER (EG. TYPE 1 DIABETES, PKU)		
4. CONGENITAL HEART DEFECT			17. PATIENT OR BABY'S FATHER HAD A CHILD WITH BIRTH DEFECTS NOT LISTED ABOVE		
5. DOWN SYNDROME					
6. TAY-SACHS (ASHKENAZI JEWISH, CAJUN, FRENCH CANADIAN)			18. RECURRENT PREGNANCY LOSS, OR A STILLBIRTH		
7. CANAVAN DISEASE (ASHKENAZI JEWISH)			19. MEDICATIONS (INCLUDING SUPPLEMENTS, VITAMINS, HERBS OR OTC DRUGS)/ILLICIT/RECREATIONAL DRUGS/ALCOHOL SINCE LAST MENSTRUAL PERIOD		
8. FAMILIAL DYSAUTONOMIA (ASHKENAZI JEWISH)					
9. SICKLE CELL DISEASE OR TRAIT (AFRICAN)			IF YES, AGENT(S) AND STRENGTH/DOSAGE		
10. HEMOPHILIA OR OTHER BLOOD DISORDERS			20. ANY OTHER		
11. MUSCULAR DYSTROPHY					
12. CYSTIC FIBROSIS					

COMMENTS/COUNSELING _____

INFECTION HISTORY	YES	NO	
1. LIVE WITH SOMEONE WITH TB OR EXPOSED TO TB			4. HEPATITIS B, C YES ☐ NO ☐
2. PATIENT OR PARTNER HAS HISTORY OF GENITAL HERPES			5. HISTORY OF STD, GONORRHEA, CHLAMYDIA, HPV, HIV, SYPHILIS (CIRCLE ALL THAT APPLY)
3. RASH OR VIRAL ILLNESS SINCE LAST MENSTRUAL PERIOD			6. OTHER (SEE COMMENTS)

COMMENTS _____

_____ INTERVIEWER'S SIGNATURE _____

INITIAL PHYSICAL EXAMINATION

DATE ____ / ____ / ____   WEIGHT _____   HEIGHT _____   BMI _____   BP _____

1. HEENT	☐ NORMAL	☐ ABNORMAL	12. VULVA	☐ NORMAL	☐ CONDYLOMA	☐ LESIONS
2. FUNDI	☐ NORMAL	☐ ABNORMAL	13. VAGINA	☐ NORMAL	☐ INFLAMMATION	☐ DISCHARGE
3. TEETH	☐ NORMAL	☐ ABNORMAL	14. CERVIX	☐ NORMAL	☐ INFLAMMATION	☐ LESIONS
4. THYROID	☐ NORMAL	☐ ABNORMAL	15. UTERUS SIZE	____ WEEKS		☐ FIBROIDS
5. BREASTS	☐ NORMAL	☐ ABNORMAL	16. ADNEXA	☐ NORMAL	☐ MASS	
6. LUNGS	☐ NORMAL	☐ ABNORMAL	17. RECTUM	☐ NORMAL	☐ ABNORMAL	
7. HEART	☐ NORMAL	☐ ABNORMAL	18. DIAGONAL CONJUGATE	☐ REACHED	☐ NO	____ CM
8. ABDOMEN	☐ NORMAL	☐ ABNORMAL	19. SPINES	☐ AVERAGE	☐ PROMINENT	☐ BLUNT
9. EXTREMITIES	☐ NORMAL	☐ ABNORMAL	20. SACRUM	☐ CONCAVE	☐ STRAIGHT	☐ ANTERIOR
10. SKIN	☐ NORMAL	☐ ABNORMAL	21. SUBPUBIC ARCH	☐ NORMAL	☐ WIDE	☐ NARROW
11. LYMPH NODES	☐ NORMAL	☐ ABNORMAL	22. GYNECOID PELVIC TYPE	☐ YES	☐ NO	

COMMENTS (Number and explain abnormals) _____

_____ EXAM BY _____

ACOG ANTEPARTUM RECORD (FORM B)

Patient Addressograph

NAME _____
         LAST   FIRST   MIDDLE

DRUG ALLERGY_____ | LATEX ALLERGY   ☐ YES   ☐ NO

IS BLOOD TRANSFUSION ACCEPTABLE?   ☐ YES   ☐ NO | ANTEPARTUM ANESTHESIA CONSULT PLANNED   ☐ YES   ☐ NO

PROBLEMS/PLANS

1. _____

2. _____

3. _____

4. _____

5. _____

6. _____

MEDICATION LIST
(Include Dosage)   Start date   Stop date

1. _____   ___/___/___   ___/___/___

2. _____   ___/___/___   ___/___/___

3. _____   ___/___/___   ___/___/___

4. _____   ___/___/___   ___/___/___

5. _____   ___/___/___   ___/___/___

6. _____   ___/___/___   ___/___/___

EDD CONFIRMATION		**18–20-WEEK EDD UPDATE**	
INITIAL EDD		QUICKENING ___/___/___ +22 WKS = ___/___/___	
LMP ___/___/___ = EDD ___/___/___		FUNDAL HT	
INITIAL EXAM ___/___/___ = ___ WKS = EDD ___/___/___		AT UMBIL ___/___/___ +20 WKS = ___/___/___	
ULTRASOUND ___/___/___ = ___ WKS = EDD ___/___/___		ULTRASOUND ___/___/___ = ___ WKS = ___/___/___	
INITIAL EDD ___/___/___ INITIALED BY _____		FINAL EDD ___/___/___ INITIALED BY _____	

PREPREGNANCY WEIGHT
_____

WEEKS GEST (BEST EST.)	FUNDAL HEIGHT (CM)	PRESENTATION	FHR	FETAL MOVEMENT	PRETERM LABOR SIGNS/SYMPTOMS +=PRESENT 0=ABSENT	CERVIX EXAM (DIL./EFF./STA.) ULTRASOUND LENGTH	BLOOD PRESSURE	WEIGHT	URINE (ALBUMIN/GLUCOSE)	EDEMA	PAIN SCALE (0-10)	NEXT APPOINTMENT	PROVIDER (INITIALS)	COMMENTS

PROBLEMS _____

COMMENTS _____

*Describe the intensity of discomfort ranging from 0 (no pain) to 10 (worst possible pain).

ACOG ANTEPARTUM RECORD (FORM C)

Patient Addressograph

LABORATORY AND EDUCATION

INITIAL LABS	DATE	RESULT	REVIEWED
BLOOD TYPE	/ /	A B AB O	
D (Rh) TYPE	/ /		
ANTIBODY SCREEN	/ /		
HCT/HGB/MCV	/ /	_____ % _____ g/dL	
PAP TEST	/ /	NORMAL/ABNORMAL/_____	
VARICELLA	/ /		
RUBELLA	/ /		
VDRL	/ /		
URINE CULTURE/SCREEN	/ /		
HBsAg	/ /		
HIV COUNSELING/TESTING*	/ /	POS. NEG. DECLINED	

OPTIONAL LABS	DATE	RESULT	
HEMOGLOBIN ELECTROPHORESIS	/ /	AA AS SS AC SC AF ↑A₂ POS. NEG. DECLINED	
PPD	/ /		
CHLAMYDIA	/ /		
GONORRHEA	/ /		
CYSTIC FIBROSIS	/ /	POS. NEG. DECLINED	
TAY-SACHS	/ /	POS. NEG. DECLINED	
FAMILIAL DYSAUTONOMIA	/ /	POS. NEG. DECLINED	
HEMOGLOBIN			
GENETIC SCREENING TESTS (SEE FORM B)	/ /		
OTHER			

8–20-WEEK LABS (WHEN INDICATED/ELECTED)	DATE	RESULT	
ULTRASOUND	/ /		
1ST TRIMESTER ANEUPLOIDY RISK ASSESSMENT	/ /	POS. NEG. DECLINED	
MSAFP/MULTIPLE MARKERS	/ /	POS. NEG. DECLINED	
2ND TRIMESTER SERUM SCREENING	/ /	POS. NEG. DECLINED	
AMNIO/CVS	/ /		
KARYOTYPE	/ /	46,XX OR 46,XY/OTHER_____	
AMNIOTIC FLUID (AFP)	/ /	NORMAL_____ ABNORMAL_____	
ANTI-D IMMUNE GLOBULIN (RHIG)	/ /		

COMMENTS/ADDITIONAL LABS

*Check state requirements before recording results.   (CONTINUED)

PROVIDER SIGNATURE (AS REQUIRED) _____

ACOG ANTEPARTUM RECORD (FORM D)

LABORATORY AND EDUCATION *(continued)*

24–28-WEEK LABS (WHEN INDICATED)	DATE	RESULT		COMMENTS/ADDITIONAL LABS
HCT/HGB/MCV	/ /	_____ % _____ g/dL		
DIABETES SCREEN	/ /	1 HOUR_____		
GTT (IF SCREEN ABNORMAL)	/ /	_____FBS _____1 HOUR		
		_____2 HOUR _____3 HOUR		
D (Rh) ANTIBODY SCREEN	/ /			
ANTI-D IMMUNE GLOBULIN (RhIG) GIVEN (28 WKS OR GREATER)	/ /	SIGNATURE _____		

32–36-WEEK LABS	DATE	RESULT	
HCT/HGB	/ /	_____ % _____ g/dL	
ULTRASOUND (WHEN INDICATED)	/ /		
HIV (WHEN INDICATED)*			
VDRL (WHEN INDICATED)	/ /		
GONORRHEA (WHEN INDICATED)	/ /		
CHLAMYDIA (WHEN INDICATED)	/ /		
GROUP B STREP	/ /		

*Check state requirements before recording results.

COMMENTS

_____
_____
_____
_____
_____
_____

ACOG ANTEPARTUM RECORD (FORM D, *continued*)

PROVIDER SIGNATURE (AS REQUIRED) _____

Patient Addressograph

NAME _____
      LAST   FIRST   MIDDLE

PLANS/EDUCATION
(COUNSELED ☐)—BY TRIMESTER. INITIAL AND DATE WHEN DISCUSSED.

FIRST TRIMESTER	COMPLETED	NEED FOR FURTHER DISCUSSION
☐ HIV AND OTHER ROUTINE PRENATAL TESTS		☐ FOLLOW-UP IN 3RD TRIMESTER, IF NEEDED
☐ RISK FACTORS IDENTIFIED BY PRENATAL HISTORY		
☐ ANTICIPATED COURSE OF PRENATAL CARE		
☐ NUTRITION AND WEIGHT GAIN COUNSELING; SPECIAL DIET		
☐ TOXOPLASMOSIS PRECAUTIONS (CATS/RAW MEAT)		
☐ SEXUAL ACTIVITY		
☐ EXERCISE		
☐ INFLUENZA VACCINE		
☐ SMOKING COUNSELING		
☐ ENVIRONMENTAL/WORK HAZARDS		
☐ TRAVEL		
☐ TOBACCO (ASK, ADVISE, ASSESS, ASSIST, AND ARRANGE)		
☐ ALCOHOL		
☐ ILLICIT/RECREATIONAL DRUGS		
☐ USE OF ANY MEDICATIONS (INCLUDING SUPPLEMENTS, VITAMINS, HERBS, OR OTC DRUGS)		
☐ INDICATIONS FOR ULTRASOUND		
☐ DOMESTIC VIOLENCE		
☐ SEAT BELT USE		
☐ CHILDBIRTH CLASSES/HOSPITAL FACILITIES		
SECOND TRIMESTER		
☐ SIGNS AND SYMPTOMS OF PRETERM LABOR		
☐ ABNORMAL LAB VALUES		
☐ INFLUENZA VACCINE		
☐ SELECTING A NEWBORN CARE PROVIDER		
☐ SMOKING COUNSELING		
☐ DOMESTIC VIOLENCE		
☐ POSTPARTUM FAMILY PLANNING/TUBAL STERILIZATION		

(CONTINUED)

COMMENTS

ACOG ANTEPARTUM RECORD (FORM E)

PLANS/EDUCATION *(continued)*
(COUNSELED ☐)—BY TRIMESTER. INITIAL AND DATE WHEN DISCUSSED.

THIRD TRIMESTER	COMPLETED	NEED FOR FURTHER DISCUSSION
☐ ANESTHESIA/ANALGESIA PLANS		
☐ FETAL MOVEMENT MONITORING		
☐ LABOR SIGNS		
☐ VBAC COUNSELING		
☐ SIGNS AND SYMPTOMS OF PREGNANCY-INDUCED HYPERTENSION		
☐ POSTTERM COUNSELING		
☐ CIRCUMCISION		
☐ BREAST OR BOTTLE FEEDING		
☐ POSTPARTUM DEPRESSION		
☐ INFLUENZA VACCINE		
☐ SMOKING COUNSELING		
☐ DOMESTIC VIOLENCE		
☐ NEWBORN EDUCATION (NEWBORN SCREENING, JAUNDICE, SIDS, CAR SEAT)		
☐ FAMILY MEDICAL LEAVE OR DISABILITY FORMS		

REQUESTS

TUBAL STERILIZATION CONSENT SIGNED   DATE   INITIALS
                                          ___/___/___   _____

HISTORY AND PHYSICAL HAVE BEEN SENT TO HOSPITAL, IF APPLICABLE.   DATE   INITIALS
                                          ___/___/___   _____

COMMENTS

ACOG ANTEPARTUM RECORD (FORM E, *continued*)

Plans/Education Notes

_____
_____
_____
_____
_____
_____
_____
_____
_____
_____
_____
_____
_____
_____
_____
_____
_____
_____
_____
_____
_____
_____
_____
_____
_____
_____
_____
_____
_____
_____
_____

ACOG ANTEPARTUM RECORD (FORM E, *continued*)

Patient Addressograph

NAME ____
LAST FIRST MIDDLE

ID # ____

EDD ____________________

Supplemental Visits

PREPREGNANCY WEIGHT ________

	WEEKS GEST. (BEST EST.)	FUNDAL HEIGHT (CM)	PRESENTATION	FHR	FETAL MOVEMENT	PRETERM LABOR SIGNS/SYMPTOMS: +=PRESENT o=ABSENT	CERVIX EXAM (DIL/EFF/STA.) ULTRASOUND LENGTH	BLOOD PRESSURE	WEIGHT	URINE (ALBUMIN/GLUCOSE)	EDEMA	PAIN SCALE* (0-10)	NEXT APPOINTMENT	PROVIDER (INITIALS)

COMMENTS

*Describe the intensity of discomfort ranging from 0 (no pain) to 10 (worst possible pain).

Progress Notes

PROVIDER SIGNATURE (AS REQUIRED) ______________________________

ACOG ANTEPARTUM RECORD (FORM F)

Patient Addressograph

NAME _____
        LAST   FIRST   MIDDLE

ID # _____

EDD _____

Supplemental Visits

PREPREGNANCY
WEIGHT
_____

Column headers (angled): WEEKS GEST (BEST EST.) | FUNDAL HEIGHT (CM) | PRESENTATION | FHR | FETAL MOVEMENT | PRETERM LABOR SIGNS/SYMPTOMS (+) PRESENT (0=) ABSENT | CERVIX EXAM (DIL./EFF./STA.) ULTRASOUND LENGTH | BLOOD PRESSURE | WEIGHT | URINE (ALBUMIN/GLUCOSE) | EDEMA | PAIN SCALE* (0–10) | NEXT APPOINTMENT | PROVIDER (INITIALS)

COMMENTS

*Describe the intensity of discomfort ranging from 0 (no pain) to 10 (worst possible pain).

Progress Notes

PROVIDER SIGNATURE (AS REQUIRED)_____

ACOG ANTEPARTUM RECORD (FORM F, continued)

NAME _____
　　　LAST　　　　　　　　　　　FIRST　　　　　　　　　MIDDLE

ID # _____

Progress Notes

_____
_____
_____
_____
_____
_____
_____
_____
_____
_____
_____
_____
_____
_____
_____
_____
_____
_____
_____
_____
_____
_____
_____
_____
_____
_____
_____
_____
_____
_____
_____
_____

PROVIDER SIGNATURE (AS REQUIRED)_____

ACOG ANTEPARTUM RECORD (FORM G)

Patient Addressograph

NAME _____
         LAST   FIRST   MIDDLE

ID # _____

Progress Notes

_____
_____
_____
_____
_____
_____
_____
_____
_____
_____
_____
_____
_____
_____
_____
_____
_____
_____
_____
_____
_____
_____
_____
_____
_____
_____
_____
_____
_____
_____
_____

PROVIDER SIGNATURE (AS REQUIRED)_____

ACOG ANTEPARTUM RECORD (FORM G, *continued*)

POSTPARTUM FORM

NAME _____
LAST   FIRST   MIDDLE

DELIVERY DATE _____   HOSPITAL _____

DISCHARGE DATE _____

DELIVERY INFORMATION

DELIVERY AT_____WEEKS

			LABOR	ANESTHESIA
☐ VAGINAL	☐ CESAREAN	TUBAL STERILIZATION ☐ YES ☐ NO	☐ NONE	☐ NONE
☐ SVD	☐ PRIMARY (For_____)	NOTES _____	☐ SPONTANEOUS	☐ LOCAL/PUDENDAL
☐ VACUUM	☐ REPEAT - ELECTIVE	_____	☐ INDUCED	☐ EPIDURAL
☐ FORCEPS	☐ REPEAT - UNSUCCESSFUL VBAC	_____	☐ AUGMENTED	☐ SPINAL
☐ EPISIOTOMY	☐ INCISION	_____		☐ GENERAL
☐ LACERATIONS	☐ LOW TRANSVERSE	_____		☐ OTHER
☐ VBAC	☐ LOW VERTICAL	_____		
	☐ CLASSICAL	DELIVERED BY_____		

POSTPARTUM INFORMATION

COMPLICATIONS

☐ NONE   ☐ HEMORRHAGE   ☐ INFECTION   ☐ HYPERTENSION   ☐ DIABETES   ☐ OTHER _____

DISCHARGE INFORMATION

NEONATAL INFORMATION

NAME OF BABY _____

SEX
☐ FEMALE   ☐ MALE
            CIRCUMCISION ☐ YES ☐ NO

BIRTH WEIGHT _____

DISPOSITION
☐ HOME WITH MOTHER   ☐ IN HOSPITAL
☐ TRANSFER   ☐ NEONATAL DEATH
☐ STILLBIRTH   ☐ OTHER

COMPLICATIONS/ANOMALIES _____
_____
_____

NEWBORN CARE PROVIDER _____

MATERNAL INFORMATION

☐ NONSMOKER   ☐ QUIT SMOKING DURING PREGNANCY

☐ CURRENT SMOKER

HGB/HCT LEVEL _____

MEDICATIONS _____
_____

FEEDING METHOD   ☐ BREAST   ☐ BOTTLE

CONTRACEPTIVE METHOD (IF APPLICABLE) _____
_____

DIAGNOSTIC STUDIES PENDING _____
_____
_____

SECONDARY DIAGNOSIS/PREEXISTING CONDITIONS
☐ ASTHMA   ☐ HYPERTENSION
☐ DIABETES   ☐ OTHER _____

IMMUNIZATIONS GIVEN
☐ ANTI-D IMMUNE GLOBULIN
☐ RUBELLA
☐ OTHER _____
_____

FOLLOW-UP APPT
DATE _____
LOCATION _____
OTHER _____
_____
_____
_____

INTERIM CONTACTS

DATE	COMMENT
_____	_____
_____	_____
_____	_____
_____	_____
_____	_____
_____	_____
_____	_____
_____	_____

PROVIDER SIGNATURE (AS REQUIRED)_____

DATE _____

LAB STUDIES REQUESTED _____

_____

HGB/HCT _____ LAST PAP TEST _____

FEEDING METHOD _____

CONTRACEPTIVE METHOD _____

POSTPARTUM DEPRESSION SCREENING _____

INTIMATE PARTNER VIOLENCE SCREENING _____

DIABETES _____

DISCUSS PREVENTION OF
RELAPSE TO SMOKING TECHNIQUES _____

INTERIM HISTORY

_____

_____

_____

_____

PHYSICAL EXAM

BP _____   WT _____

BREASTS   ☐ NORMAL _____

ABDOMEN   ☐ NORMAL _____

EXTERNAL GENITALS ☐ NORMAL _____

VAGINA   ☐ NORMAL _____

CERVIX   ☐ NORMAL _____

UTERUS   ☐ NORMAL _____

ADNEXA   ☐ NORMAL _____

RECTAL-VAGINAL   ☐ NORMAL _____

PAP TEST   ☐ YES   ☐ NO

COMMENT

_____

_____

_____

_____

_____

_____

_____

_____

_____

_____

_____

_____

_____

_____

_____

_____

_____

_____

_____

_____

ALLERGIES _____

_____

MEDICATIONS/CONTRACEPTION _____

_____

_____

_____

☐ DISPENSED

INTERVAL CARE RECOMMENDATIONS

FOR GENERAL HEALTH PROMOTION _____

_____

_____

_____

_____

_____

FOR REPRODUCTIVE HEALTH PROMOTION _____

_____

_____

_____

_____

_____

RETURN VISIT _____

REFERRALS _____

_____

EXAMINED BY _____

PROVIDER SIGNATURE (AS REQUIRED)_____

appendix B

Early Pregnancy Risk Identification for Consultation

Risk Factor	Recommended Consultation*
Medical history and conditions	
Asthma	
Symptomatic on medication	Obstetrician-gynecologist
Severe (multiple hospitalizations)	MFM subspecialist
Cardiac disease	
Cyanotic, prior MI, aortic stenosis, pulmonary hypertension, Marfan syndrome, prosthetic valve, AHA Class II or greater	MFM subspecialist
Other	Obstetrician-gynecologist
Diabetes mellitus	
Class A-C	Obstetrician-gynecologist
Class D or greater	MFM subspecialist
Drug and alcohol use	Obstetrician-gynecologist
Epilepsy (on medication)	Obstetrician-gynecologist
Family history of genetic problems (Down syndrome, Tay-Sachs disease, PKU)	MFM subspecialist
Hemoglobinopathy (SS, SC, S-thal)	MFM subspecialist
Hypertension	
Chronic, with renal or heart disease	MFM subspecialist
Chronic, without renal or heart disease	Obstetrician-gynecologist
Prior pulmonary embolus or deep vein thrombosis	Obstetrician-gynecologist
Psychiatric illness	Obstetrician-gynecologist
Pulmonary disease	
Severe obstructive or restrictive	MFM subspecialist
Moderate	Obstetrician-gynecologist

(continued)

Early Pregnancy Risk Identification for Consultation (*continued*)

Risk Factor	Recommended Consultation*
Renal disease	
Chronic, creatinine ≥3 with or without hypertension	MFM subspecialist
Chronic, other	Obstetrician–gynecologist
Requirement for prolonged anticoagulation	MFM subspecialist
Severe systemic disease	MFM subspecialist
Obstetric history and conditions	
Age ≥35 at delivery	Obstetrician–gynecologist
Cesarean delivery, prior classical or vertical incision	Obstetrician–gynecologist
Incompetent cervix	Obstetrician–gynecologist
Prior fetal structural or chromosomal abnormality	MFM subspecialist
Prior neonatal death	Obstetrician–gynecologist
Prior fetal death	Obstetrician–gynecologist
Prior preterm delivery or preterm PROM	Obstetrician–gynecologist
Prior low birth weight (<2,500 g)	Obstetrician–gynecologist
Second-trimester pregnancy loss	Obstetrician–gynecologist
Uterine leiomyomata or malformation	Obstetrician–gynecologist
Initial laboratory tests	
HIV	
Symptomatic or low CD4 count	MFM subspecialist
Other	Obstetrician–gynecologist
CDE (Rh) or other blood group isoimmunization (excluding ABO, Lewis)	MFM subspecialist
Initial examination—condylomata (extensive, covering vulva or vaginal opening)	Obstetrician–gynecologist

Abbreviations: AHA, American Heart Association; HIV, human immunodeficiency virus; MFM, maternal–fetal medicine; MI, myocardial infarction; PKU, phenylketonuria; PROM, premature rupture of membranes.

*At the time of consultation, continued patient care should be determined to be by collaboration with the referring care provider or by transfer of care.

Modified from March of Dimes Birth Defects Foundation, Committee on Perinatal Health. Toward improving the outcome of pregnancy: the 90s and beyond. White Plains, New York: March of Dimes Birth Defects Foundation, 1993.

Ongoing Pregnancy Risk Identification for Consultation

Risk Factor	Recommended Consultation*
Medical history and conditions	
Drug/alcohol use	Obstetrician–gynecologist
Proteinuria (≥2+ by catheter sample, unexplained by urinary tract infection)	Obstetrician–gynecologist
Pyelonephritis	Obstetrician–gynecologist
Severe systemic disease that adversely affects pregnancy	MFM subspecialist
Obstetric history and conditions	
Blood pressure elevation (diastolic ≥90 mm Hg), no proteinuria	Obstetrician–gynecologist
Fetal growth restriction suspected	Obstetrician–gynecologist
Fetal abnormality suspected by ultrasonography	
Anencephaly	Obstetrician–gynecologist
Other	MFM subspecialist
Fetal demise	Obstetrician–gynecologist
Gestational age 41 weeks (to be seen by 42 weeks)	Obstetrician–gynecologist
Gestational diabetes mellitus	Obstetrician–gynecologist
Herpes, active lesions 36 weeks	Obstetrician–gynecologist
Hydramnios by ultrasonography	Obstetrician–gynecologist
Hyperemesis, persisting beyond first trimester	Obstetrician–gynecologist
Multiple gestation	Obstetrician–gynecologist
Oligohydramnios by ultrasonography	Obstetrician–gynecologist
Preterm labor, threatened, <37 weeks	Obstetrician–gynecologist
Premature rupture of membranes	Obstetrician–gynecologist
Vaginal bleeding ≥14 weeks	Obstetrician–gynecologist

(continued)

Ongoing Pregnancy Risk Identification for Consultation *(continued)*

Risk Factor	Recommended Consultation*
Examination and laboratory findings	
Abnormal MSAFP (low or high)	Obstetrician–gynecologist
Abnormal Pap test result	Obstetrician–gynecologist
Anemia (Hct <28%, unresponsive to iron therapy)	Obstetrician–gynecologist
Condylomata (extensive, covering labia and vaginal opening)	Obstetrician–gynecologist
HIV	
Symptomatic or low CD4 count	MFM subspecialist
Other	Obstetrician–gynecologist
CDE (Rh) or other blood group isoimmunization (excluding ABO, Lewis)	MFM subspecialist

Abbreviations: Hct, hematocrit; HIV, human immunodeficiency virus; MFM, maternal–fetal medicine; MSAFP, maternal serum alpha-fetoprotein.

*At the time of consultation, continued patient care should be determined to be by collaboration with the referring care provider or by transfer of care.

Modified from March of Dimes Birth Defects Foundation, Committee on Perinatal Health. Toward improving the outcome of pregnancy: the 90s and beyond. White Plains, New York: March of Dimes Birth Defects Foundation, 1993.

appendix D

Standard Terminology for Reporting of Reproductive Health Statistics in the United States*

The adoption of standard definitions and reporting requirements for reproductive health statistics will provide an improved basis for standardization and uniformity in the design, implementation, and evaluation of intervention strategies. The reduction of maternal and infant mortality and the improvement of the health of our nation's women and infants are the ultimate goals. The collection and analysis of reliable statistical data are an essential part of in-depth investigations and incorporate case finding, individual review, and analysis of risk factors. These studies could then yield valuable clinical information for practitioners, aiding them in improved case management for patients at high risk, which would result in decreased morbidity and mortality.

Both the collection and the use of statistics have been hampered by lack of understanding of differences in definitions, statistical tabulations, and reporting requirements among state, national, and international bodies. Misapplication and misinterpretation of data may lead to erroneous comparisons and conclusions. For example, specific requirements for reporting of fetal deaths often have been misinterpreted as implying a weight or gestational age for viability. Distinctions can and should be made among: 1) the definition of an event, 2) the reporting requirements for the event, and 3) the statistical tabulation and interpretation of the data. The definition indicates the meaning of a term (eg, live birth, fetal death, or maternal death). A reporting requirement

---

*Different states use different birth weight and gestational age criteria to define fetal death. The Committee on Obstetric Practice of the American College of Obstetricians and Gynecologists recommends that perinatal mortality statistics be based on a gestational weight of 500 g.

is that part of the defined event for which reporting is mandatory or desired. Statistical tabulations connote the presentation of data for the purpose of analysis and interpretation of existing and future conditions. The data should be collected in a manner that will allow them to be presented in different ways for different users. Adjustments should be made for variations in reporting before comparisons among data are attempted.

If information is collected and presented in a standardized manner, comparisons between the new data and the data obtained by previous reporting requirements can be delineated clearly and can contribute to improved public understanding of reproductive health statistics. For ease in assimilating this information, it is divided into three sections: 1) definitions, 2) statistical tabulations, and 3) reporting requirements and recommendations. Some of the definitions and recommendations are a departure from those currently or historically accepted; however, these recommendations were agreed on by an interorganizational group that was brought together in the mid 1980s to review terminology related to reproductive health issues.

Definitions

Live birth: The complete expulsion or extraction from the mother of a product of human conception, irrespective of the duration of pregnancy, which, after such expulsion or extraction, breathes or shows any other evidence of life, such as beating of the heart, pulsation of the umbilical cord, or definite movement of voluntary muscles, whether or not the umbilical cord has been cut or the placenta is attached. Heartbeats are to be distinguished from transient cardiac contractions; respirations are to be distinguished from fleeting respiratory efforts or gasps.

Birth weight: The weight of a neonate determined immediately after delivery or as soon thereafter as feasible. It should be expressed to the nearest gram.

Gestational age: The number of weeks that have elapsed between the first day of the last normal menstrual period (not the presumed time of conception) and the date of delivery, irrespective of whether the gestation results in a live birth or a fetal death.

Neonate:

Low birth weight—Any neonate, regardless of gestational age, whose weight at birth is less than 2,500 g.

Preterm*—Any neonate whose birth occurs through the end of the last day of the 37th week (259th day) following the onset of the last menstrual period.

Term—Any neonate whose birth occurs from the beginning of the first day (260th day) of the 38th week through the end of the last day of the 42nd week (294th day) following the onset of the last menstrual period.

Postterm—Any neonate whose birth occurs from the beginning of the first day (295th day) of the 43rd week following the onset of the last menstrual period.

Fetal death: Death before the complete expulsion or extraction from the mother of a product of human conception, fetus and placenta, irrespective of the duration of pregnancy; the death is indicated by the fact that, after such expulsion or extraction, the fetus does not breathe or show any other evidence of life, such as beating of the heart, pulsation of the umbilical cord, or definite movement of voluntary muscles. Heartbeats are to be distinguished from transient cardiac contractions; respirations are to be distinguished from fleeting respiratory efforts or gasps. This definition excludes induced termination of pregnancy.

Neonatal death: Death of a liveborn neonate before the neonate becomes age 28 days (up to and including 27 days, 23 hours, and 59 minutes from the moment of birth).

Infant death: Any death at any time from birth up to, but not including, 1 year of age (364 days, 23 hours, and 59 minutes from the moment of birth).

Maternal death†: The death of a woman from any cause related to or aggravated by pregnancy or its management (regardless of the duration or site of pregnancy), but not from accidental or incidental causes.

---

*These definitions are for statistical purposes and are not intended to affect clinical management. Appropriate assessment of fetal maturity for purposes of clinical management is delineated in Chapter 4.

Statisticians making a determination of the status of a neonate, namely preterm or term, should define preterm as less than 259 days and term as 259 days to less than 294 days to ensure comparable calculations with the medical community. Statisticians, by formula, subtract the date of the first day of the last menstrual period from the date of birth, whereas physicians include the first day, thus accounting for the difference.

†Death occurring to a woman during pregnancy or after its termination from causes not related to the pregnancy or to its complications or management is not considered a maternal death. Nonmaternal deaths may result from accidental causes (eg, auto accident or gunshot wound) or incidental causes (eg, concurrent malignancy).

Direct obstetric death—The death of a woman resulting from obstetric complications of pregnancy, labor, or the puerperium; from interventions, omissions, or treatment; or from a chain of events resulting from any of these.

Indirect obstetric death—The death of a woman resulting from a previously existing disease or a disease that developed during pregnancy, labor, or the puerperium that did not have direct obstetric causes, although the physiologic effects of pregnancy were partially responsible for the death.

In 1987, the Centers for Disease Control and Prevention (CDC) collaborated with the Maternal Mortality Special Interest Group of the American College of Obstetricians and Gynecologists (ACOG), the Association of Vital Records and Health Statistics, and state and local health departments to initiate the National Pregnancy Mortality Surveillance System. The CDC–ACOG Maternal Mortality Study Group introduced two new terms, which are being used by the CDC and increasingly by some states and researchers. The study group differentiates between pregnancy-associated and pregnancy-related deaths.

Pregnancy-associated death: The death of any woman, from any cause, while pregnant or within 1 calendar year of termination of pregnancy, regardless of the duration and the site of pregnancy.

Pregnancy-related death: A pregnancy-associated death resulting from: 1) complications of the pregnancy itself, 2) the chain of events initiated by the pregnancy that led to death, or 3) aggravation of an unrelated condition by the physiologic or pharmacologic effects of the pregnancy that subsequently caused death.

Induced termination of pregnancy: The purposeful interruption of an intrauterine pregnancy with the intention other than to produce a liveborn infant, and which does not result in a live birth. This definition excludes management of prolonged retention of products of conception following fetal death.

Statistical Tabulations

Statistical tabulations for vital events related to pregnancy provide the medical and statistical community with valuable information on reproductive health and generate data on trends apparent in this country and worldwide. This information often is disaggregated and used to examine specific events over time or within selected geographic locations. In informing the public about health issues, media sources often report various statistical measures. Heightened public interest in health-related issues makes it essential that the medical community understand and have the capacity to interpret these statistics.

The following explanations of statistical tabulations are intended to provide the reader with a better understanding of the measures used for events related to reproduction.

Rate: A measure of the frequency of some event in relation to a unit of population during a specified time period, such as a year; events in the numerator of the rate occur to individuals in the denominator. Rates express the risk of the event in the specified population during a particular time. Rates generally are expressed as units of population in the denominator (eg, per 1,000, per 100,000). For example, the 1982 teenage birth rate was 52.9 live births per 1,000 women aged 15–19 years.

Ratios: A term that expresses a relationship of one element to a different element (where the numerator is not necessarily a subset of the denominator). A ratio generally is expressed per 1,000 of the denominator element. For example, the sex ratio of live births for 1982 was 1,051 males per 1,000 females.

In the formulae that follow, *period* refers to a calendar year.

Live Birth Measures

These measures are designed to show the rate at which childbearing is occurring in the population. The crude birth rate, which relates the total number of births to the total population, indicates the impact of fertility on population growth. The general fertility rate is a more specific measure of fertility because it relates the number of births to the population at risk, namely, women of childbearing age (assumed to be ages 15–44 years). An even more specific set of rates, the age-specific birth rate, relates the number of births to women of specific ages directly to the total number of women in that age group. Formulae for these measures are:

$$\text{Crude birth rate} = \frac{\text{Number of live births to women of all ages during a calendar year} \times 1{,}000}{\text{Total estimated mid-year population}}$$

$$\text{General fertility rate} = \frac{\text{Number of live births to women of all ages during a calendar year} \times 1{,}000}{\text{Estimated mid-year population of women aged 15–44 years}}$$

$$\text{General pregnancy rate} = \frac{\begin{array}{c}\text{Number of live births} + \text{number of fetal}\\ \text{deaths} + \text{number of induced terminations of}\\ \text{pregnancy during a calendar year} \times 1{,}000\end{array}}{\begin{array}{c}\text{Estimated mid-year population}\\ \text{of women aged } 15\text{-}44 \text{ years}\end{array}}$$

$$\text{Age-specific birth rate} = \frac{\begin{array}{c}\text{Number of live births to women in a specific}\\ \text{age group during a calendar year} \times 1{,}000\end{array}}{\begin{array}{c}\text{Estimated mid-year population}\\ \text{of women in same age group}\end{array}}$$

$$\text{Total fertility rate} = \frac{\text{The sum of age-specific birth rates of women}}{\text{at each age group } 10\text{-}14 \text{ through } 45\text{-}49.}$$

Five-year age groups are used; therefore, the sum is multiplied by 5. This rate also can be computed by using single years of age.

Because the birth weight of the infant is included on the birth certificate, it is possible to tabulate and focus an analysis on selected groups of live births, for example, those weighing 500 g or more. Births can be tabulated by where they occur. Therefore, they can be shown by place of occurrence, by place of residence, and by kind of setting of delivery, such as at a hospital or home. Most tabulations of vital statistics are routinely calculated by place of residence of the mother, but they could be tabulated on another basis as well. What is essential, however, is that the classification be the same for all events under consideration for a specific measure.

Fetal Mortality Measures

The population at risk for fetal mortality is the number of live births plus the number of fetal deaths in a year. Fetal death indices, defined by a minimum weight and gestational age, indicate the magnitude of late pregnancy losses.

It is recognized that most states report fetal deaths on the basis of gestational age. However, birth weight can be more accurately measured than can gestational age. Therefore, it is recommended that states adopt minimum reporting requirements of fetal deaths based on and labeled as specific birth weight rather than gestational age (see "Fetal Death" under "Reporting Requirements and Recommendations," as follows). In addition, statistical tabulations of fetal deaths should include, at a minimum, fetal deaths of those weighing 500 g or more.

It is recognized that states will not be able to immediately translate data from gestational age to weight, and, for comparative purposes, it may be desirable to know fetal death rates for various gestational periods. Therefore, the collection of both weight and gestational age is recommended to allow for these comparisons. When calculating fetal death rates based on gestational age, the number of weeks or more of stated or presumed gestation can be substituted for weight in the previous formulae.

$$\text{Fetal death rate} = \frac{\substack{\text{Number of fetal deaths} \\ \text{(x weight or more) during a period} \times 1,000}}{\substack{\text{Number of fetal deaths (x weight or more)} + \\ \text{number of live births during the same period}}}$$

$$\text{Fetal death ratio} = \frac{\substack{\text{Number of fetal deaths} \\ \text{(x weight or more) during a period} \times 1,000}}{\text{Number of live births during the same period}}$$

Perinatal Mortality Measures

Indices of perinatal mortality combine fetal deaths and live births with only brief survival (up to a few days or weeks) on the assumption that similar factors are associated with these losses. The population at risk is the total number of live births plus fetal deaths, or alternatively, the number of live births. Perinatal mortality indices can vary as to age of the fetus and the infant who is included in the particular tabulation. However, the concept itself cuts across all the calculations.

It is recommended that perinatal mortality measures be based on and labeled with specific weight rather than gestational age (see "Reporting Requirements and Recommendations," as follows).

$$\text{Perinatal mortality rate} = \frac{\substack{\text{Number of infant deaths of less than x days} \\ + \text{ number of fetal deaths (with stated or} \\ \text{presumed weight of y or more)} \\ \text{during the same period} \times 1,000}}{\text{Number of live births during the same period}}$$

It is recognized that states will not be able to immediately translate data from gestational age to weight, and for purposes of comparability, knowledge of gestational age (based on last menstrual period) may be required and should be collected. When perinatal death rates based on gestational age are calculated, the number of weeks of a stated or presumed gestational age can be substituted for weight in the formulae. When comparisons based on gestational age are desired, the generally accepted breakdown is:

- Perinatal period I includes infant deaths occurring at less than 7 days and fetal deaths with a stated or presumed period of gestation of 28 weeks or more.

- Perinatal period II includes infant deaths occurring at less than 28 days and fetal deaths with a stated or presumed period of gestation of 20 weeks or more.

- Perinatal period III includes infant deaths occurring at less than 7 days and fetal deaths with a stated or presumed gestation of 20 weeks or more.

Perinatal measures can be specific for race and other characteristics. Perinatal events can be tabulated by where they occur. Therefore, they can be shown by place of occurrence, by place of residence, and by place of delivery, such as at a hospital or home. Most tabulations of vital statistics are routinely calculated by place of residence of the woman, but they could be tabulated by place of occurrence. What is essential, however, is that the classification be the same for all events under consideration for a specific measure.

Indices of infant mortality are designed to show the likelihood that live births with certain characteristics will survive the first year of life or, conversely, will die during the first year of life. For infant mortality, the "population at risk" is approximated by live births that occur in a calendar year. One can compare the infant mortality rate of different population groups, such as that between white and black infants. Interest sometimes focuses on two different periods in the first year of an infant's life, such as the very early period when the infant is younger than 28 days (up through 27 days, 23 hours, and 59 minutes from the moment of birth), called the neonatal period; and the later period starting at the end of the 28th day up to, but not including, age 1 year (364 days, 23 hours, and 59 minutes), called the postneonatal period. Accordingly, two indices reflect these differences, namely, the neonatal mortality rate and the postneonatal mortality rate. The neonatal period can be divided further for statistical tabulations:

- Neonatal period I is from the moment of birth through 23 hours and 59 minutes.

- Neonatal period II starts at the end of the 24th hour of life through 6 days, 23 hours, and 59 minutes.

- Neonatal period III starts at the end of the 7th day of life through 27 days, 23 hours, and 59 minutes.

The denominator for the postneonatal mortality rate also can be calculated by subtracting the number of neonatal deaths from the number of live births. This denominator more accurately defines the population at risk of death in the postneonatal period. In addition, it should be noted that infant deaths can be broken down into birth weight categories, if desired, for comparative purposes when birth and death records are linked (see "Reporting Requirements and Recommendations," as follows).

$$\text{Infant mortality rate} = \frac{\text{Number of infant deaths (neonatal and postneonatal) during a period} \times 1{,}000}{\text{Number of live births during the same period}}$$

$$\text{Neonatal mortality rate} = \frac{\text{Number of neonatal deaths during a period} \times 1{,}000}{\text{Number of live births during the same period}}$$

$$\text{Postneonatal mortality rate} = \frac{\text{Number of postneonatal deaths during a period} \times 1{,}000}{\text{Number of live births during the same period}}$$

Maternal Mortality Measures

Measures of maternal mortality are designed to indicate the likelihood that a pregnant woman will die from complications of pregnancy, childbirth, or the puerperium. Accordingly, the population at risk is an approximation of the population of pregnant women in a year; the approximation usually is taken to be the number of live births. Maternal mortality can be examined in terms of characteristics of the woman, such as age, race, and cause of death. The maternal mortality rate measures the risk of death from deliveries and complications of pregnancy, childbirth, and the puerperium.

The group exposed to risk consists of all women who have been pregnant at some time during the period. Therefore, the population at risk should theoretically include all fetal deaths (reported and unreported), all induced terminations of pregnancy, and all live births. Because most states do not require the reporting of all fetal deaths and a large number of states still do not require reporting of induced terminations of pregnancy, the entire population at risk cannot be included in the denominator. Therefore, the total number of live births has become the generally accepted denominator. It is recommended that when complete ascertainment of the denominator (ie, the number of pregnant women) is achieved, a modified maternal mortality rate should be defined, in addition to the traditional rate. The rate is most frequently expressed per 100,000 live births:

$$\text{Maternal mortality rate} = \frac{\text{Number of deaths attributed to maternal conditions during a period} \times 100,000}{\text{Number of live births during the same period}}$$

Death rates for specified maternal causes are computed by restricting the numerator to the specified cause. The maternal mortality rates specific for race and age groups are computed by appropriately restricting both the numerator and the denominator to the specified group. Caution should be used in interpreting rates in small geographic areas; it may not be possible to generate race- and age-specific rates.

For statistical comparisons with the World Health Organization (WHO), it is recommended that two tabulations of statistics be prepared: 1) maternal deaths within 42 days of the end of pregnancy (WHO); and 2) maternal deaths with no time limitation for comparison within the United States.

The CDC uses the following statistical measures of pregnancy-related mortality:

$$\text{Pregnancy mortality ratio} = \frac{\text{Number of pregnancy-related deaths during a period} \times 100,000}{\text{Number of live births during the same period}}$$

$$\text{Pregnancy mortality rate} = \frac{\text{Number of pregnancy-related deaths during a period} \times 100,000}{\text{Number of pregnancies (live births, fetal deaths, induced and spontaneous abortions, ectopic pregnancies, and molar pregnancies)}}$$

Measures of Induced Termination of Pregnancy

Measures of induced pregnancy termination parallel those of fetal deaths but refer to "induced" events. The population at risk for induced termination of pregnancy is taken to be live births in a year, which is used as a surrogate measure of pregnancies. Because this is not actually the total population at risk, this measure generally is considered to be a ratio.

$$\text{Induced termination of pregnancy ratio I} = \frac{\text{Number of induced terminations occurring during a period} \times 1{,}000}{\text{Number of live births occurring during the same period}}$$

Another measure is one that, by also including an estimate of pregnancies that do not result in live births, more closely approximates the population at risk:

$$\text{Induced termination of pregnancy ratio II} = \frac{\text{Number of induced terminations occurring during a period} \times 1{,}000}{\text{Number of induced terminations of pregnancies + live births + reported fetal deaths during the same period}}$$

Still a third measure is a rate that provides information on the probability that a woman of a certain age or race will have an induced termination of pregnancy:

$$\text{Induced termination of pregnancy rate} = \frac{\text{Number of induced terminations occurring during a period} \times 1{,}000}{\text{Female population aged 15–44 years}}$$

Sometimes indices for induced termination are specific for certain characteristics of the woman; that is, they can refer to women of particular age or race groups.

Reporting Requirements and Recommendations

Reporting requirements for vital events related to reproductive health enable the collection of data that are essential to the calculation of statistical tabulations to examine trends and changes at the local, state, and national levels. The data used in statistical tabulations may be only a portion of those collected, because of the need for consistency in a tabulation and because of the variations in reporting requirements from state to state. For instance, although a few states require that all fetal deaths, regardless of length of gestation, be reported, statistical tabulations of fetal death rates by the National Center for Health Statistics use only those fetal deaths occurring at 20 weeks or more of gestation.

Live Birth

It generally is recognized that all states report all live births, as defined in the definitions section of this document. It is recommended that all live births be reported, regardless of birth weight, length of gestation, or survival time.

Fetal Death

Reporting requirements for fetal deaths now vary from state to state. At present, most states require reporting of fetal deaths by gestational age. It generally is recognized that birth weight can be measured more accurately than can gestational age. The 1992 revision of the Model State Vital Statistics Act and Regulations recommends reporting of all spontaneous losses occurring at 20 weeks or more of gestation or weighing 350 g or more. It must be emphasized that a specific birth weight criterion for reporting of fetal deaths does not imply a point of viability and should be chosen instead for its feasibility in collecting useful data.

Current statistical tabulations of fetal deaths include, at a minimum, fetal deaths at 500 g or more. Furthermore, 27 states have adopted the requirement of reporting deaths of more than 20 weeks of gestation. Therefore, it is recommended that all state fetal death report forms include birth weight and gestational age.

Perinatal Mortality

Perinatal mortality indices generally combine fetal deaths and live births that survive only briefly (up to a few days or weeks). Because reporting requirements of fetal deaths vary from state to state, perinatal mortality reporting also will vary (see definitions of perinatal periods in "Perinatal Mortality Measures" in this appendix).

As with fetal deaths, it is recommended that perinatal mortality be weight specific. However, for purposes of comparability, knowledge of gestational age (based on last menstrual period) should be collected.

Infant Mortality

All states require that all infant deaths (neonatal plus postneonatal), as defined in the section "Definitions" in this document, be reported. Infant deaths by birth weight are not routinely available for the United States as a whole because birth weight information is not collected on the death certificate. However, because birth weight is reported on the birth certificate, it is possible to obtain information on infant deaths by birth weight by linking together the birth certificate and the death certificate for the same infant. At present, most states link birth and death certificates. A national linked birth certificate and infant death certificate file is now available.

In addition, it is recommended that infant death reports include the exact interval from birth rather than categories such as "neonatal" or "postneonatal." This, too, will allow for more specific age-related death analyses.

Maternal Mortality

Every state is required to report all maternal deaths. Because the number of annual deaths attributed to maternal mortality is approximately only 300, emphasis must be placed on in-depth investigations. Case finding, together with individual review and analysis of risk factors contributing to maternal deaths, is of the highest importance. Collection of data regarding these rare events is critical, when combined, as it should be, with educational review by those closest to the case, usually the obstetrician–gynecologists in the hospital and the surrounding region. Such analysis can yield clinical information about risk factors associated with, for example, detection and treatment of ectopic pregnancies or with anesthesia. This clinical information can then be gathered and exchanged to help practitioners identify risk factors that contribute to maternal death and associated conditions.

The CDC–ACOG Maternal Mortality Study Group also has designed a new system of classifying pregnancy-related deaths after review of the case. This system differentiates between the immediate and underlying causes of death as stated on the death certificate, associated obstetric and medical conditions or complications, and the outcome of pregnancy. For example, if a woman died of a hemorrhage that resulted from a ruptured ectopic pregnancy, the immediate cause of death would be classified as "hemorrhage," the associated obstetric condition would be classified as "ruptured fallopian tube," and the outcome of pregnancy would be "ectopic pregnancy." This classification scheme allows analysis of the chain of events that led to the death.

Induced Termination of Pregnancy

The United States has no national system for reporting induced termination of pregnancy. State health departments vary greatly in their approaches to the compilation of these data, from compiling no data to: 1) periodically requesting hospitals, clinics, and physicians performing the procedures to voluntarily report total number of procedures performed; 2) requiring (by legislative or regulatory authority) hospitals, clinics, and physicians to periodically report aggregate level data on number or number and characteristics of procedures; or 3) requiring (by legal or regulatory authority) hospitals, clinics, and physicians to periodically report individual data on each procedure performed.

Since 1969, the CDC Division of Reproductive Health has published an annual Abortion Surveillance Report based on data provided from state health departments, when available, and from data voluntarily provided to the CDC from hospitals and clinics in states with no data available from health departments. In addition to information on the number and characteristics of induced terminations of pregnancy, the Abortion Surveillance Report contains information from the CDC abortion mortality surveillance, which was begun with the cooperation of state health departments in 1972. Investigation and review of each related death by epidemiologists in the Division of Reproductive Health result in improved detailed nosological identification of abortion mortality by type of risk.*

Since 1977, the National Center for Health Statistics has analyzed the induced terminations of pregnancy occurring in up to 13 states in which individual reports of induced termination are submitted to state vital registration offices. In addition, the Alan Guttmacher Institute, a private organization, publishes information on induced termination that it obtains from a nationwide survey of providers of induced termination.

Collecting information on the number of induced terminations of pregnancy, the characteristics of women having such procedures, and the number and characteristics of all deaths related to induced termination of pregnancy would be extremely valuable in identifying and evaluating risk factors for specific population groups and for the public in general. By gathering these data, studies could be instituted that would examine clinical issues and then results could be shared with practitioners. Knowing the outcomes could further the body of knowledge and ultimately reduce the risks.

Therefore, state health departments are urged to compile statistics on induced termination of pregnancy to evaluate and improve the quality of their data. Furthermore, state health departments that do not compile such statistics are urged to explore mechanisms for initiating their collection.

Rates of Vaginal Births After Cesarean Delivery

Two methods for defining vaginal birth after cesarean delivery (VBAC) rates are proposed:

$$1.\ \text{VBAC rate} = \frac{\text{Total number of VBACs}}{\begin{array}{c}\text{Total number of women with prior cesarean}\\ \text{deliveries, including women who were}\\ \text{candidates for a trial of labor but declined}\\ \text{and women who were not candidates}\end{array}} \times 100$$

---

*The CDC Abortion Surveillance Report includes information on events categorized by the CDC as abortions (legal, illegal, and spontaneous). Although this terminology predates the recommendations in this document and is at variance with the definition herein, it has been commonly used and understood to include induced termination of pregnancy.

2. Trial of labor
success rate =

$$\frac{VBAC}{\text{Number of women who had a trial of labor after cesarean delivery}} \times 100$$

Clearly, these rates are interrelated. However, calculations based on the rates as defined allow a more accurate comparison of practice between providers and between institutions.

Current Reporting Requirements

The following general fetal death reporting requirements, as of 1997, should be brought into conformity with the recommendations in this report:

Gestation of ≥20 weeks:

Alabama	Maryland*	Oklahoma
Alaska	Minnesota	Oregon
California	Nebraska	Texas
Connecticut	Nevada	Utah
Florida	New Jersey	Vermont*
Illinois	North Carolina	Washington
Indiana	North Dakota	West Virginia
Iowa	Ohio	Wyoming

Gestation of ≥20 weeks or birth weight of ≥500 g:
District of Columbia

Gestation of ≥20 weeks or birth weight of ≥350 g:

Arizona	Kentucky	Missouri
Delaware	Louisiana	New Hampshire
Guam	Massachusetts	South Carolina
Idaho	Mississippi	Wisconsin

Birth weight of >350 g:
Kansas

Gestation of ≥20 weeks or birth weight of ≥400 g:
Michigan

Birth weight of ≥500 g:
New Mexico
South Dakota
Tennessee*

*Modifiers apply.

Gestation of ≥5 months:
   Puerto Rico

Gestation of ≥16 weeks:
   Pennsylvania

All products of human conception:

American Samoa	Hawaii	Northern Mariana Islands
Arkansas	Maine	Rhode Island
Colorado	New York City	Virginia
Georgia	New York State	Virgin Islands

Web Site Resources

Agency for Healthcare Research and Quality	www.ahrq.gov
American Academy of Pediatrics	www.aap.org
The American College of Obstetricians and Gynecologists	www.acog.org
American College of Pathologists	www.cap.org
American Medical Association (Practice Guidelines Partnership)	www.ama-assn.org
Association for Professionals in Infection Control and Epidemiology	www.apic.org
Association of Women's Health, Obstetric and Neonatal Nurses	www.awhonn.org
The Centers for Disease Control and Prevention	www.cdc.gov
Cochrane Collaboration	www.cochrane.org
HIV/AIDS Treatment Information Service	www.hivatis.org
Joint Commission	www.jointcommission.org
March of Dimes	www.marchofdimes.com
Medem	www.medem.com
The National Academies	www.nas.edu
National Center for Health Statistics	www.cdc.gov/nchswww/index.htm
National Institutes of Health	www.nih.gov
National Patient Safety Foundation	www.npsf.org
Occupational Safety and Health Administration	www.osha.gov
Organization of Teratology Information Services	www.otispregnancy.org
Pediatric Infectious Diseases Society	www.pids.org

U.S. Environmental Protection Agency   www.epa.gov
U.S. Food and Drug Administration   www.fda.gov
U.S. Public Health Service   www.usphs.gov
Commissioned Corps

appendix F

Federal Requirements for Patient Screening and Transfer

In 1986, the United States Congress first enacted legal requirements specifying how Medicare-participating hospitals with emergency services must handle individuals with emergency medical conditions or women who are in labor. Since then, the patient screening and transfer law has undergone numerous refinements and revisions. Physicians should expect that this law will continue to evolve and that there will be additional modifications to it in the future.

Requirements for an Appropriate Medical Screening Examination

Federal law requires that all Medicare-participating hospitals with a dedicated emergency department must provide an "appropriate medical screening examination" for any individual who comes to the emergency department for medical treatment or examination to determine whether the patient has an emergency medical condition. This examination must be made within the capability of the hospital's emergency department, including ancillary services routinely available to the emergency department. For example, "[i]f a hospital has a department of obstetrics and gynecology, the hospital is responsible for adopting procedures under which the staff and resources of that department are available to treat a woman in labor who comes to its emergency department."

Medical screening examinations also must "...be conducted by individuals determined qualified by hospital by-laws or rules and regulations." Therefore, it is up to a hospital to designate who is a "qualified medical person" to provide an appropriate medical screening examination. The law does not require that physicians perform all screening examinations. Therefore, a hospital can determine under what circumstances a physician is required to provide medical screening and when screening can be done by a nonphysician.

Determining Whether a Patient Has an Emergency Medical Condition

The legal definition of "emergency medical condition" is not the same as the medical one. Under the law, it is defined as:

"A medical condition manifesting itself by acute symptoms of sufficient severity (including severe pain, psychiatric disturbances and/or symptoms of substance abuse) such that the absence of immediate attention could reasonably be expected to result in—

(A) Placing the health of the individual (or, with respect to a pregnant woman, the health of the woman or her unborn child) in serious jeopardy;

(B) Serious impairment to bodily functions; or

(C) Serious dysfunction of any bodily organ or part."

It is important to note that, in the case of a pregnant woman, the health of the fetus also must be considered in determining whether an "emergency medical condition" exists.

Special Determination of Emergency Medical Conditions for Pregnant Women

The definition of an emergency medical condition also makes specific reference to a pregnant woman who is having contractions. It provides that an emergency medical condition exists if a pregnant woman is having contractions and "…there is inadequate time to effect a safe transfer to another hospital before delivery; or that transfer may pose a threat to the health or safety of the woman or the unborn child." An emergency medical condition does not exist, even when a woman is having contractions, as long as there is adequate time to effect a safe transfer before delivery and the transfer will not pose a threat to the health or safety of the mother or the fetus. Labor is defined as:

…the process of childbirth beginning with the latent phase of labor or early phase of labor and continuing through delivery of the placenta. A woman experiencing contractions is in true labor unless a physician, certified nurse-midwife, or other qualified medical person acting within his or her scope of practice as defined in hospital medical staff bylaws and State law, certifies that, after a reasonable time of observation, the woman is in false labor.

Under this definition, a qualified medical person must certify that a woman is in false labor before she can be released.

Patients With Emergency Medical Conditions

Once a patient comes to an emergency department, is appropriately screened, and is determined to have an emergency medical condition, the physician may:

1. Treat the patient and stabilize her condition.
2. Transfer the patient to another medical facility in accordance with specific procedures outlined later.

In situations in which a pregnant woman is in true labor, her condition will be considered stabilized once the child and the placenta are delivered.

Patients Can Refuse to Consent to Treatment

If a patient refuses to consent to treatment, the hospital has fulfilled its obligations under the law. If a patient refuses to consent to treatment, however, the following steps must be taken:

1. The patient must be informed of the risks and benefits of the examination or treatment or both.
2. The medical record must contain a description of the examination and treatment that was refused by the patient.
3. The hospital must take all reasonable steps to secure the patient's written informed refusal. The written document must indicate that the person has been informed of the risks and benefits of the examination or treatment or both.

Procedures for Transferring a Patient to Another Medical Facility

In general, a patient who meets the criteria of an emergency medical condition may not be transferred until he or she is stabilized. There are, however some exceptions to this prohibition.

The patient may request a transfer, in writing, after being informed of the hospital's obligations under the law and the risks of transfer. The unstabilized patient's written request for transfer must indicate the reasons for the request and that the patient is aware of the risks and benefits of transfer.

An unstabilized patient also may be transferred if a physician signs a written certification that:

> ... based upon the information available at the time of transfer, the medical benefits reasonably expected from the provision of appropriate medical treatment at another medical facility outweigh the increased risks to the individual or, in the case of a woman in labor, to the woman or the unborn child, from being transferred.

The certification must contain a summary of the risks and benefits of transfer.

If a physician is not physically present in the emergency department at the time of the transfer of a patient, a qualified medical person can sign the certification described previously after consulting with a physician who authorizes the transfer. The physician must countersign the certification as contemporaneously as possible.

Patients Can Refuse to Consent to Transfer

If the hospital offers to transfer a patient, in accordance with the appropriate procedures, and the patient refuses to consent to transfer, the hospital also has fulfilled its obligations under the law. When a patient refuses to consent to the transfer, the hospital must take the following steps:

1. The patient must be informed of the risks and benefits of the transfer.

2. The medical record must contain a description of the proposed transfer that was refused by the patient.

3. The hospital must take all reasonable steps to secure the patient's written informed refusal. The written document must indicate that the person has been informed of the risks and benefits of the transfer and the reasons for the patient's refusal.

Additional Requirements of the Transferring and Receiving Hospitals

The transferring hospital must comply with the following requirements to ensure that the transfer was appropriate:

1. The receiving hospital must have space and qualified personnel to treat the patient and must have agreed to accept the transfer. A hospital with

specialized capabilities, such as a neonatal intensive care unit, may not refuse to accept patients if space is available.

2. The transferring hospital must minimize the risks to the patient's health, and the transfer must be executed through the use of qualified personnel and transportation equipment.

3. The transferring hospital must send to the receiving hospital all medical records related to the emergency condition that are available at the time of transfer. These records include available history, records related to the emergency medical condition, observations of signs or symptoms, preliminary diagnosis, results of diagnostic studies or telephone reports of the studies, treatment provided, results of any tests and informed written consent or certification, and the name of any on-call physician who has refused or failed to appear within a reasonable time to provide necessary stabilizing treatment. Other records not yet available must be sent as soon as possible.

General Requirements

The following general requirements should be met:

1. Medical records related to transfers must be retained by both the transferring and receiving hospitals for 5 years from the date of the transfer.

2. Hospitals are required to report to the Centers for Medicare and Medicaid Services or the state survey agency within 72 hours from the time of the transfer any time they have reason to believe they may have received a patient who was transferred in an unstable medical condition.

3. Hospitals are required to post signs in areas such as entrances, admitting areas, waiting rooms, and emergency departments with respect to their obligations under the patient screening and transfer law.

4. Hospitals also are required to post signs stating whether the hospital participates in the Medicaid program under a state-approved plan. This requirement applies to all hospitals, not only those that participate in Medicare.

5. Hospitals must keep a list of physicians who are on call after the initial examination to provide treatment to stabilize a patient with an emergency medical condition.

6. Hospitals must keep a central log of all individuals who come to the emergency department seeking assistance and the result of each individual's visit.

7. A hospital may not delay providing appropriate medical screening to inquire about payment method or insurance status.

Enforcement and Penalties

Physicians and hospitals violating these federal requirements for patient screening and transfer are subject to civil monetary penalties of up to $50,000 for each violation and to termination from the Medicare program. Hospitals are prohibited from penalizing physicians who report violations of the law or who refuse to transfer an individual with an unstabilized emergency medical condition.

Scope of Services for Uncomplicated Obstetric Care

Global obstetric care comprises services normally provided in uncomplicated obstetric care. These include antepartum care, intrapartum care, and postpartum care:

- Antepartum Care
  - The first prenatal visit with initial history and physical examination
  - Generally, a woman with an uncomplicated pregnancy is examined every 4 weeks for the first 28 weeks of gestation, every 2 weeks until 36 weeks of gestation, and weekly thereafter. The frequency of follow-up visits is determined by the individual needs of the woman and the assessment of her risks.

- Intrapartum Care
  - Supervision of uncomplicated labor
  - Uncomplicated vaginal delivery (with or without episiotomy, forceps, or vacuum delivery)

- Postpartum Care
  - Hospital visits
  - Outpatient (office, routine, uncomplicated visits)

appendix H

Occupational Safety and Health Administration Regulations on Occupational Exposure to Bloodborne Pathogens*

In 1970, the U.S. Congress enacted the Occupational Safety and Health Act to protect workers from unsafe and unhealthy conditions in the workplace. To oversee this effort, the law also created the Occupational Safety and Health Administration (OSHA) within the U.S. Department of Labor. The Occupational Safety and Health Administration has the responsibility for developing and implementing job safety and health standards and regulations. Its standards and regulations apply to all employers and employees. To promote and ensure compliance with its standards, OSHA has the authority to conduct unannounced workplace inspections. It also maintains a reporting and record-keeping system to monitor job-related injuries and illnesses. Failure to comply with OSHA standards may result in the assessment of civil or criminal penalties.

In December 1991, OSHA issued new regulations on occupational exposure to bloodborne pathogens that are designed to minimize the transmission of human immunodeficiency virus (HIV), hepatitis B virus (HBV), and other potentially infectious materials in the workplace. The regulations cover all employees in physician offices, hospitals, medical laboratories, and other health care facilities where workers could be "reasonably anticipated" as a result of performing their job duties to come into contact with blood and other potentially infectious materials. The regulations were revised, effective April 2001, to comply with the Needlestick Safety and Prevention Act of 2000.

---

*Modified from Kaminetzky HA, Rutledge P. OSHA regulations and medical practice. Prim Care Update Ob Gyns 1995;2:143–9.

Approved State Plans

Under the federal law that created OSHA, states are encouraged to develop and operate—under OSHA guidance—state job safety and health plans. Currently, 24 states and 2 territories have OSHA-approved plans, which require them to provide standards and enforcement programs that are at least as effective as the federal standards. They are:

Alaska	Michigan	South Carolina
Arizona	Minnesota	Tennessee
California	Nevada	Utah
Connecticut*	New Jersey*	Vermont
Hawaii	New Mexico	Virgin Islands*
Indiana	New York*	Virginia
Iowa	North Carolina	Washington
Kentucky	Oregon	Wyoming
Maryland	Puerto Rico	

A list of these state OSHA offices is available on the OSHA web site at http://www.osha.gov/oshdir/states.html; call the number listed to receive a copy of the state's standards on occupational exposure to bloodborne pathogens. In Connecticut, New Jersey, New York and the Virgin Islands, the state plans cover state and local government employees only; the private sector is covered by the federal OSHA standard. In addition, states with an OSHA-approved state plan must comply with the federal OSHA standard.

Complying with the Regulations

Exposure Control Plan

To comply with the regulations, health care employers are required to prepare a written "Exposure Control Plan" designed to eliminate or minimize employee exposure to bloodborne pathogens. This plan must list all job classifications in which employees are likely to be exposed to infectious materials and the relevant tasks and procedures performed by these employees. Infectious materials include blood, semen, vaginal secretions, peritoneal fluid, amniotic fluid, any body fluid visibly contaminated with blood, all body fluids in which it is impossible to differentiate between the body fluids, any unfixed human tissue or organ (living or dead), as well as HIV-containing cell or tissue cultures, organ cultures, and HIV- or HBV-containing culture medium or other solutions.

*The state OSHA plan covers state and local government employees only.

Under the plan, employers are required to adopt universal precautions, engineering and work practice controls, and personal protective equipment requirements. Employers must also establish a schedule for implementing:

- Housekeeping requirements
- Employee training and record-keeping requirements
- Hepatitis B virus vaccination for employees and postexposure evaluation and follow-up procedures
- Communication of hazards

A detailed discussion of each of these requirements follows. The plan must be accessible to employees and made available to OSHA on request. The Exposure Control Plan must be reviewed annually and updated to reflect changes in technology that eliminate or reduce exposure to bloodborne pathogens. The employer must document this annual consideration and the use of appropriate effective safer medical procedures and devices that are commercially available. In designing and reviewing the Exposure Compliance Plan, the employer must solicit input from nonmanagerial employees who are potentially exposed to injuries from contaminated sharps. Employers must document, in the Exposure Control Plan, how they received input from employees.

Mandatory Universal Precautions

The regulations require that universal precautions must be used to prevent contact with blood or other potentially infectious materials. It is OSHA's intention to follow the Centers for Disease Control and Prevention's guidelines on universal precautions. As defined by the Centers for Disease Control and Prevention, the concept of universal precautions requires the employer and employee to assume that blood and other body fluids are infectious and must be handled accordingly.

Engineering and Work Practice Controls

Specific engineering and work practice controls for the workplace must be implemented and examined for effectiveness on a regular schedule. These controls include the following guidelines:

1. Employers are required to provide handwashing facilities that are readily accessible to employees; when this is not feasible, employees must be provided with an antiseptic hand cleanser with clean cloth or paper towels or antiseptic towelettes. It is the employer's responsibility to

ensure that employees wash their hands and any other skin immediately after gloves and other protective garments are removed.

2. Contaminated needles and other contaminated sharp objects shall not be bent, recapped, or removed unless the employer can demonstrate that no alternative is feasible or that a specific medical procedure requires such action. Shearing or breaking of contaminated needles is prohibited. Recapping or needle removal must be accomplished by a mechanical device or a one-handed technique. Contaminated reusable sharp objects shall be placed in appropriate containers until properly reprocessed; these containers must be puncture resistant, leakproof, and labeled or color coded in accordance with the regulations for easy identification.

3. Eating, drinking, smoking, applying cosmetics or lip balm, and handling contact lenses are prohibited in work areas where there is a reasonable likelihood of exposure to potentially infectious materials.

4. Food and drink must not be kept in refrigerators, freezers, shelves, cabinets, or on countertops where blood or other potentially infectious materials are present.

5. All procedures involving blood or other infectious materials shall be performed in a manner to minimize splashing, spraying, spattering, and creating droplets; mouth pipetting or suctioning of blood or other potentially infectious materials is prohibited.

6. Specimens of blood or other potentially infectious materials must be placed in closed containers that prevent leakage during collection, handling, processing, storage, transport, or shipping; containers must be labeled or color coded in accordance with the regulations for easy identification. However, when a facility uses universal precautions in the handling of all specimens, the required labeling or color coding of specimens is not necessary as long as containers are recognizable as containing specimens; this exemption applies only while the specimens and containers remain in the facility. If outside contamination of the primary container occurs, it must be placed within a second container that is leakproof, puncture resistant, and labeled or color coded accordingly.

7. Equipment that could be contaminated with blood or other infectious materials must be examined before servicing or shipping and shall be decontaminated as necessary, unless the employer can demonstrate that decontamination of the equipment or parts of the equipment is not feasible. A visible label must be attached to the equipment stating which parts remain contaminated. The employer must ensure that this infor-

mation is conveyed to all affected employees, the servicing representative, and the manufacturer before handling, servicing, or shipping so that the necessary precautions will be taken.

Personal Protective Equipment

The regulations also stress the importance of appropriate personal protective equipment that employers are required to provide at no cost to employees whose job duties expose them to blood and other infectious materials. Appropriate personal protective equipment includes but is not limited to gloves, gowns, laboratory coats, face shields or masks, eye protection, mouthpieces, resuscitation bags, pocket masks, or other ventilation devices. As defined by OSHA, personal protective equipment is considered "appropriate" if it prevents blood or other potentially infectious materials from reaching an employee's work clothes and skin, eyes, mouth, or other mucous membranes under normal conditions of use.

Employers must ensure that the employee uses appropriate personal protective equipment unless the employer can demonstrate that the employee temporarily declined to use the equipment, when under rare and extraordinary circumstances, it was the employee's professional judgment that use of personal protective equipment would have prevented the delivery of health care services or would have posed an increased hazard to the safety of the worker or co-worker. When an employee makes this judgment, the circumstances shall be investigated and documented to determine whether changes can be made to prevent such situations in the future.

Personal protective equipment in the appropriate sizes must be accessible at the worksite or issued to employees. Hypoallergenic gloves, glove liners, powderless gloves, or other similar alternatives shall be readily accessible to those employees who are allergic to the gloves normally provided. The employer shall provide for laundering and disposal of personal protective equipment, as well as repair and replace this equipment when necessary to maintain its effectiveness, at no cost to the employee. If a garment(s) is penetrated by blood or other infectious materials, it must be removed immediately or as soon as feasible. All personal protective equipment must be removed before leaving the work area, whereupon it shall be placed in a designated area or storage container for washing or disposal.

Gloves must be worn when it can reasonably be anticipated that the employee may have hand contact with blood, other potentially infectious materials, mucous membranes, and nonintact skin; when performing vascular access procedures; and when handling or touching contaminated surfaces. Disposable gloves shall be replaced as soon as practical when contaminated or when torn or punctured; they shall not be washed or decontaminated for reuse. Utility gloves may be decontaminated for reuse but must be discarded if a glove is cracked, peeling, torn, punctured, or shows other signs of deterioration.

Masks in combination with goggles or protective eye shields must be worn whenever splashes, spray, spatter, or droplets of blood may be created and eye, nose, or mouth contamination can reasonably be anticipated. Gowns and other protective body clothing such as, but not limited to, gowns, aprons, laboratory coats, clinic jackets, or similar outer garments, shall be worn in occupational exposure situations. The type and characteristics will depend on the task and degree of exposure anticipated. Surgical caps or hoods or shoe covers must be worn in situations in which "gross contamination" can reasonably be anticipated (eg, autopsies or orthopedic surgery).

Housekeeping

Employers must ensure that the worksite is maintained in a clean and sanitary condition and shall develop and implement a written schedule for cleaning and method of decontamination based on the location within the facility, type of surface to be cleaned, type of soil present, and tasks or procedures being performed in the area. All equipment and working surfaces shall be cleaned and decontaminated after contact with blood or other potentially infectious materials.

Contaminated work surfaces shall be decontaminated with an appropriate disinfectant after tasks and procedures are completed; immediately or as soon as feasible when surfaces are contaminated or after any spill of blood or other potentially infectious materials; and at the end of the work shift if the surface may have become contaminated since the last cleaning. Protective covering (eg, plastic wrap, aluminum foil, or imperviously backed absorbent paper used to cover equipment and environmental surfaces) must be removed and replaced as soon as feasible upon contamination or at the end of the work shift if they may have become contaminated during the shift. All bins, pails, cans, and similar containers intended for reuse shall be inspected and decontaminated on a regularly scheduled basis and cleaned immediately or as soon as feasible on visible contamination.

Broken glassware that may be contaminated must not be picked up directly with the hands; it must be cleaned up using a brush and dustpan, tongs, or forceps. Contaminated reusable sharp objects must not be stored or processed in a manner that requires employees to reach by hand into the containers in which these sharp objects have been placed. Containers for contaminated sharp objects must be closable, puncture resistant, leakproof on the sides and bottom, and labeled or color coded in accordance with the regulations. During use, containers for contaminated sharp objects shall be easily accessible to personnel and located as close as possible to the immediate area where sharp objects are used. Additionally, these containers must be maintained upright throughout use, replaced routinely, and not be allowed to be overfilled. Reusable containers shall not be opened, emptied, or cleaned manually or in any other manner that would expose employees to the risk of percutaneous injury. Containers of contaminated disposable sharp objects and personal protective equipment are defined as regulated waste; such containers must prevent the spillage or protrusion of contents during handling, storage, transport, or shipping.

Contaminated laundry shall be handled as little as possible and must be placed in bags or containers at the location where it was used; it must not be sorted or rinsed in the location of use. Contaminated laundry shall be transported in clearly labeled or color-coded bags or containers in accordance with the regulations. Employers shall ensure that employees who have contact with contaminated laundry wear protective gloves and other appropriate personal protective equipment. When a facility ships contaminated laundry offsite to a second facility that does not use universal precautions in handling all laundry, the facility generating the contaminated laundry must clearly mark or color code the bags or containers with appropriate biohazard labels.

Hepatitis B Vaccination

Employers are required to provide the vaccination for HBV free of charge to all employees who are at risk for occupational exposure. The vaccine must be provided within 10 days of an employee's initial assignment, except in the following cases:

- The employee has previously received the complete HBV vaccination series.
- Antibody testing has revealed that the employee is immune.
- The vaccine is contraindicated for medical reasons.

The regulations prohibit employers from making employees participate in a prescreening program as a prerequisite for receiving the vaccination. Employees who refuse the vaccination must sign a "Hepatitis B Vaccine Declination" form stating that they have declined the vaccine. If the U.S. Public Health Service ever recommends booster doses of HBV vaccine, they also must be provided to employees free of charge. The employee, however, is allowed to change his or her mind and elect to receive the vaccine at any time at the employer's expense.

Postexposure Evaluation and Follow-up

Following a report of an employee exposure incident, the employer must make immediately available to the exposed employee a confidential medical evaluation and follow-up, including at least the following information:

1. Documentation of the route(s) of exposure and the circumstances under which the exposure occurred

2. Identification and documentation of the individual who is the source of the blood or potentially infectious material, unless the employer can establish that such identification is not feasible or is prohibited by state or local law. The source individual's blood shall be tested as soon as possible and after consent is obtained, to determine HBV or HIV infectivity. If consent is not obtained, the employer must document that legally required consent cannot be obtained. If the source individual's consent is not required by law, the source individual's blood if available shall be tested and the results documented. However, when the source individual is already known to be infected with HBV or HIV, blood testing for HBV or HIV is not required. Results of the source individual's blood test shall be made available to the exposed employee, and the employee shall be informed of all applicable laws concerning the disclosure of the source individual's identity and infectious status.

3. Collection and testing of the exposed employee's blood for HBV and HIV serologic status as soon as feasible after the employee gives consent. If the employee consents to baseline blood collection but does not give consent at that time for HIV serologic testing, the sample shall be preserved for 90 days. Testing of the blood shall take place within the 90 days if the employee decides to do so.

4. Postexposure prophylaxis when medically indicated, as recommended by the U.S. Public Health Service

5. Counseling

6. Evaluation of reported illnesses

The employer must ensure that the health professional responsible for the employee's HBV vaccination is provided a copy of the OSHA regulation on bloodborne pathogens. In the case of a health professional evaluating an exposed employee, the employer shall ensure that the health professional is provided the following information:

- A copy of the OSHA bloodborne pathogens regulations
- A description of the exposed employee's duties as they relate to the exposure incident
- Documentation of the routes of exposure and circumstances under which exposure occurred
- Results of the source individual's blood testing, if available
- All medical records relevant to the appropriate treatment of the exposed employee, including vaccination status, which is the employer's responsibility to maintain

The employer must obtain and provide the employee with a copy of the evaluating health professional's written opinion within 15 days of completion. The health professional's written opinion for HBV vaccination shall be limited to whether HBV vaccination is indicated for the employee and if the employee has received such vaccination. The health professional's written opinion for postexposure evaluation and follow-up shall be limited to the following information:

- The employee has been informed of the results of the evaluation.
- The employee has been told about any medical conditions resulting from exposure to blood or other potentially infectious materials that require further evaluation or treatment.

All other findings or diagnoses must remain confidential and shall not be included in the written report.

Communications of Hazards to Employees

Warning Labels and Signs

The regulations require warning labels on containers of regulated waste and refrigerators and freezers containing blood or other potentially infectious materials. Warning labels also must be affixed to containers used to store, transport, or ship blood or other potentially infectious materials. The warnings must be fluorescent orange or orange-red; however, red bags or red containers may be substituted for labels.

Employee Training

Employers must ensure that all employees at risk for occupational exposure participate in a training program at no cost to employees and during working hours. Training shall take place at the time of an employee's initial assignment to tasks that risk exposure and at least annually thereafter. Annual training for employees shall be provided within 1 year of their previous training. Additional training must be provided when changes such as modifications of tasks or procedures or introduction of new tasks and procedures affect the worker's exposure risk. The training must be conducted by a person knowledgeable about the subject matter, and the material shall be presented at an educational level appropriate to the employees. The training program at a minimum must include:

1. A copy of the bloodborne pathogens regulations and an explanation of their contents

2. A general explanation of the epidemiology and symptoms of bloodborne diseases

3. An explanation of the modes of transmission of bloodborne diseases

4. An explanation of the employer's Exposure Control Plan and information on how the employee can obtain a copy of the plan

5. An explanation of the appropriate methods for identifying tasks and other activities that may involve exposure

6. An explanation of the methods that will prevent or reduce exposure (including appropriate engineering controls, work practices, and personal protective equipment)

7. Information on the types, proper use, location, removal, handling, decontamination, and disposal of personal protective equipment

8. An explanation of the basis for selection of personal protective equipment

9. Information on the HBV vaccine (efficacy, safety, method of administration, benefits of being vaccinated, and that the vaccine will be offered free of charge)

10. Information on the appropriate actions to take and persons to contact in an emergency involving blood or other infectious materials

11. An explanation of the procedure for follow-up if an exposure incident occurs (including the method for reporting incident and the medical follow-up that may be available)

12. Information on the postexposure evaluation and follow-up that the employer is required to provide for the employee

13. An explanation of the signs and labels and/or color-coding requirements

14. An opportunity for interactive questions and answers with the person conducting the training session

Record-Keeping Requirements

The employer shall maintain an accurate record for each employee at risk for occupational exposure that includes the following information:

- The name and social security number of employee

- The employee's HBV vaccination status (dates and any medical information relative to the employee's ability to receive the vaccination)

- The results of examinations, medical testing, and follow-up procedures

- The employer's copy of the health professional's written evaluation as required following an exposure incident

- A copy of the information provided to the health professional as required following an exposure incident

The employer shall ensure the confidentiality of employee records; information shall not be disclosed without the employee's written consent. The employer is required to maintain records for the duration of employment plus 30 years. The employer also must maintain records of the training sessions that include the contents or a summary of the training sessions, the dates, the names and qualifications of persons who conducted training sessions, and the names and job titles of employees who attended sessions. These records shall be maintained for 3 years from the date the training session occurred.

All records shall be made available to the assistant secretary of OSHA for examination and copying, including employee medical records, for which the employee's consent is not needed. In the event of an employer going out of business, these records must be transferred to the new owner or must be offered to the National Institute for Occupational Safety and Health.

Sharps Injury Log

An employer with more than 10 employees shall maintain a "sharps injury log" to record percutaneous injuries from contaminated sharps. The information in the log shall be kept in a way to protect the confidentiality of the injured employee. The log must contain:

- The type and brand of device involved in the incident
- The department or work area where the exposure incident occurred
- An explanation of how the incident occurred

The bloodborne pathogens regulations are just one of the OSHA standards that physician offices must follow to be in compliance. Other OSHA regulations include standards on the hazards of chemicals in the workplace, compressed gases, office equipment, and an action plan in case of fire. An emergency hotline number has been established by OSHA to report emergencies: 800-321-OSHA.

American Academy of Pediatrics Policy Statements and American College of Obstetricians and Gynecologists Committee Opinions, Educational Bulletins, and Practice Bulletins

American Academy of Pediatrics Policy Statements

Ad Hoc Task Force on Definition of the Medical Home

American Academy of Pediatrics. Ad Hoc Task Force on Definition of the Medical Home: The medical home. Pediatrics 1992;90:774.

Committee on Adolescence

Adolescent pregnancy: current trends and issues. American Academy of Pediatrics. Committee on Adolescence. Pediatrics 2005;116:281–6.

Counseling the adolescent about pregnancy options. American Academy of Pediatrics. Committee on Adolescence. Pediatrics 1998;101:938–40.

Committee on Bioethics

Guidelines on foregoing life-sustaining medical treatment. American Academy of Pediatrics. Committee on Bioethics. Pediatrics 1994;93:532–6.

Committee on Children with Disabilities

Guidelines for home care of infants, children, and adolescents with chronic disease. American Academy of Pediatrics. Committee on Children with Disabilities. Pediatrics 1995;96:161–4.

Committee on Drugs

Guidelines for monitoring and management of pediatric patients during and after sedation for diagnostic and therapeutic procedures: an update. American Academy of Pediatrics, American Academy of Pediatric Dentistry. Pediatrics 2006;118:2587–602.

Neonatal drug withdrawal [published erratum appears in Pediatrics 1998;102:660]. American Academy of Pediatrics. Committee on Drugs. Pediatrics 1998;101:1079–88.

Committee on Fetus and Newborn

Noninitiation or withdrawal of intensive care for high risk newborns. American Academy of Pediatrics. Committee on Fetus and Newborn. Pediatrics 2007;119:401–3.

Prevention and management of pain in the neonate: an update. American Academy of Pediatrics. Committee on Fetus and Newborn; American Academy of Pediatrics. Section on Surgery, Canadian Paediatric Society, Fetus and Newborn Committee. Pediatrics 2006;118:2231–41.

Advanced practice in neonatal nursing. American Academy of Pediatrics. Committee on Fetus and Newborn. Pediatrics 2003;111:1453–4.

Hospital stay for healthy term newborns. American Academy of Pediatrics. Committee on Fetus and Newborn. Pediatrics 2004;113:1434–6.

Noninitiation or withdrawal of intensive care for high-risk newborns. American Academy of Pediatrics. Committee on Fetus and Newborn. Pediatrics 2007;119:401–3.

Perinatal care at the threshold of viability. American Academy of Pediatrics. Committee on Fetus and Newborn. Pediatrics 2002;110:1024–7.

Surfactant replacement therapy for respiratory distress syndrome. American Academy of Pediatrics. Committee on Fetus and Newborn. Pediatrics 1999;103:684–5.

The Apgar score. American Academy of Pediatrics. Committee on Fetus and Newborn, and American College of Obstetricians and Gynecologists. Pediatrics 2006;117:1444–7.

Apnea, sudden infant death syndrome, and home monitoring. American Academy of Pediatrics. Committee on Fetus and Newborn. Pediatrics 2003;111:914–7.

Controversies concerning Vitamin K and the newborn. American Academy of Pediatrics. Committee on Fetus and Newborn. Pediatrics 2003;112:191–2.

Levels of neonatal care [published erratum appears in Pediatrics 2005;115:1118]. American Academy of Pediatrics. Committee on Fetus and Newborn. Pediatrics 2004;114:1341–7.

Age terminology during the perinatal period. American Academy of Pediatrics. Committee on Fetus and Newborn. Pediatrics 2004;114:1362–4.

Committee on Genetics

Folic acid for the prevention of neural tube defects. American Academy of Pediatrics. Committee on Genetics. Pediatrics 1999;104:325–7.

Maternal phenylketonuria. American Academy of Pediatrics. Committee on Genetics. Pediatrics 2001;107:427–8.

Newborn screening fact sheets. American Academy of Pediatrics. Committee on Genetics. Pediatrics 2006;118:e934–63.

Prenatal screening and diagnosis for pediatricians. American Academy of Pediatrics. Committee on Genetics. Pediatrics 2004; 114:889–94.

Committee on Infectious Diseases

American Academy of Pediatrics. Red book: 2006 report of the Committee on Infectious Diseases. 27th ed. Elk Grove Village (IL): AAP; 2006.

Revised guidelines for prevention of early-onset group B streptococcal (GBS) infection. American Academy of Pediatrics. Committee on Infectious Diseases and Committee on Fetus and Newborn. Pediatrics 1997;99:489–96.

Committee on Injury and Poison Prevention

Safe transportation of newborns at hospital discharge. American Academy of Pediatrics. Committee on Injury and Poison Prevention. Pediatrics 1999;104:986–7.

Safe transportation of premature and low birth weight infants. American Academy of Pediatrics. Committee on Injury and Poison Prevention and Committee on Fetus and Newborn. Pediatrics 1996; 97:758–60.

Committee on Nutrition

Hypoallergenic infant formulas. American Academy of Pediatrics. Committee on Nutrition. Pediatrics 2000;106:346–9.

Iron fortification of infant formulas. American Academy of Pediatrics. Committee on Nutrition. Pediatrics 1999;104:119–23.

American Academy of Pediatrics Committee on Nutrition. Pediatric nutrition handbook. 5th ed. Elk Grove Village (IL): AAP; 2004.

Soy protein-based formulas: recommendations for use in infant feeding. American Academy of Pediatrics. Committee on Nutrition. Pediatrics 1998;101:148–53.

Committee on Pediatric AIDS

Human milk, breastfeeding, and transmission of human immunodeficiency virus type 1 in the United States. American Academy of Pediatrics. Committee on Pediatric AIDS. Pediatrics 2003;112:1196–205.

Technical report: perinatal human immunodeficiency virus testing and prevention of transmission. American Academy of Pediatrics. Committee on Pediatric AIDS. Pediatrics 2000;106:e88.

Committee on Practice and Ambulatory Medicine

Eye examination and vision screening in infants, children, and young adults by pediatricians. American Academy of Pediatrics. Committee on Practice and Ambulatory Medicine and Section on Ophthalmology; American Association of Certified Orthoptists; American Association for Pediatric Ophthalmology and Strabismus; American Academy of Ophthalmology. Pediatrics 2003;111:902–7.

Recommendations for preventive pediatric health care. American Academy of Pediatrics. Committee on Practice and Ambulatory Medicine. Pediatrics 2000;105:645–6.

Committee on Psychosocial Aspects of Child and Family Health

American Academy of Pediatrics. Guidelines for health supervision III. 3rd ed, updated 2002. Elk Grove Village (IL): AAP; 2002.

The prenatal visit. American Academy of Pediatrics. Committee on Psychosocial Aspects of Child and Family Health. Pediatrics 2001;107:1456–8.

Committee on Substance Abuse

Alcohol use and abuse: a pediatric concern. American Academy of Pediatrics. Committee on Substance Abuse. Pediatrics 2001;108:185–9.

Joint Committee on Infant Hearing

Year 2000 position statement: principles and guidelines for early hearing detection and intervention programs. Joint Committee on Infant Hearing; American Academy of Audiology; American Academy of Pediatrics; American Speech-Language-Hearing Association; Directors of Speech and Hearing Programs in State Health and Welfare Agencies. Pediatrics 2000;106:798–817.

Neonatal Resuscitation Steering Committee

American Academy of Pediatrics, American Heart Association. Textbook of neonatal resuscitation. 5th ed. Elk Grove Village (IL): AAP; Dallas (TX): AHA; 2006.

Subcommittee on Hyperbilirubinemia

Management of hyperbilirubinemia in the newborn infant 35 or more weeks of gestation [published erratum appears in Pediatrics 2004;114:1138]. American Academy of Pediatrics. Subcommittee on Hyperbilirubinemia. Pediatrics 2004;114:297–316.

Section on Endocrinology

Update of newborn screening and therapy for congenital hypothyroidism. American Academy of Pediatrics. Section on Endocrinology and Committee on Genetics; American Thyroid Association. Public Health Committee; Pediatric Endocrine Society. Pediatrics 2006;117:2290–2303.

Section on Home Care

American Academy of Pediatrics. Guidelines for pediatric home health care. Elk Grove Village (IL): AAP; 2002.

Section on Ophthalmology

Screening examination of premature infants for retinopathy of prematurity [published erratum appears in Pediatrics 2006;118:1324]. American Academy of Pediatrics; American Academy of Ophthalmology; American Association for Pediatric Ophthalmology; and Strabismus. Pediatrics 2006;117:572–6.

Section on Breast-Feeding

Breastfeeding and the use of human milk. American Academy of Pediatrics. Section on Breastfeeding. Pediatrics 2005;115:496–506.

Task Force on Circumcision

Circumcision policy statement. American Academy of Pediatrics. Task Force on Circumcision. Pediatrics 1999;103:686–93.

Task Force on Infant Positioning and SIDS

The changing concept of sudden infant death syndrome: diagnostic coding shifts, controversies regarding the sleep environment, and new variables to consider in reducing risk. American Academy of Pediatrics; Task Force on Sudden Infant Death Syndrome. Pediatrics 2005;116:1245–55.

Section on Transport Medicine

American Academy of Pediatrics. Guidelines for air and ground transport of neonatal and pediatric patients. 3rd ed. Elk Grove Village (IL): AAP; 2006.

American College of Obstetricians and Gynecologists Committee Opinions

Committee on Ethics

297   Nonmedical use of Obstetric Ultrasonography. Obstet Gynecol 2004;104:423–4. (August 2004)

321 Maternal Decision Making, Ethics, and the Law. Obstet Gynecol 2005;106: 1127–37. (November 2005)

368 Adoption. Obstet Gynecol 2007;109:1507–10. (June 2007)

Committee on Genetics

183 Routines Storage of Umbilical Cord Blood for Potential Future Transplantation (joint with Committee on Obstetric Practice). (April 1997; reaffirmed 2004)

212 Screening for Canavan Disease. Obstet Gynecol Vol. 92, No. 5. (November 1998, reaffirmed 2004)

230 Maternal Phenylketonuria. Obstet Gyneol Vol. 94, No. 1. (January 2000; reaffirmed 2004)

257 Genetic Evaluation of Stillbirths and Neonatal Deaths. Obstet Gynecol Vol. 97, No. 5. (May 2001)

287 Newborn Screening. Obstet Gynecol 2003;102:887–9. (October 2003)

298 Prenatal and Preconceptional Carrier Screening for Genetic Diseases in Individuals of Eastern European Jewish Descent. Obstet Gynecol 2004;104:425–8. (August 2004; reaffirmed 2006)

318 Screening for Tay–Sachs Disease. Obstet Gynecol 2005;106:893–4. (October 2005)

324 Perinatal Risks Associated With Assisted Reproductive Technology (joint with Committees on Obstetric Practice and Gynecologic Practice). Obstet Gynecol 2005;106:1143–6. (November 2005)

325 Update on Carrier Screening for Cystic Fibrosis. Obstet Gynecol 2006;106: 1465–8. (December 2005)

338 Screening for Fragile X Syndrome. Obstet Gynecol 2006;107:1483–5. (June 2006)

Committee on Health Care for Underserved Women

316 Smoking Cessation During Pregnancy (joint with Committee on Obstetric Practice). Obstet Gynecol 2005;106:883–8. (October 2005)

343 Psychosocial Risk Factors: Perinatal Screening and Intervention. Obstet Gynecol 2006;108:469–77. (August 2006)

361 Breastfeeding: Maternal and Infant Aspects (joint with Committee on Obstetric Practice). Obstet Gynecol 2007;109:479–80. (February 2007)

Committee on Obstetric Practice

125 Placental Pathology. (July 1993; reaffirmed 2006)

183 Routine Storage of Umbilical Cord Blood for Potential Future Transplantation (joint with Committee on Genetics). (April 1997; reaffirmed 2004)

228   Induction of Labor with Misoprostol. Obstet Gynecol Vol. 94, No. 5. (November 1999; reaffirmed 2006)

234   Scheduled Cesarean Delivery and the Prevention of Vertical transmission of HIV Infection. Obstet Gynecol Vol. 95, No. 5. (May 2000; reaffirmed 2006)

240   Statement on Surgical Assistants (joint with Committee on Gynecologic Practice). Obstet Gynecol Vol. 96, No. 2. (August 2000; reaffirmed 2006)

248   Response to Searle's Drug Warning on Misoprostol. Obstet Gynecol Vol. 96, No. 6. (December 2000; reaffirmed 2006)

256   Optimal Goals for Anesthesia Care in Obstetrics (joint with American Society of Anesthesiologists). Obstet Gynecol Vo. 97, No. 5. (May 2001; reaffirmed 2006)

258   Fetal Pulse Oximetry. Obstet Gynecol 2001;98:523–4. (September 2001; reaffirmed 2004)

260   Circumcision. Obstet Gynecol 2001;98:707–8. (October 2001; reaffirmed 2004)

264   Air Travel During Pregnancy. Obstet Gynecol 2001;98:1187–8. (December 2001; reaffirmed 2006)

267   Exercise During Pregnancy and the Postpartum Period. Obstet Gynecol 2002;99:171–3. (January 2002; reaffirmed 2005)

268   Management of Asymptomatic Pregnant or Lactating Women Exposed to Anthrax. Obstet Gynecol 2002;99:366–8. (February 2002; reaffirmed 2005)

273   Antenatal Corticosteroid Therapy for Fetal Maturation. Obstet Gynecol 2002;99:871–3. (May 2002; reaffirmed 2005)

275   Obstetric Management of Patients with Spinal Cord Injuries. Obstet Gynecol 2002;100:625–7. (September 2002; reaffirmed 2005)

276   Safety of Lovenox in Pregnancy. Obstet Gynecol 2002;100:845–6. (October 2002; reaffirmed 2005)

279   Prevention of Early-Onset Group B Streptococcal Disease in Newborns. Obstet Gynecol 2002;100:1405–12. (December 2002; reaffirmed 2005)

281   Rubella Vaccination. Obstet Gynecol 2002;100:1417. (December 2002; reaffirmed 2005)

282   Immunization During Pregnancy. Obstet Gynecol 2003;101:207–12. (January 2003; reaffirmed 2005)

283   New U.S. Food and Drug Administration Labeling on Cytotec (Misoprostol) Use and Pregnancy. Obstet Gynecol 2003;101:1049–50. (May 2003; reaffirmed 2006)

284   Nonobstetric Surgery in Pregnancy. Obstet Gynecol 2003;102:431. (August 2003; reaffirmed 2006)

288   Professional Liability and Gynecology-Only Practice (joint with Committee on Gynecologic Practice and Professional Liability). Obstet Gynecol 2003;102:981. (October 2003; reaffirmed 2006)

291 Use of Progesterone to Reduce Preterm Birth. Obstet Gynecol 2003;102:1115–6. (November 2003; reaffirmed 2006)

295 Pain Relief During Labor (joint with American Society of Anesthesiologists). Obstet Gynecol 2004;104:213. (July 2004; reaffirmed 2006)

299 Guidelines for Diagnostic Imaging During Pregnancy. Obstet Gynecol 2004;104: 647–512. (September 2004; reaffirmed 2006)

304 Prenatal and Perinatal Human Immunodeficiency Virus Testing: Expanded Recommendations. Obstet Gynecol 2004;104:1119–24. (November 2004; reaffirmed 2006)

305 Influenza Vaccination and Treatment During Pregnancy. Obsetet Gynecol 2004; 104:1125–6. (November 2004; reaffirmed 2006)

315 Obesity in Pregnancy. Obstet Gynecol 2005:106:671–5. (September 2005)

316 Smoking Cessation During Pregnancy (joint with Committee on Health Care for Underserved Women). Obstet Gynecol 2005;106:883–8. (October 2005)

324 Perinatal Risks Associated with Assisted Reproductive Technology (joint with Committees on Genetics and Gynecologic Practice). Obstet Gynecol 205;106: 1143–6. (November 2005)

326 Inappropriate Use of the Terms Fetal Distress and Birth Asphyxia. Obstet Gynecol 2005;106:1469–70. (December 2005)

333 The Apgar Score (joint with American Academy of Pediatrics Committee on Fetus and Newborn). Obstet Gynecol 2006;107:1209–12. (May 2006)

339 Analgesia and Cesarean Delivery Rates. Obstet Gyencol 2006;107:1487–8. (June 2006)

340 Mode of Term Singleton Breech Delivery. Obstet Gynecol 2006;108:235–7. (July 2006)

342 Induction of Labor for Vaginal Birth After Cesarean Delivery. Obstet Gyencol 2006;108:465–7. (August 2006)

346 Amnioinfusion Does Not Prevent Meconium Aspiration Syndrome. Obstet Gynecol 2006;108:1053–5. (August 2006)

348 Umbilical Cord Blood Gas and Acid Base Analysis. Obstet Gynecol 2006;108: 1319–22. (November 2006)

354 Treatment with Selective Serotonin Reuptake Inhibitors During Pregnancy. Obstet Gynecol 2006;108:1601–3. (December 2006)

361 Breastfeeding: Maternal and Infant Aspects (joint with Committee on Health Care for Underserved Women). Obstet Gynecol 2007;109:479–80. (February 2007)

Committee on Quality Improvement and Patient Safety

286 Patient Safety in Obstetrics and Gynecology. Obstet Gynecol 2003;102:883–5. (October 2003)

Practice Bulletins

38   Perinatal Care at the Threshold of Viability. Obstet Gynecol 2002;100:617–24. (September 2002; reaffirmed 2006)

40   Shoulder Dystocia. Obstet Gynecol 2002;100:1045–50. (November 2002; reaffirmed 2006)

43   Management of Preterm Labor. Obstet Gynecol 2003;101:1039–47. (May 2003; reaffirmed 2006)

44   Neural Tube Defects. Obstet Gynecol 2003;102:203–13. (July 2003; reaffirmed 2006)

47   Prophylactic Antibiotics in Labor and Delivery. Obstet Gynecol 2003;102:875–82. (October 2003; reaffirmed 2006)

48   Cervical Insufficiency. Obstet Gynecol 203;102:1091–9. (November 2003; reaffirmed 2006)

49   Dystocia and Augmentation of Labor. Obstet Gynecol 2003;102:1445–54. (December 2003; reaffirmed 2006)

52   Nausea and Vomiting of Pregnancy. Obstet Gynecol 2004;103:803–15. (April 2004; reaffirmed 2007)

54   Vaginal Birth After Previous Cesarean Delivery. Obstet Gynecol 2004;104:203–12. (July 2004; reaffirmed 2007)

55   Management of Postterm Pregnancy. Obstet Gynecol 2004;104:639–46. (September 2004; reaffirmed 2007)

56   Multiple Gestation: Complicated Twin, Triplet, and High-Order Multifetal Pregnancy (joint with Society for Maternal–Fetal Medicine). Obstet Gynecol 2004;104:869–83. (October 2004; reaffirmed 2007)

58   Ultrasonography in Pregnancy. Obstet Gynecol 2004;104:1449–58. (December 2004; reaffirmed 2007)

60   Pregestational Diabetes Mellitus. Obstet Gynecol 2005;105:675–86. (March 2005; reaffirmed 2007)

68   Antiphospholipid Syndrome. Obstet Gynecol 2005;106;1113–21. (November 2005)

70   Intrapartum Fetal Heart Rate Monitoring. Obstet Gynecol 2005;106:1453–61. (December 2005)

71   Episiotomy. Obstet Gynecol 2006;107:957–62. (April 2006)

75   Management of Alloimmunization During Pregnancy. Obstet Gynecol 2006;108:457–64. (August 2006)

76   Postpartum Hemorrhage. Obstet Gynecol 2006;108:1039–47. (October 2006)

77   Screening for Fetal Chromosomal Abnormalities (joint with Society for Maternal–Fetal Medicine). Obstet Gynecol 2007;109:217–27. (January 2007)

78   Hemoglobinopathies in Pregnancy. Obstet Gynecol 2007;109:229–37. (January 2007)

80   Premature Rupture of Membranes. Obstet Gynecol 2007;109:1007–19. (April 2007)

82   Management of Herpes in Pregnancy. Obstet Gynecol 2007;109:1489–98 (June 2007)

Educational and Technical Bulletins

230   Assessment of Fetal Lung Maturity (November 1996; reaffirmed 2005)

248   Viral Hepatitis in Pregnancy. Obstet Gynecol Vol. 92, No. 1. (July 1998; reaffirmed 2006)

251   Obstetric Aspects of Trauma Management. Obstet Gynecol Vol. 92, No. 3. (September 1998; reaffirmed 2006)

Technology Assessments in Obstetrics and Gynecology

1   Genetics and Molecular Diagnostic Testing. Obstet Gynecol 2002;100:193–211. (July 2002)

index

Page numbers followed by italicized letters *b*, *f*, and *t* indicate boxes, figures, and tables, respectively.